Hans-Ludwig Spohr

Fetal alcohol syndrome

Hans-Ludwig Spohr

Fetal alcohol syndrome

A lifelong challenge

In collaboration with Heike Wolter

Translated by Betteke Maria van Noort, Heike Wolter and
Hans-Ludwig Spohr

DE GRUYTER

Author
FASD-Zentrum, Berlin
Prof. Dr. med. Hans-Ludwig Spohr in cooperation with Charité – Universitätsmedizin Berlin
Department of Child and Adolescent Psychiatry, Psychosomatic Medicine and Psychotherapy
Campus Virchow Clinical Complex
Augustenburger Platz 1
Mittelallee 5a, 13353 Berlin, Germany
hans-ludwig.spohr@charite.de

ISBN 978-3-11-044207-6
e-ISBN (PDF) 978-3-11-043656-3
e-ISBN (EPUB) 978-3-11-043387-6

Library of Congress Cataloging-in-Publication Data
A CIP catalog record for this book has been applied for at the Library of Congress.

Bibliographic information published by the Deutsche Nationalbibliothek
The Deutsche Nationalbibliothek lists this publication in the Deutsche Nationalbibliografie;
detailed bibliographic data are available on the Internet at http://dnb.dnb.de.

© 2018 Walter de Gruyter GmbH, Berlin/Boston
Cover image: istockfoto/kdshutterman
Typesetting: le-tex publishing services GmbH, Leipzig
Printing and binding: CPI books GmbH, Leck
♾ Printed on acid-free paper
Printed in Germany

www.degruyter.com

Dedication

This exceptional book gives a comprehensive overview of the field of Fetal Alcohol Syndrome, ranging from basic science and diagnosis all the way to prevention and management. The book is beautifully written in clear language, such that it is a pleasure to read and will be comprehensible to a wide range of readers. A unique feature of the book is that balanced attention is given to the diagnosis and management of FAS at all ages, from newborns to adults. The text is supported by numerous case studies and photographs of children and adults with FAS, and ends with a series of real-life stories from families living with FASD. This book is highly recommended for clinicians and other health care workers, for parents and caregivers, and indeed, for anyone who needs to know more about FAS.

November 19, 2017

Diane Black

Diane Black, Ph. D.
Chairperson of the Board of the European FASD Alliance

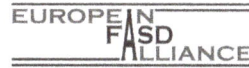

EUROPEAN
FASD
ALLIANCE

Preface

Following the German original edition of 2013 and an early second edition of 2015, De Gruyter has decided to publish an English edition of the textbook "Fetal alcohol syndrome – A lifelong challenge".

Discovered in 1973 by David Smith and Kenneth Jones, fetal alcohol syndrome today constitutes one of the most common causes of congenital brain damage worldwide. While prevalence rates are still rising, the diagnostic focus today is increasingly directed at affected adult patients.

This book intends to not only describe fetal alcohol spectrum disorder comprehensively from a historical, clinical and scientific perspective but also to provide guidance to patients, foster and adoptive parents and other caregivers in diagnosis and support. The numerous biographies described shall contribute to a better understanding of what is still known to be the "silent disease".

I would like to express my deepest gratitude to Dr. Cynthia Morton, Medical Geneticist, Professor of Pathology, Harvard Medical School, Boston for her generous and untiring effort in helping us to translate this book.

When we finished she wrote to me
"It is a priviledge to live my life now with a profound appreciation of the numerous selfless families who have devoted themselfes to the care of other human beings, who through no fault of their own live with disabilities. Despite what Thomas Jefferson stated in the Declaration of Independence: *All men a created equal. . .* it is simply not true; and it is the duty of those of us who are more fortunate with our health to help those who are less fortunate."

Berlin, November 2017   H.-L. Spohr

https://doi.org/10.1515/9783110436563-201

Contents

List of authors

Author

Prof. Dr. med. Hans-Ludwig Spohr
FASD-Zentrum Berlin
in cooperation with
Department of Child and Adolescent Psychiatry,
Psychosomatic Medicine and Psychotherapy
Charité – Universitätsmedizin Berlin
Augustenburger Platz 1, 13353 Berlin
hans-ludwig.spohr@charite.de

Editorial assistance

Heike Wolter, MD
Department of Child and Adolescent Psychiatry,
Psychosomatic Medicine and Psychotherapy
Sozialpädiatrisches Zentrum
Charité – Universitätsmedizin Berlin
Augustenburger Platz 1, 13353 Berlin
heike.wolter@charite.de

With contributions from

Appendix A
Dipl. Psych. Gela Becker
Evangelical Children's home Sonnenhof e. V.
Neuendorfer Straße 60, 13585 Berlin
sonnenhof-ev@t-online.de

Chapter 16
Dipl. Soz. Päd. Manuela Nagel
Department of Obstetrics
Charité – Universitätsmedizin Berlin
Augustenburger Platz 1, 13353 Berlin
manuela.nagel@charite.de

Dr. med. Jan-Peter Siedentopf
Department of Obstetrics
Charité – Universitätsmedizin Berlin
Augustenburger Platz 1, 13353 Berlin
jan-peter.siedentopf@charite.de

Chapter 4
Betteke Maria van Noort, MSc
Department of Child and Adolescent Psychiatry,
Psychosomatic Medicine and Psychotherapy
Charité – Universitätsmedizin Berlin
Augustenburger Platz 1, 13353 Berlin
betteke.van-noort@charite.de

Chapter 17
Martha Krijgsheld
Chair of the FAS Foundation of the Netherlands
Postbus 13
9980 AA Uithuizen

Susan Fleisher
Founder and former executive director of
National Organisation for Foetal Alcohol Syndrome-UK (NOFAS-UK)
Susan.Fleisher@nofas-uk.org

Sandra Ionno Butcher
Chief Executive of NOFAS-UK
022 Southbank House
Black Prince Road, Lambeth
London SE1 7SJ
info@nofas-uk.org

Part I: **The fetal alcohol syndrome and its diagnosis**

1 The syndrome

1.1 First description of FAS

When in 1973 the renowned medical journal the *Lancet* published an article by Jones and Smith entitled "Pattern of malformation in offspring of chronic alcohol mothers" [1], it was met with much scepticism and head shaking, since chronic alcoholism had always been, and was widely accepted as such by society, a male problem.

Following their first description the authors published a paper called "Recognition of the fetal alcohol syndrome in early infancy" [2]. With the term fetal alcohol syndrome (FAS)they described a new syndrome, which in the following 40 years radically changed our knowledge about "alcohol in utero" and the long lasting cerebral disturbance of children.

Ann Streissguth was a young clinical psychotherapist and psychiatrist back then, who worked in the Dysmorphology Unit of the University of Washington, which was led by David Smith. She examined children with dysmorphic abnormalities both neurologically and psychiatrically, and remembered that she could hardly believe that these children with their similar features were damaged only by the alcohol use of their mothers during pregnancy. However, because they recognised that the singular overlap between these children was, indeed, the chronic alcohol abuse of their mothers during pregnancy, this had to be the reason for their morphological abnormalities and cognitive impairments.

At once Streissguth [3] started an extensive literature search in the medical library of the University of Washington and was surprised when she realised that until 1973 there had been not a single scientific paper suggesting damaging effects from prenatal alcohol exposure.

This is difficult to understand nowadays. Despite all the professional scepticism, only a few years after the first *Lancet* article, FAS was described as a congenital "birth defect" worldwide. It became one of the most common causes for congenital psychomental developmental disorders with a higher incidence than trisomy 21 or spina bifida.

However, Lemoine et al. had already reported about a large number of children in France damaged by maternal alcoholism during pregnancy in 1968. Unfortunately, this article was published in a regional French medical journal (*Quest medicale*) and stayed unnoticed until the publication of D. Smith et al. in the *Lancet* [4].

1.2 History of FAS in the United States of America and Canada

In the following years, FAS was described and studied scientifically worldwide. The incidences of the syndrome and the different manifestations, as well as the potential pathomechanism were targets of intensive research.

https://doi.org/10.1515/9783110436563-001

In 1981, only a few years after discovery of the syndrome the Surgeon General of the United States [5] gave a nationwide warning against alcohol consumption during pregnancy. As a consequence of this warning, not only alcohol-dependent women were alarmed, but also especially women who had drunk occasionally (i.e. a glass of champagne in the very early and often still unknown pregnancy) were terrified.

Due to a lot of uncertainty in the initial years surrounding this new syndrome, which is moreover difficult to diagnose there were probably over-diagnoses of children with FAS.

In 1978, Clarren and Smith [6] published the first major study of 65 children affected by FAS in the *New England Journal of Medicine*. In this publication, the authors showed the wide range and variability in the clinical presentation of FAS.

The syndrome was commonly not recognised at birth or in the first months of life due to missing specific clinical symptoms, in particular craniofacial dysmorphia. Therefore, especially obstetricians and neonatologists continued to question the existence of FAS [7].

The first eight children described by Jones and Smith in 1973 [1] were infants not older than 5 years of age. Subsequently, the "typical FAS face", which allows a prima vista diagnosis, was just focused on young children for the first years. It was only much later that the diagnosis was extended from newborns to adolescents and even to adult patients.

Soon after Jones and Smith [1] defined FAS numerous animal studies were established that examined the harmful effects of alcohol exposure during pregnancy especially on the developing brain. These studies were able to show a relationship between alcohol exposure and several types of impairments. These findings successfully counteracted the initial scepticism of doctors regarding the teratogenic effects of alcohol [8].

In 1981 Sulik et al. [9] published a convincing mouse model showing disrupted and altered embryogenesis in mice offspring under laboratory conditions. After feeding pregnant mice with alcohol the fetal mice showed characteristic craniofacial dysmorphic signs compared to controls, with significant similarities to craniofacial features of children suffering from FAS (Fig. 1.1).

Furthermore, animal studies in rats showed long-term behavioural effects in offspring after intrauterine alcohol exposure [10, 11].

1.3 History of FAS in Europe and Germany

In 1968, Lemoine et al. [4] presented a detailed description of impairment in 127 children after prenatal alcohol exposure. Other European publications examining FAS followed from Sweden, Finland, England and Germany.

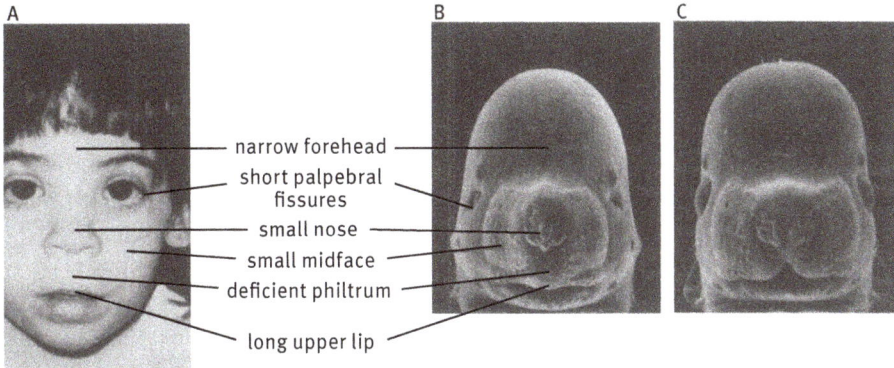

Fig. 1.1: K. Sullik et al., craniofacial dysmorphia shown in animal experiments. A) Human FAS patient, B) 14-day-old mouse fetus exposed to alcohol, C) control mouse fetus [9].

As early as 1976, Bierich and Majewski described the clinical manifestation of FAS in Germany [12]. Majewski, a human geneticist in Düsseldorf, introduced the term "alcohol embryopathy", which continued to be used for a long time in Germany. In 1981, he described his first speculations regarding the pathogenesis of FAS [13] and in 1993 he was able to report his experience with 200 patients with FAS [14].

In the year 1976, the paediatric cardiologist Hermann Löser and his colleagues described the cardiovascular malformations seen in FAS [15, 16]. In addition, in 1976 the French epidemiologist Kaminski described the relationship between prenatal alcohol exposure and intrauterine damage relating to disruption of neonatal development and, especially, disturbance of growth and maturation [17].

In Sweden, Olegard et al. were the first to publish a case-report about FAS in 1979 [18]. A few years later, in 1987, Larsson et al. demonstrated that children, whose alcoholic mothers were able to stop drinking alcohol during pregnancy and underwent a therapeutic intervention, had a more positive developmental outcome. This positive developmental effect continued even when the intervention was implemented in late pregnancy [19].

In 1996, Strömland, an ophthalmologist from Stockholm, and her colleagues described the tortuositas of retinal vessels as a characteristic ocular defect seen in children prenatally exposed to alcohol [20]. After a first case report in Finland, in 1979, Autti–Rämö published a prospective 3-year follow-up study of 24 children with FAS in 1993 [21].

In 1992, the European Union (EU) initiated the large multi-centre study "European Maternal Alcohol Consumption Study" (EUROMAC-Study) in six European countries (Denmark, the Netherlands, Spain, Portugal, Great Britain and Germany).

In each study centre, 1000 healthy pregnant women were examined prospectively, regarding their history of alcohol consumption during pregnancy. The time of exploration was during pregnancy or at the latest shortly after delivery, and all newborns were examined extensively at birth.

The amount of alcohol consumed by the mothers during pregnancy was divided into different groups, starting at 0 g of absolute alcohol per week and going up to 150 g per week in intervals of 30 g.

In summary, it was found that a consumption of 120 g of absolute alcohol per week or more, i.e. one glass of wine per day, caused a small but significant adverse effect on growth in the newborns examined [22].

In addition, in three centres (Dundee, UK; Arhus, Denmark; Berlin, Germany) although several hundred children were examined neurologically to determine the stage of teratogenicity, no significant delay in the infant's development was detected.

Since 1977, numerous children had been examined and diagnosed as having FAS by Spohr and Steinhausen in Berlin. With the support of the German Research Foundation (Deutsche Forschungsgemeinschaft, DFG) they were able to examine 60 children prospectively.

After a 4-year follow-up, published in 1987 [23], a 10-year follow-up study was published in *The Lancet* in 1993 [24]. Results from these patients at adolescence, were presented in 1994 [25].

After patients reached adulthood a cohort of 37 of them was re-examined and permanent damage due to prenatal alcohol exposure was demonstrated [26].

In 1993, Steinhausen and colleagues described the long-term consequencesof FAS. They were able to show that psychopathological abnormalities and cognitive impairments persisted into adolescence and did not diminish over time [28]. In 1996, the book *Alcohol, pregnancy, and the developing child* was edited by Spohr und Steinhausen [29].

In summary, fetal alcohol syndrome (FAS) was first introduced as a teratogenic syndrome only existing in childhood with an incidence of 1–2/1000 newborns.

However, today we know that this classification was just the "tip of the iceberg". It took several years to understand the full magnitude of this syndrome. In the meantime, FAS has changed from a purely dysmorphic syndrome to a highly complex neurological and psychiatric disease in affected patients, who are likely to suffer lifetime consequences of intrauterine alcohol exposure.

1.4 Current incidence and prevalence of FAS

Incidence is the rate of new cases or newly diagnosed cases of a disease per population in a given time period, usually based on 1000 live births per year.

In the first comprehensive study, Abel and Sokol examined the incidence of FAS in 1987. They found 18 studies published in the USA and Europe. A total of 163 cases of FAS was identified based on 88 236 births, corresponding to an incidence of 1.9/1000 live births [30]. The authors indicated that the incidence rate varied significantly depending on study design, study population and whether the study was prospective (lower incidence) or retrospective (higher incidence). The study population were women with a low socioeconomic status, mostly African-American or Native American who were treated in city hospitals. This resulted in significantly higher incidence rates compared to studies investigating Caucasian middle-class women. The incidence rate in this population was much lower (0.26/1000 live births) [31].

These early incidence studies were all focussed on "classical" FAS with typical cranio-facial features. It took a couple of years until the full dimension and variation of prenatal alcohol exposure became apparent.

Since more and more alcohol exposed children were identified without the characteristic dysmorphic features of FAS, but often with severe cognitive and psychopathological impairments, the term fetal alcohol spectrum disorder (FASD) was introduced as an "umbrella" term used to describe these cases.

In 1991, we examined the incidence of FAS in a women's hospital in Berlin, using intrauterine growth retardation as one of the characteristic symptoms. A population of 1002 newborns was consecutively screened for intrauterine growth retardation by ultrasound during pregnancy [33]. Growth retardation was found in 62 of these 1002 newborns.

One newborn received the FAS diagnosis directly at birth; the child's mother was heavily intoxicated at delivery and the newborn suffered from strong withdrawal symptoms. Of the 62 newborns showing growth retardation, 47 were re-examined between the ages of 8 and 19 months; 15 mothers refused to participate. Partial FAS (pFAS) was diagnosed in five children at follow-up. In conclusion, this study revealed an incidence of 6/1000 births (one FAS and five pFAS) [33]. Based on 662712 births in 2011, an approximate annual rate of 3000–4000 children affected by FAS was predicted for Germany. Stratton reported an incidence of 1–3(5)/1000 newborns in the USA in 1996 [32].

In 2014, a more recent epidemiological study from Alberta, Canada, reported clearly higher incidence rates of 14.2-to 43.8 per 1000 births [39].

The term prevalence describes the proportion of individuals in a population with a certain condition, i.e. disease or risk factors in a given time period. Prevalence is usually expressed as a percentage or as a number of cases (i.e. 1000 people) in a defined population. In contrast, incidence is usually reported as an annual rate within 1000 live births.

Early prevalence studies for FAS were published by May et al. in a population community in South Africa [34, 35]. They performed an extensive examination, including a neuropsychological evaluation in school children aged 6–7 years diagnosed with FAS, and the biological mothers were interviewed regarding their drinking behaviour during pregnancy. As expected, current prevalence rates were higher than the incidence rates based on newborns, since FASD often is not diagnosed before school age.

Prevalence studies in school children have been conducted in South Africa, in Italy and in the USA. In South Africa, the prevalence rate for FAS and pFAS was 7%

of school children; in Italy, the prevalence rate was 3% of school children and in the USA 1–2%. The authors, however, remarked that these prevalence rates are based on children with FAS or pFAS only. To date, the total degree of damage of FASD is still unknown [34, 35, 39].

The amount of maternal alcohol consumption during pregnancy is described in the literature with the so-called QFT factor. *Quantity* is the amount of alcohol consumed during pregnancy. *Frequency* refers to how often alcohol was consumed, and *timing* stands for when the alcohol was consumed. Unfortunately, in addition to the amount, frequency and timing of alcohol consumption, there are several other factors that make it difficult to give accurate prevalence estimates for FASD [32, 34]. There are, for example, several maternal risk factors for the development of FASD, such as diet during pregnancy, genetic factors (in particular an alcohol dehydrogenase polymorphism), ethnicity, as well as demographic, socioeconomic and psychosocial factors. In order to obtain a somewhat accurate estimate of the prevalence of FASD, all of these factors need to be taken into account.

Currently, the prevalence rate of all forms of FAS is generally estimated at 2–4%, depending on the definition and study design [35].

A recent epidemiological study from Canada in 2014 found an average prevalence of 11.7 (8.2–51.1) per 1000 individuals for the year 2012. These rates are clearly even higher than the previously estimated population prevalence of 1%. In addition, the study showed that males were more often affected than females, and a young age of exposure was more affected than an old age one [39].

In a further study from 2014, May and colleagues examined the prevalence of FASD in first graders living in a representative midwestern community in the USA. In line with earlier studies, prevalence rates were higher than assumed previously: the prevalence estimate for FAS was 6–9 per 1000 children, for pFAS 11–17 per 1000 and for ARND 6–22 per 1000 children. These rates lead to an estimated prevalence rate of 24–48 per 1000 children for FASD [40].

In 2008, Clarren and Lutke found a more conservative prevalence rate of FASD in Canada of 1% [36]. This would imply that of the 33 million people living in Canada, 330000 are affected by FAS or pFAS. However, only a small number of these patients, i.e. so far less than 20000, are diagnosed using the Canadian Guidelines [38]. If this prevalence rate from Canada were transferred to the German population of 80 million people, this would result in the unimaginable high number of 800000 potentially affected patients; similarly to Canada, only a marginal amount of these patients is currently identified.

In a very recent meta-analysis from 2016, Roozen et al. report the worldwide prevalence of FASD following a systematic literature review [41]. The authors conclude that the prevalence estimates are higher than previously assumed. These varying results can be explained by geography and descent. However, the prevalence studies included in this meta-analysis often suffered from poor methodological quality. The authors, therefore, concluded that the reported pooled estimates must be interpreted with caution. They emphasise the urgent need for clear guidelines on estimating prevalence rates for FASD.

In summary, it should be concluded that these increasing prevalence rates leave clinicians bewildered because of the complexity of making a clinical diagnosis. Usually, an interdisciplinary team is necessary, which consists of a dysmorphologist, paediatrician, child neurologist, psychologist and social worker, to determine the final diagnosis cooperatively. The high prevalence rate contrasts heavily with the relatively low number of diagnosed patients in the USA, Canada and Europe.

Bibliography

[1]   Jones KL, Smith DW, Ulleland CN, Streissguth AP. Pattern of malformation in offspring of chronic alcoholic mothers. Lancet 1973, 1(815), 1267–71.
[2]   Jones KL, Smith DW. Recognition of the fetal alcohol syndrome in early infancy, Lancet 1973, 2(836), 999–1001.
[3]   Streissguth AP. Fetal Alcohol Syndrome. Paul H. Brookes Publishing Co, Baltimore, Maryland 1997.
[4]   Lemoine P, Harousseau H, Borteyru JP, Menuet JC. Les enfants des parents alcooliques: anomalies observées à propos de 127 cas. Quest Medicale (Paris) 1968, 21, 476–82.
[5]   Surgeon General's Advisory on Alcohol in Pregnancy. FDA Drug Bulletin 1981, 11(2), 9–10.
[6]   Clarren SK, Smith DW. The fetal alcohol syndrome: experience with 65 patients and a review of the world literature. The New England Journal of Medicine 1978, 298(19), 1063–7.
[7]   Little BB, Snell LM, Rosenfeld CR, Gilstrap LC, Grant NF. Failure to recognize fetal alcohol syndrome in newborn infants. American Journal of Diseases of children 1990, 144(10), 1142–46.
[8]   Hannigan JH, Abel EL. Animal models for the study of alcohol-related birth defects. In: Spohr HL, Steinhausen HC (eds). Alcohol, pregnancy and the developing child. Cambridge University Press, UK 1996, 77–102.
[9]   Sulik KK, Johnson MC, Webb MA. Fetal alcohol syndrome: Embryogenesis in a mouse model. Science 1981, 214, 936–38.
[10] Riley EP, Hannigan JH, Balaz-Hannigan MA. Behavioral teratology on the study of early brain damage: considerations for the assessment of neonates. Neurobehavioral Toxicology and Teratology 1985, 7, 635–8.
[11] Riley EP. The longterm behavioral effects of prenatal alcohol exposure in rats. Alcohol: Clinical and experimental research 1990, 14, 670–3.
[12] Bierich JR, Majeski F, Michaelis R, Tillner I. Über das embryo-fetale Alkoholsyndrom. European Journal of Pediatrics 1976, 121, 155–77.
[13] Majewski F. Alcohol embryopathy: some facts and speculations about pathogenesis. Neurobehavioral Toxicology and Teratology 1981, 3(2), 129–44.
[14] Majewski F. Alcohol embryopathy: experience with 200 patients. Developmental Brain Dysfunction 1993, 6, 248–65.
[15] Löser H, Majewski F, Apitz J, Bierich JR. Kardiovaskuläre Fehlbildungen bei embryofetalen Alkohol-Syndrom. Klinische Pädiatrie 1976, 188, 233–40.
[16] Löser H, Majewski F. Type and frequency of cardiac defects in embryofetal alcohol syndrome: Report of 16 cases. British Heart Journal 1977, 39, 1374–79.

[17] Kaminski M, Rumeau-Rouquette C, Schwartz D. Consommation d'alcool chez les femmes en-
ceintes et issue de la grossesse. Revue Epidemiologique Médicale Sociale Santé Publique
1976, 24(1), 27–40.
[18] Olegard R, Sabel KG, Aronsson M. et al. Effects on the child of alcohol abuse during pregnancy.
Acta paediatrica Scandinavia 1979, 275(Suppl), 112–121.
[19] Larsson G, Bohlin AB. Fetal Alcohol syndrome and preventative strategies. Pediatrician 1987,
14, 51–6.
[20] Strömland K, Miller M, Cook C. Ocular teratology. Survey of Ophthalmology 1991, 35(6), 429–
46.
[21] Autti-Rämö I. The outcome of children exposed to alcohol in utero: A prospective follow-up
study during the first three years. University of Helsinki, Department of Child Neurology, Helsinki Finland 1993.
[22] Florey CduV, Tailor D, Bolumar F, Kaminski M, Olsen J (eds). European Maternal Alcohol Consumption Study (EUROMAC). Journal of Epidemiology 1992, 21 (Suppl X9).
[23] Spohr HL, Steinhausen HC. Follow-up studies of children with fetal alcohol syndrome. Neuropediatrics 1987, 18(1), 13–17.
[24] Spohr HL, Willms J, Steinhausen HC. Prenatal alcohol exposure and long-term developmental
consequences. Lancet 1993, 341(8850), 907–10.
[25] Spohr HL, Willms J, Steinhausen HC. The fetal alcohol syndrome in adolescence. Acta Paediatrica Scand. 1994, 83 (404), 19–26.
[26] Spohr HL, Willms J, Steinhausen HC. Fetal Alcohol Spectrum Disorders in Young Adulthood.
J. Pediatr 2007, 150, 175–179.
[27] Steinhausen HC, Gobel D, Nestler V. Psychopathology in the offspring of alcoholic parents.
Journal of the American Academy of Child and adolescent Psychiatry 1984, 23(4), 465–471.
[28] Steinhausen HC, Willms J, Spohr HL. Long-term psychopathological and cognitive outcome of
children with fetal alcohol syndrome. Journal of the American Academy of Child and Adolescent
Psychiatry 1993, 32(5), 990–994.
[29] Spohr HL, Steinhausen HC (eds). Alcohol, pregnancy and the developing child. Cambridge
University Press, Cambridge 1996.
[30] Abel EL, Sokol RJ. Incidence of fetal alcohol syndrome and economic impact of FAS-related
anomalies. Drug Alcohol Depend 1987, 19, 51–70.
[31] Abel EL. An update on incidence of FAS: FAS is not an equal opportunity birth defect. Neurotoxicol Teratol 1995, 17(4), 437–443.
[32] Institute of Medicine (IOM), Stratton KR, Howe CJ, Battaglia FC (eds). Fetal alcohol Syndrome:
Diagnosis, Epidemiology, Prevention, and Treatment. National Academy Press, Washington,
D.C. 1996.
[33] Schöneck U, Spohr HL, Willms J, Steinhausen HC. Alkoholkonsum und intrauterine Dystrophie.
Auswirkungen und Bedeutung im Säuglingsalter. Monatschr Kinderheilk 1992, 140, 34–41.
[34] May PA, Gossage JP, Marais AS, Adnams CM, Hoyme HG, Jones KL et al. The epidemiology of
fetal alcohol syndrome and partial FAS in a South African Community. Drug Alcohol Depend
2007, 88 (2–3), 259–271.
[35] May PA, Gossage JP, Kalberg WO, Robinson LK, Buckley D, Manning M et al. Prevalence and
epidemiologic characteristics of FASD from various research methods with an emphasis from
recent in-school studies. Dev. Disabil. Res. Rev. 2009, 15, 176–92.
[36] Clarren SK, Lutke J. Building clinical capacity for fetal alcohol spectrum disorder diagnoses in
western and northern Canada. Can. J. Clin. Pharmacol 2008, 15, 2223–237.
[37] Clarren S, Salmon A, Jonsson E. Introduction: How common is FASD. In: Clarren S, Salmon A,
Jonsson E (eds). Prevention of Fetal Alcohol Spectrum Disorder (FASD). Wiley-Blackwell, New
Jersey 2011.

[38] Chudley AE, Conry J, Cook JL, Cook C, Rosales T, LeBlanc N. Fetal alcohol spectrum disorder: Canadian guidelines for diagnosis. CMAJ 2005, 172(5suppl), S1–S21.
[39] Than NX, Jonsson E, Salmon A, Sebastianski M. Incidence and Prevalence of Fetal Alcohol Spectrum disorder by Sex and Age Group in Alberta, Canada. J Popul Ther Clin Pharmacol 2014, 21(3), e395–e404.
[40] May PA, Baete A, Russo J, Elliott AJ, Blankenship J, Kalberg WO et al. Prevalence and characteristics of fetal alcohol spectrum disorders. Pediatrics 2014, 134(5), 855–66.
[41] Roozen S, Peters G-JY, Kok G, Townend D, Nijhuis J, Curfs L. Worldwide Prevalence of Fetal Alcohol Spectrum Disorders: A Systematic Literature Review Including Meta-Analysis. Alcohol Clin Exp Res 2016, 40(1), 18–32.

2 Diagnosis of fetal alcohol syndrome

2.1 Definition

Fetal alcohol spectrum disorders (FASD)is a term that describes a variety of syndrome manifestations characterised by physical and mental abnormalities, as well as behavioural and learning difficulties, associated with prenatal alcohol exposure during pregnancy and presumably lasting a lifetime.

2.1.1 Fetal alcohol syndrome (FAS)

FAS is the "classic" version of the syndrome with typical characteristics such as growth deficiency, dystrophy, microcephaly, facial dysmorphic features, mental retardation, and psychiatric, cognitive and social abnormalities associated with a confirmed or suspected maternal alcohol consumption during pregnancy (Fig. 2.1).

The first children described by Jones and Smith in 1973 [1] belonged to this category. A "prima vista diagnosis" is generally possible with the presence of typical dysmorphic features, even when information on maternal alcohol consumption of the mother during pregnancy is unknown.

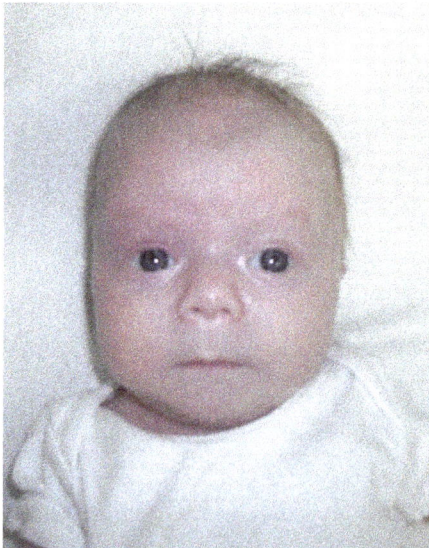

Fig. 2.1: Fetal alcohol syndrome (FAS).

https://doi.org/10.1515/9783110436563-002

2.1.2 Partial fetal alcohol syndrome (pFAS)

Soon after the first description of FAS, it was recognised that even children with confirmed prenatal alcohol exposure did not necessarily present with a "prima vista" manifestation of the disorder and full-blown dysmorphic features (i.e. the single pathognomonic diagnostic criteria for FAS), but these patients nevertheless had clear cognitive, social and emotional abnormalities (Fig. 2.2), and were classified as having pFAS.

　　Follow-up examinations in adulthood confirmed that pFAS is not less severe or a harmless variation of the syndrome. Those affected by pFAS suffer from the same difficulties in their everyday lives as FAS-patients, but they often have even greater problems because pFAS is diagnosed less often [2].

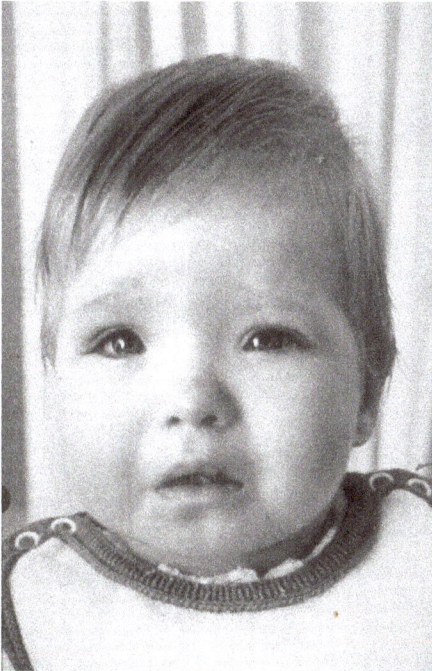

Fig. 2.2: Partial fetal alcohol syndrome (pFAS).

2.1.3 Alcohol-related neurodevelopmental disorder (ARND)

The term ARND was introduced by the National Academy of Medicine (NAM, formerly the Institute of Medicine, 1996) [7]. ARND describes a group of patients with confirmed maternal alcohol consumption during pregnancy and evidence of neurodevelopmental abnormalities, i.e. decreased cranial size at birth or structural brain abnormalities or neurological hard and soft signs and evidence of a complex pattern of developmental delay, behavioural abnormalities and cognitive impairments that cannot be explained by familial background or environment alone (Fig. 2.3).

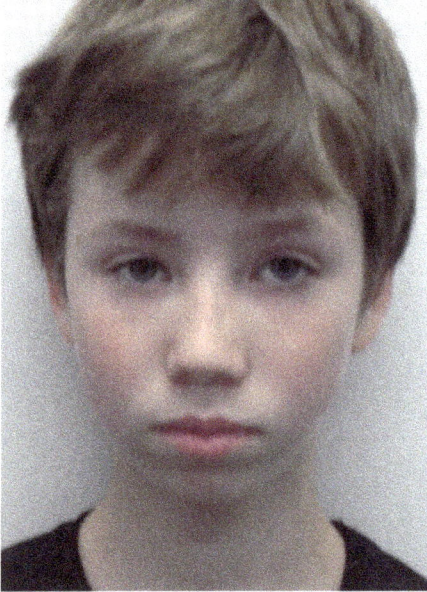

Fig. 2.3: Alcohol-related neurodevelopmental disorder (ARND).

2.1.4 Alcohol-related birth defect (ARBD)

The term ARBD was introduced to describe congenital malformations of other organ systems as a direct consequence of teratogenic effects of alcohol including cardiac, skeletal, renal, ocular or auditory malformations and dysplasia. In currently used guidelines this term is no longer a diagnostic criterion.

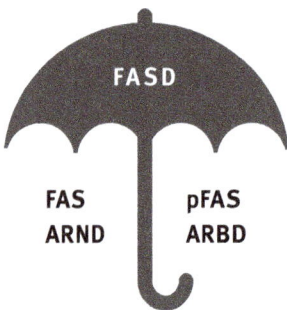

Fig. 2.4: Overview of FASD.
FAS: fetal alcohol syndrome; pFAS: partial fetal alcohol syndrome; ARND: alcohol-related neurodevelopmental disorder; ARBD: alcohol-related birth defects.

2.2 Clinical picture of FAS in a historical context

With the discovery of FAS in 1973 a new syndrome emerged, and the "medical world" reacted highly discomforted to the news. However, in a historical context, this syndrome was not a new phenomenon. Women have always consumed alcohol, perhaps not as openly and socially accepted as for men, but there are sufficient sources supporting this statement, as far back as in the Bible. In the Book of Judges (Chapter 13:3–5) the birth of Samson is prophesised to his mother by an angel as follows:

> "You are barren and childless, but you are going to become pregnant and give birth to a son. Now see to it that you drink no wine or other fermented drink and that you do not eat anything unclean. You will become pregnant and have a son whose head is never to be touched by a razor because the boy is to be a Nazirite, dedicated to God from the womb."

It seems rather unlikely that this biblical quotation really represents an archaic knowledge about the damaging effects of alcohol. The interpretation by Abel [2] probably holds true, i.e. that Samson was supposed to lead a pure life as a Nazirite from the moment of his conception.

There is a similar situation with a well-known quote from the Roman era, which was mentioned by Jones and Smith in their first publication [1]. In Plato's laws (nomoi), a Carthaginian law is discussed, which states that it is not proper for a bride and bridegroom to drink wine, since they should have their wits about them and make sure their offspring are born from reasonable beings.

The source is not clearly preserved, and Plato might have meant it merely as a desirable attitude; not only thinking of the female and her imminent pregnancy, but also referring to the damaging effects of wine on the male. However, the possible intrauterine damaging effects on the newly conceived child were surely not implied [2].

In one of the first scientific examinations of this disorder, the British physician William Sullivan mentioned in 1899 that the mortality rate of children born to chronic alcoholic women in prison compared to their non-alcoholic inmates was twice as high [3].

In a steel engraving by William Hogarth, the horrors of uncontrolled alcoholism are artistically depicted (Fig. 2.5). In "Gin Lane" (1756), the horrific consequences of unbounded alcoholism are dramatically and powerfully depicted, which was the result of a royal edict that freely allowed the existence of gin distilleries in England in the 18th century. As described by Abel, this "gin epidemic" in England cannot be expressed better than by the clear increase in the yearly gin consumption which went from 2 million gallons in the year 1714 to 11 million gallons in the year 1750. Already in the year 1736, there were apparently 7000 "gin houses" in London alone, which means that every sixth house in London must have been a "gin house" [2].

In the middle of the picture of William Hogarth, a completely wasted, deliriously smiling woman is seen, who symbolically dropped her poor, neglected baby from her

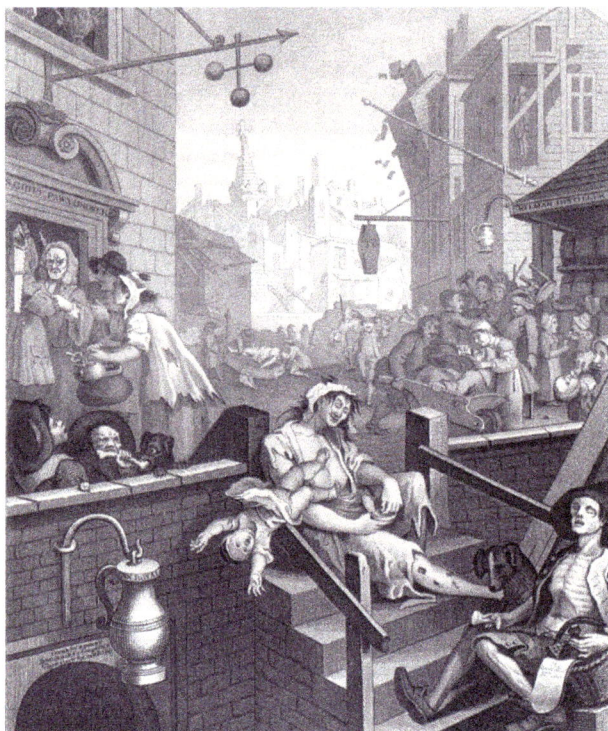

Fig. 2.5: "Gin Lane" steel engraving on paper by William Hogarth in 1756 (public domain).

arms into the depths of social misfortune. Instead of holding her child, she is taking a pinch of snuff from a can. She is therefore, most likely the first historical documentation of an alcohol-dependent woman with a child with probable intrauterine alcohol damage and, moreover, she is the first "prototype" of a polysubstance-dependent woman; not a chronically alcoholic woman without additional consumption of nicotine; something that Hogarth already recognised 250 years ago.

In the first description of the syndrome in Seattle [1], the authors only described children. At that time, FAS was thought to be a paediatric disorder, only being of interest to paediatricians and maybe child and adolescent psychiatrists. Many people believed that symptoms would normalise over time with the help of intensive treatment, a type of delayed biological maturation. At first, we also thought that this was the case, but a clear and long-lasting improvement happened rarely; the older the affected children became, the more the wide spectrum of clinical impairments became apparent, which lead to the fundamental finding that this syndrome also affects older adolescents and adults. Unfortunately, even today this disorder is still largely unknown to neurologists and psychiatrists.

2.3 Development of the diagnostic criteria for FAS

2.3.1 Diagnostic criteria according to Sokol and Clarren

After the initial description of the syndrome in 1973, Sokol and Clarren were the first to develop diagnostic criteria in the USA in 1989 [5]:
1. Prenatal and postnatal growth deficiency
   Dysfunctional central nervous system (CNS):
   (a) neurological
   (b) development
   (c) intelligence
2. Characteristic craniofacial dysmorphia
   (a) microcephaly
   (b) short palpebral fissures
   (c) thin upper lip
   (d) elongated, flattened maxilla zone (midface)
   (e) ill-defined philtrum

Only in those children whose growth deficiencies and weight abnormalities are evident, whose head circumference is microcephalic, who have mental retardation and who show very typical facial abnormalities is it not necessary for a diagnosis to confirm maternal alcohol consumption during pregnancy.

For all other patients, who represent the overwhelming majority of patients, the maternal alcohol consumption during pregnancy must be confirmed as a crucial criterion for the diagnosis. During the diagnostic process it is often necessary to search meticulously for any information regarding alcohol use during pregnancy. This is often very difficult because information from the birthmother is not available or – if known by the child services – not communicated with adoptive or foster parents for reasons of data privacy. If there is contact with the biological mother, alcohol use is often denied. Therefore, the most important anamnestic information for a diagnosis remains uncertain, and subsequently, the most frequent diagnosis nowadays is: "suspicion of FAS".

This is not helpful for the affected children, adolescents or adults, because neither the authorities nor social services will grant someone disability status with its accompanying social benefits when a diagnosis is only suspected. Moreover, appropriate support in school, as well as support by the Federal Employment Agency is often not available without a clear diagnosis.

2.3.2 The Majewski score

In addition to the American diagnostic guidelines by Sokol and Clarren as of 1989, Majewski published in 1981 a catalogue compiling 25 single symptoms of the "alcohol embryopathy," a term used in Germany for a couple of years to describe FAS.

All single symptoms were scored in a so named "Majewski score", and the final diagnosis, alcohol embryopathy, was divided into different categories of severity, ranging from category III (very severe syndrome) to category I (mild syndrome).

In 1993, Majewski examined 200 patients and based on his score he described the large heterogeneity of this disorder [6]. However, for many reasons, particularly the low retest-reliability in follow-up examinations, the Majewski score did not establish itself as a routine diagnostic instrument internationally or in Germany.

2.3.3 Institute of Medicine [now the National Academy of Medicine (NAM)]

In the year 1996, the Institute of Medicine (IOM) gave a comprehensive description of the different degrees of manifestation of fetal alcohol damage, summarised by the overall term FASD, used interchangeably with the term FAS and subdivided into the diagnoses FAS, pFAS, ARND (Alcohol-Related Neurodevelopmental Disorder) and ARBD (Alcohol-Related Birth Defects) [7], see Table 2.1.

Tab. 2.1: IOMdescription in 1996 (modified from [7]).

FASD	
FAS	*pFAS*
– Pre- and postnatal growth deficiency (length/weight below the 10th percentile). – Facial abnormalities (small eyes, smooth philtrum, thin upper lip). – CNS-damage (structural, neurological and functional damage).	– Two or more facial abnormalities. – Two or more other characteristics. – A complex pattern of cognitive impairments and behavioural abnormalities, who are not in line with normal development and cannot be explained genetically.
ARND	*ARBD*
– Symptoms and abnormalities resulting from CNS-damage associated with FAS without the typical facial abnormalities of the syndrome.	– Malformations of other organ systems, as a consequence of the teratogenic effect of intrauterine alcohol exposition (e.g. heart failures, bone- and kidney malformations, visual- and hearing impairments)

Note by the author: The terms FAS and FASD have not been defined clearly and are often used interchangeably, encompassing the other terms.

2.3.4 Clarification of IOM criteria

In 2005, Hoyme and colleagues published this practical clinical guidelinein the journal *Paediatrics* for the diagnosis of FASD with the aim of specifying the IOM-criteria from 1996 more precisely [8].

The syndrome was divided into
1. FAS with confirmed maternal alcohol exposure
2. FAS without confirmed maternal alcohol exposure
3. partial FAS with confirmed maternal alcohol exposure
4. partial FAS without confirmed maternal alcohol exposure
5. alcohol-related birth defects (ARBD)
6. alcohol-related neurodevelopmental disorder (ARND)

1. FAS with confirmed maternal alcohol consumption
A. Confirmed maternal alcohol exposure
B. Characteristic pattern of facial abnormalities ($\rightarrow$ 2 of the following)
   1. short palpebral fissures
   2. thin upper lip (Likert scale score 4 or 5)
   3. smooth philtrum (Likert scale score 4 or 5)
C. Evidence of pre- and postnatal growth deficiency
   1. height and weight $\leq$ 10th percentile (when possible, corrected with racial norms)
D. Evidence of decreased cranial size or abnormal morphogenesis
   1. structural brain abnormality
   2. head circumference $\leq$ 10th percentile ($\leq$ 1 of 2 standard deviation)

2. FAS without confirmed maternal alcohol exposure
A. Characteristic pattern of facial abnormalities ($\rightarrow$ 2 of the following)
   1. short palpebral fissures
   2. thin upper lip (Likert scale score 4 or 5)
   3. smooth philtrum (Likert scale score 4 or 5)
B. Evidence of pre- and postnatal growth deficiency
   1. height and weight $\leq$ 10th percentile (when possible, corrected with racial norms)
C. Evidence of decreased cranial size or abnormal morphogenesis
   1. structural brain abnormality
   2. head circumference $\leq$ 10th percentile ($\leq$ 1 of 2 standard deviation)

3. Partial FAS with confirmed maternal alcohol exposure
A. Confirmed maternal alcohol exposure
B. Characteristic pattern of facial abnormalities ($\rightarrow$ 2 of the following)

   1. short palpebral fissures (≤ 10th percentile)
   2. thin upper lip (Likert scale score 4 or 5)
   3. smooth philtrum (Likert scale score 4 or 5)
C. One of the following characteristics:
   1. Evidence of pre- and postnatal growth deficiency
      a. height and weight ≤ 10th percentile (when possible, corrected with racial norms)
   2. Evidence of decreased cranial size or abnormal morphogenesis
      a. structural brain abnormality
      b. head circumference ≤ 10th percentile
   3. Evidence of a complex pattern of behavioural or cognitive abnormalities that cannot be explained by genetic disposition, familial background or environment alone*

4. Partial FAS without confirmed maternal alcohol exposure
B. Characteristic pattern of facial abnormalities (→ 2 of the following)
   1. short palpebral fissures (≤ 10th percentile)
   2. thin upper lip (Likert scale score 4 or 5)
   3. smooth philtrum (Likert scale score 4 or 5)
C. One of the following characteristics:
   1. evidence of pre- and postnatal growth deficiency
      a. height and weight ≤ 10th percentile (when possible, corrected with racial norms)
   2. evidence of decreased cranial size or abnormal morphogenesis
      a. structural brain abnormality
      b. head circumference ≤ 10th percentile
   3. evidence of a complex pattern of behavioural or cognitive abnormalities that cannot be explained by genetic disposition, familial background or environment alone*

5. Alcohol-related neurodevelopmental disorder (ARND)
A. Confirmed maternal alcohol exposure
B. Evidence for at least one of the following:
   1. Evidence of decreased cranial size or abnormal morphogenesis
      a. structural brain abnormality
      b. head circumference ≤ 10th percentile
   2. Evidence of a complex pattern of behavioural or cognitive abnormalities that cannot be explained by genetic disposition, familial background or environment alone*

*impairments in the execution of more complex tasks (planning, judgement, abstract thinking, metacognition, mathematical skills, motor dysfunction, poor school performance and impaired social skills)

2.3.5 Development of diagnostic guidelines by the Canadian Medical Association

Independently of the US guidelines, in 2005 the Canadian Medical Association developed diagnostic criteria and guidelines for FASD and detailed comments were added [9].

The guidelines are made up of seven sections:
1. screening and transferal to a specialised centre;
2. physical examination and differential diagnosis;
3. neuropsychological examination;
4. treatment and follow-up examinations;
5. collection of information on maternal alcohol consumption during pregnancy;
6. diagnostic criteria for FAS, pFAS and other neurodevelopmental disorders caused by alcohol exposition during pregnancy (ARND);
7. harmonisation of the Canadian data with the IOM-criteria and the 4-Digit Diagnostic Code from the USA

When compared in more detail, the same criteria are used in the Canadian guidelines [9] as in the 4-Digit Diagnostic Code [10], which is described extensively in Chapter 3. In contrast to the 4-Digit Diagnostic Code, the 10th percentile is used instead the 3rd percentile, as a cut-off for weight, height and head circumference. Ranking of typical facial features is in accordance with the criteria described by Astley in the 4-Digit Diagnostic Code [10].

The Canadian guidelines propose a multidisciplinary team for the diagnostic process, comprising of following professional groups:
- physician familiar with diagnosing FAS
- case manager (nurse, social worker)
- psychologist
- occupational therapist
- logopedist

In 2004, the 3rd edition of the 4-Digit Diagnostic Code from Astley [10] was published, and today it is widely used as an international guideline for FAS (see Chapter 3).

2.3.6 Development of diagnostic guidelines in Germany

In Germany, the evidence-based S3 guideline for the diagnosis of FAS was established in 2013 and supplemented and adjusted for the diagnoses of pFAS and ARND in 2016.

A multidisciplinary guideline group has issued recommendations for the diagnosis of FAS after assessment of the available scientific evidence. This information was derived from pertinent literature (2001–2011) retrieved by a systematic search in PubMed and the Cochrane Library, along with the US-American and Canadian guidelines and additional literature retrieved by a manual search.

Of the 1383 publications retrieved by the searches, 178 were analysed for the evidence they contained. It was concluded that the fully developed clinical syndrome of FAS should be diagnosed on the basis of the following criteria: Patients must have at least one growth abnormality, e.g. short stature, as well as all three characteristic facial abnormalities – short palpebral fissure length, a thin upper lip, and a smooth philtrum. They must also have at least one diagnosed structural or functional abnormality of the central nervous system, e.g. microcephaly or impaired executive function. Confirmation of intrauterine exposure to alcohol.

Conclusion: Practical, evidence-based criteria have now been established for the diagnosis of the fully-developed FAS syndrome. The improved clarity and specificity will guide clinicians in accurate diagnosis of infants and children prenatally exposed to alcohol [11, 14].

2.3.7 The difficulty of comparing different diagnostic methods

In May 2016, Claire Coles et al. [15] published a comparison of five methods for the clinical diagnosisof FASD. Through this comparison with highly varying results between the different diagnostic methods, the dilemma surrounding the heterogeneous nature of FASD became clear.

The following methods were compared:
1. Emory FAS Clinic (2000)
2. 4-Digit-Diagnostic Code, Seattle (2000)
3. Centres for Disease Control and Prevention (Fetal Alcohol Syndrome: Guidelines for referral and Diagnosis, 2004);
4. Canadian Guidelines (2005);
5. Hoyme modifications (2005)

Without going into details on the different diagnostic methods, the results were highly divergent and not very encouraging. The incidences for an FASD diagnosis, for example, were very far apart (CDC: 4.74%, Hoyme: 59.58%). The authors concluded that the absence of an external standard makes it very difficult to determine which diagnostic system is most accurate.

Significant differences in the diagnostic process for FASD were already found in 2006 when comparing the Hoyme Diagnostic Guidelines and the 4-Digit Diagnostic Code. Besides the methodological issues, which are unresolved to this day and have become more apparent in the abovementioned article, one should ask the question why it is so difficult to diagnose FAS.

2.4 Why is it so difficult to diagnose FAS?

1. There is no pathognomonic symptom proving the diagnosis.
2. Only few patients have the full-blown syndrome with typical craniofacial features. 70–80% of affected patients have no or only mild dysmorphic features.
3. There is no distinct and disorder-specific neuropsychiatric profile.
4. Comorbid disorders often lead to misdiagnoses.
5. Poly-drug-dependent women are often additionally alcohol dependent but they mostly deny alcohol consumption.
6. Alcohol still is a taboo subject in our society.
7. Many physicians are still unfamiliar with the diagnosis of FAS.

FAS remains difficult to diagnose despite a significant increase of awareness in our society, because there are no "pathognomonic" symptoms except for the facial dysmorphic features, which are present in only 20–30% of patients. To date, no laboratory tests are available, and the diagnosis depends on the clinical experience of the physician familiar with FAS.

If characteristic facial dysmorphic features are missing, the only diagnostic indications are a small head circumference, microcephaly, impairments in executive functioning, mental retardation and growth deficiency. These symptoms are non-specific, often caused by intrauterine alcohol exposure, but also existing for different reasons.

Sometimes medical attention is mainly focussed on comorbid disorders such as organic malformations, cognitive deficits, attention deficit hyperactivity disorder (ADHD), impulse control and attention deficit disorder (ADS), attachment disorder, emotional disturbances, substance use disorders, etc., and the etiologic diagnosis remains unnoticed.

Some clinical signs occur more often in FAS, and a wide range of studies and investigations have endeavoured to detect a specific pattern that would be pathognomonic for FAS. However, so far, no sufficient validation could be established, and therefore an intensive examination and experience is needed, especially if the history of alcohol consumption during pregnancy is uncertain or unknown.

FAS is certainly not limited to the lower social class, but here it will be recognised more often, due to desolate family circumstances that sometimes lead to the need for intervention through child services and subsequently withdrawing of these children from their homes. These children then will live with foster or adoptive parents, who are faced with increasing abnormalities. They will consult a doctor or specialised FAS clinic for a diagnosis, especially when alcohol problems of the birth mother are known.

But even in these cases a clear diagnosis frequently remains difficult because social services often do not pass important information to the foster or adoptive parents, although it is generally known by now that child neglect and domestic violence in dysfunctional families is often associated with/triggered by parental alcohol problems, and thus the risk for intrauterine alcohol exposure of children of these families is very high.

Moreover, there seems to be an increase of poly-drug-dependent pregnant women. In addition to their alcohol dependency, they often have a nicotine addiction and consume illegal drugs on a daily basis, for example cannabis/marijuana and heroin, and more recently, crystal meth.

In this case to confirm a diagnosis of FAS is particularly difficult – usually the illegal drug abuse is recognised and treated by physicians, but underlying alcohol consumption often remains undisclosed or kept secret.

The diagnosticprocess is additionally difficult due to the fact that a history of alcohol consumption is difficult to verify either because drinking alcohol during pregnancy is still taboo or a history of alcohol consumption is often neglected and not expressly solicited by professionals as an important part of the medical history.

Furthermore, even today, physicians have more theoretical than practical knowledge about FAS.

In 2006, the American Academy of Pediatrics conducted a representative survey amongst about 900 paediatricians, analysing their levels of knowledge of FAS. The survey revealed that the large majority of the participants was informed about the incidence, the teratogenic effects, the lifelong brain damage and the associated psychiatric problems, but that only 50% of the respondents felt clinically capable to diagnose FAS and only 34% felt capable to treat these patients or organise therapeutic measures for them.

The following responses were given concerning their personal clinical experiences with these patients in the last 12 months: 42% had suspected the presence of FAS, 20% had diagnosed FAS and 18% had referred patients to experts to confirm the FAS diagnosis [4].

These paediatricians were well informed about FAS but largely struggled in transferring their academic knowledge into their clinical work when diagnosing and treating a child with FAS.

These results describe the main problem and difficulty with this disorder: both physicians and the general public increasingly are aware of the syndrome, but in clinical practice the affected children are still not sufficiently diagnosed and treated.

2.5 Misconceptions about FAS

After experience during the first 30 years with FAS and its great diversity and different manifestations, many prejudices and misconceptions still persist, particularly in the general public, but also amongst physicians, nurses, and in health and social services. The most common misconceptions are summarised below:

People with FAS are identifiable due to their atypical and dysmorphic faces.

Only a small number of affected children, adolescents or adults present facial ab-normalities (i.e. craniofacial dysmorphia). The "classical" FAS patients are the tip of the iceberg. About 70–80% of patients do not have the typical facial changes.

People with FAS always have mental retardation.

Not all of those affected by prenatal alcohol exposure necessarily suffer from men-tal retardation. In one of our own studies [12], 32% of adult patients had a normal IQ, and in a large American study 25% of patients also had an IQ in the average range [13]. Usually only patients with a severe form of FAS, with typical dysmorphic features, growth deficiency and microcephaly are affected by a below average intelligence level or intellectual impairment.

The behavioural problems seen in FAS are the result of bad upbringing by the par-ents, care givers or a poor social environment.

The prenatal alcohol damage often results in inflexible, inappropriate behaviour. Due to attention and hyperactivity disorder, memory deficits and impairments in so-cial perception; these affected patients are not able to behave appropriately in social settings. Parents and caregivers are often faced with incomprehension and criticism, resulting in additional stress for them.

Accepting that children with FAS may have brain damage implies that their social surroundings and the general population give up these sick children.

Some people think that accepting mental retardation as being part of FASD means that any help or support for these "hopeless" cases might be terminated. First of all, there are no "hopeless" cases and secondly, according to scientific findings, extensive support and long-term care is helpful and really improves the situation to a certain extent in these patients.

Symptoms and developmental delay in a child with FAS will vanish over time.

Unfortunately, we know nowadays that FAS is with high probability a permanent and lifelong disorder. Those affected need extensive support and assistance, partic-ularly in adolescence and adulthood. This is important to know for foster parents, because normally foster care ends at the age of 18 and, long-lasting support options have to be planned and organised.

To diagnose a child with FAS is a burden for the child and will lead to stigmatisation.

Receiving the diagnosis is the first step towards treatment and support. With a diagnosis, which is difficult to obtain and is often a lengthy journey fraught with prob-lems, foster parents and care givers have finally "arrived". The difficulties and prob-lems are not the result of a wrongful or inadequate upbringing, but are caused by an organic disease. In the absence of a diagnosis, it is very difficult to receive any form of treatment, therapy and social or governmental support.

The FAS diagnosis is useless since there is no adequate treatment.

A diagnosis is especially important if a disorder is only recognisable by clinical symptoms. A correct diagnosis explains why these affected children are so different compared to others and helps to end the search for an explanation of being different.

Those who take care of the child become knowledgeable that they are not responsible for the child's behavioural problems. A correct diagnosis facilitates organisation of appropriate support and therapy.

People with FAS are irresponsible because they are unmotivated and indifferent.

Unfortunately, this is a widespread misconception about FAS, which is far removed from the reality of those affected, because their problems are clearly created by the numerous limitations due to underlying brain damage. Adolescents and adults with pFAS/ARND are often unfairly criticised for their behaviour and mistakes because of beeing compared to healthy peers (see Streissguth [13]).

Bibliography

[1]   Jones KL, Smith DW, Ulleland CN, Streissguth AP. Pattern of malformation in offspring of chronic alcoholic mothers. Lancet 1973, 1(815), 1267–71.
[2]   Abel EL. Fetal Alcohol Syndrome and Fetal Alcohol Effects. Plenum Press, New York and London 1984.
[3]   Sullivan WC. A note on the influence of maternal inebriety on the offspring. Journal of Mental Science 1899, 45, 489–503.
[4]   Gahagan S, Sharpe TT, Brimacombe M et al. Paediatricians' Knowledge, Training, and Experience in the Care of children with Fetal Alcohol Syndrome. Pediatrics 2006, 118 (3), 657–668(e).
[5]   Sokol, RJ, Clarren SK. Guidelines for use of terminology describing the impact of prenatal alcohol in the offspring. Alcoholism: Clinical and Experimental Research 1989, 13(4), 597–598.
[6]   Majewski F. Clinical symptoms in patients with fetal alcohol syndrome. In: Spohr HL & Steinhausen HC (eds). Alcohol, pregnancy and the developing child. Cambridge University Press, Great Britain 1996, 15–39.
[7]   Institute of Medicine (IOM), Stratton KR, Howe CJ, Battaglia FC (eds). Fetal alcohol Syndrome: Diagnosis, Epidemiology, Prevention, and Treatment. National Academy Press, Washington, D.C. 1996.
[8]   Hoyme HE, May PA, Kalberg WO, Kodituwakku P, Gossage JP et al. A practical clinical approach to diagnosis of fetal alcohol syndrome spectrum disorders: clarification of the 1996 institute of medicine criteria. Pediatrics 2005, 115 (1), 39–47.
[9]   Chudley AE, Conry J, Cook JL, Cook C, Rosales T, LeBlanc N. Fetal alcohol spectrum disorder: Canadian guidelines for diagnosis. CMAJ 2005, 172(5suppl), S1–S21.
[10] Astley SJ. Diagnostic guide for Fetal Alcohol Spectrum Disorders: The 4-Digit Diagnostic Code. 3rd edn. University of Washington Publication Services, Seattle WA 2004.
[11] Landgraf MN, Notacker M, Heinen F. Diagnosis of fetal alcohol syndrome (FAS): German guideline version 2013. Eur J Paediatr Neurol. 2013, 17(5), 437–446.
[12] Spohr HL, Willms J, Steinhausen HC. Fetal Alcohol Spectrum Disorders in Young Adulthood. J. Pediatr 2007, 150, 175–179.
[13] Streissguth AP, Barr HM, Kogan J et al. Understanding the occurrence of secondary disabilities in clients with fetal alcohol syndrome (FAS) and fetal alcohol effects (FAE).Final report to the Centers for Disease Control and Prevention (CDC). University of Washington, Fetal Alcohol and Drug Unit, Seattle 1996, 96–106.
[14] Landgraf MN, Notacker M, Kopp IB, Heinen F. The diagnosis of fetal alcohol syndrome. Dtsch Arztebl Int. 2013, 110(42), 703–710.
[15] Coles CD, Gailey AR, Mulle JG, Kable JA, Lynch ME, Jones KL. A Comparison Among 5 Methods for the Clinical Diagnosis of Fetal Alcohol Spectrum Disorders. Alcohol Clin Exp Res 2016, 40(5), 1000–1009, doi: 10.1111/acer.13032.

3 The 4-Digit Diagnostic Code

3.1 Introduction

The 4-Digit Diagnostic Code is an important instrument for diagnosing FAS in the United States, and the 3rd edition from 2004 is widely used internationally as well [3]. For more than 15 years this diagnostic tool has been used exclusively in our clinic in Berlin and it was the basis for the German S3 Guidelines for Fetal Alcohol Syndrome in 2013 [1].

Years of experience using this method for diagnosing FAS in many affected children, adolescents, and more recently also in adults improved the diagnostic accuracy in individuals of all ages. Today, the strengths as well as the weaknesses of the 4-Digit Diagnostic Code are well known, in particular because Coles et al. (2016) emphasised the discrepancies and the lack of conceptual clarity in the most commonly used assessment methods [19].

We have modified the 4-Digit Code slightly, according to a more practical classification in daily clinical use. Therefore, from of a multitude of classifications suggested by the authors, we only use the diagnostic categories FAS, pFAS and ARND. Because ARND is not classified in the 4-Digit Diagnostic Code, we instead apply "neuro-behavioural disorder, alcohol exposed" as an equivalent category.

Comparing different diagnostic methods, Coles et al. (2016) [19] confirmed our experience that no diagnostic method is superior to any other, and due to the lack of a special diagnostic instrument for FAS in adults, we modified and adjusted the 4-Digit Diagnostic Code to diagnose also these affected adult patients (see Section 14.2).

3.1.1 Benefits and some disadvantages of the 4-Digit Diagnostic Code:

Benefits:
– Diagnostic precision is increased by using objective, quantitative measures as well as the option to use facial image analysis software with validated normative data.
– The presence of prenatal alcohol exposition is documented without judgement.
– Other possible pre- and postnatal factors and events influencing birth outcome and further development of the child (e.g. illnesses of the mother or birth complications) are documented.
– Although the diagnostic process seems complex and challenging at first, due to its standardised and structured methodology, it is not difficult.

Disadvantages:
– A multi-disciplinary professional team is necessary.
– Although the process is standardised, an experienced diagnostician is critical.

https://doi.org/10.1515/9783110436563-003

- To substantiate a diagnosis without characteristic facial features (i.e. pFAS, ARND) remains difficult even when using the 4-Digit Diagnostic Code.
- Presently, the diagnostic assessment method is limited to children and adolescents up to the age of 18.

3.1.2 Classification

Susan Astley, an epidemiologist, and Sterling Clarren, a paediatrician and dysmorphologist, both from the University of Washington, examined the characteristics of the phenotype of FASD. They concluded that except for a "typical face" caused by intrauterine alcohol exposure there was no characteristic feature pathognomonic to this disorder. Microcephaly, growth deficiency and developmental delay, as well as cognitive impairments and behavioural problems, seen in FAS, are common clinical symptoms non-specific to intrauterine alcohol exposure [2].

They examined the faces of thousands of children with FAS and were able to reduce the many craniofacial anomalies to three key dysmorphic facial features: small palpebral fissures, a thin upper lip and a smooth philtrum.

These facial features are the typical characteristics seen in patients with the full-blown syndrome and often allow direct diagnosis [3]. Furthermore, growth deficiency, structural and functional CNS damage and maternal alcohol abuse during pregnancy have to be evaluated, and these four domains serve as the basis for creating the 4-Digit Diagnostic Code by evaluating and ranking the level of severity.

Each diagnostic domain is ranked independently according to level of severity with a four-point scale (Likert scale) with *1 point* reflecting complete absence of symptoms, *2 points* reflecting mild presence of symptoms, *3 points* a moderate presence of symptoms or features and *4 points* reflecting a strong "classic" and definite presence of symptoms or features, indicating that the syndrome is indisputably present. Table 3.1 provides a list of the ranking of the four diagnostic domains.

Tab. 3.1: Ranking of the four diagnostic domains in the 4-Digit Diagnostic Code (modified from [3]).

Growth deficiency	none 1, mild 2, moderate 3, significant 4
facial dysmorphic features	none 1, mild 2, moderate 3, severe 4
CNS damage	none 1, mild 2, probable 3, definite 4
Prenatal alcohol consumption	none 1, unknown 2, probable 3, high risk 4

3.2 Growth deficiency

Children who are exposed to alcohol prenatally often present growth deficiency (underweight and/or short stature). Many children are small-for-date newborns and often continue to be underweight and of short stature for several years. However, a variety of potential contributing causes must be considered, including genetic factors (e.g. height of the parents), illnesses of the mother during pregnancy or postnatal influences such as deprivation and malnutrition. It is possible that a newborn of an alcoholic diabetic mother may have an almost normal weight, with dystrophy obscured due to the frequent significantly higher birth weight observed in children of diabetic mothers.

3.2.1 Clinical remarks regarding growth deficiency

Pre- and postnatal growth deficiency is defined as weight and length below the third percentile. Several variable factors warrant consideration:

- As presented by authors of the Canadian guidelines, children who are not exposed to alcohol during the third trimester may not have growth deficiency, but are still at risk for cognitive impairments, behavioural problems and developmental difficulties.
- A teratogen-induced growth deficiency is a consistent impairment over a period of time or sometimes for the entirety of life (i.e. with growth parallel to the normal developmental chart curves but at a lower level). In contrast, growth deficiency caused by postnatal influences leads to periodic fluctuations in the growth curve.

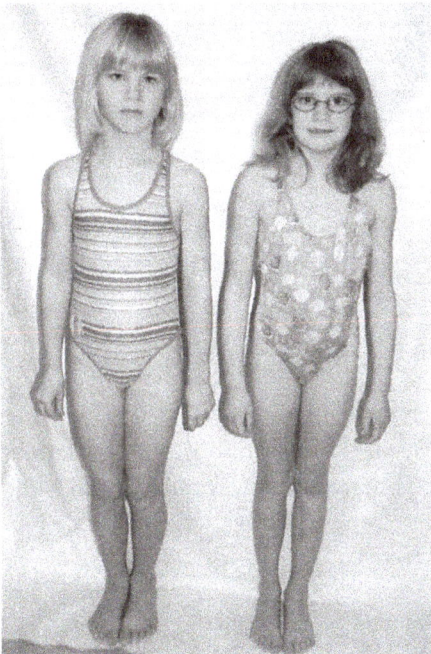

Fig. 3.1: 11-year old female with FAS (right) and healthy 7-year-old female (left).

– One of the important characteristics of a growth deficiency in FAS is the lack of catch-up growth as children age [4]. Growth disturbances seen in FAS are not the result of growth hormone deficiency, but rather a consequence of the lack of peripheral responsiveness to growth hormones [5].
– Growth deficiency does not always persist; particularly post-pubertal girls may have significantly increased weight and often become overweight or even obese.
– If a patient is not diagnosed until adulthood, data of growth development during childhood must be taken into account, but unfortunately often they are unknown.
– Additionally, standards for body length and weight for adults are not available, especially for different ethnic groups.

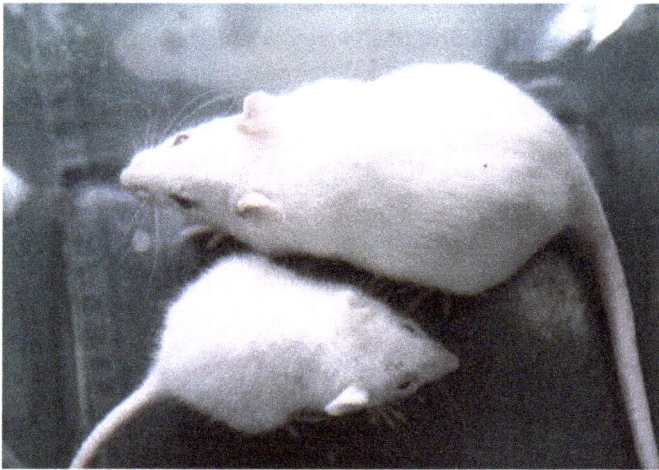

Fig. 3.2: Example of growth deficiency in a 21-day-old Wistar rat with intrauterine alcohol exposure compared to a healthy control animal (Spohr et al., 1994).

3.3 Dysmorphic facial features

David Smith, who first used the term FAS in 1973, identified three facial dysmorphic features as key criteria for diagnosis [6]. Astley and Clarren confirmed the sensitivity and specificity of these facial criteria in a large analytical study in 2010 [7] and found a remarkable correlation between the facial dysmorphic features and brain damage or brain dysfunction: the prevalence of brain damage increased linearly with an increase in severity of the dysmorphic features.

The three criteria of craniofacial dysmorphia in FAS (Fig. 3.3):
1. small palpebral fissure (≤ 3rd percentile),
2. thin upper lip (rank 4 or 5 on the Likert scale) and
3. smooth philtrum (rank 4 or 5 on the Likert scale).

Facial dysmorphology can either be assessed directly or by using facial image analysis software on a computer [9]. We assess the palpebral fissures directly with a measuring tape held as closely as possible to the eye without touching the child's eye or eyelashes (Fig. 3.5).

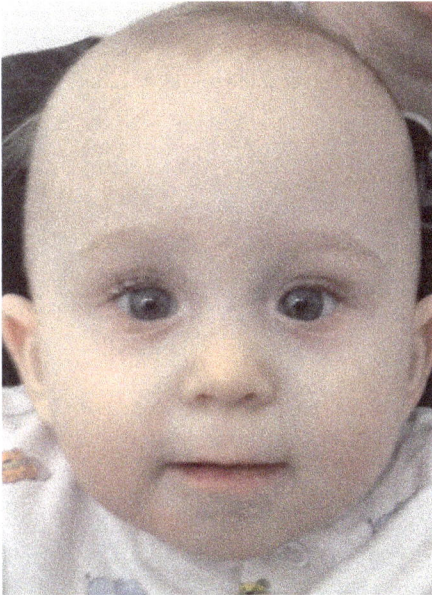

Fig. 3.3: Facial features of FAS (craniofacial dysmorphia).

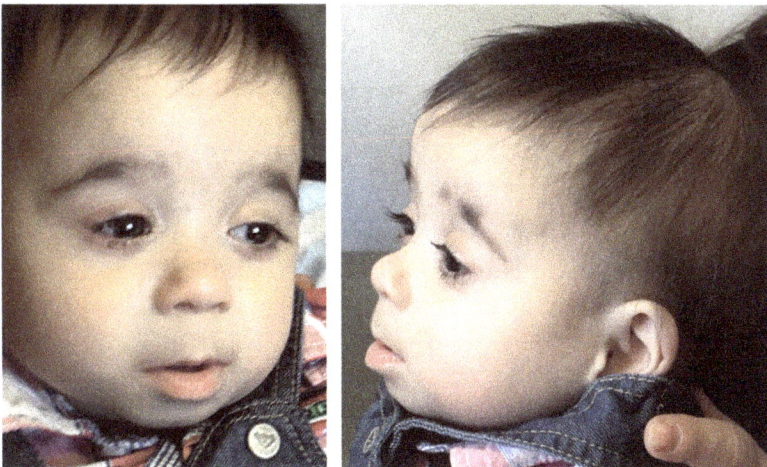

Fig. 3.4: 11-month-old boy.

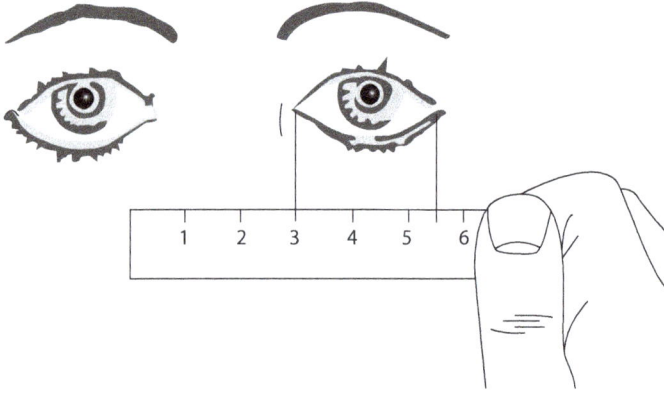

Fig. 3.5: Palpebral fissure length measurement from the inner corner of the eye (inner canthus) to the outer corner of the eye (outer canthus) [3].

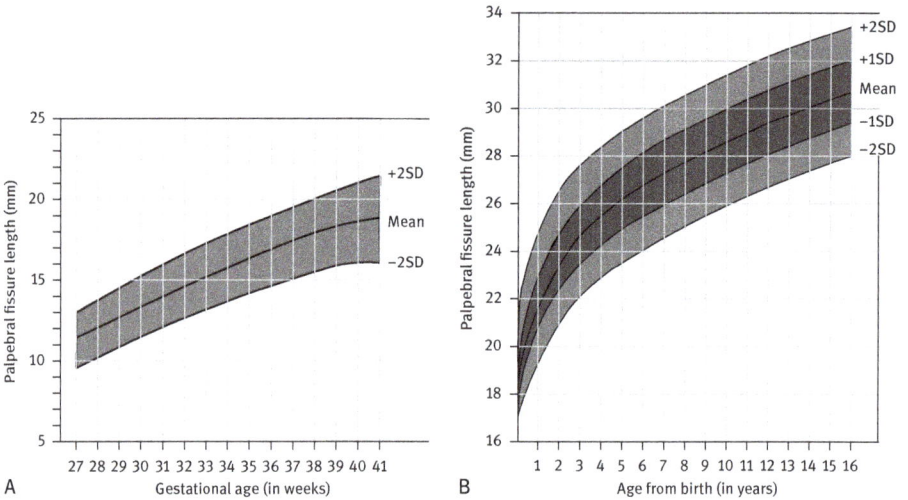

Fig. 3.6: A) Percentile curves of fetal palpebral fissure lengths from the 27th week of pregnancy until birth, and B) percentile curves of palpebral fissure lengths in girls and boys from birth until the age of 16; modified from [10].

Palpebral fissure lengths are compared to standardised male and female percentile curves from Hall et al. from 1989 [10] for Caucasian patients (Fig. 3.6 A, B). Since 2010, we use more restricted fissure length percentiles for boys and girls between the ages of 6 and 18 (Fig. 3.7) [11].

The upper lip and the philtrum are assessed with the Lip-Philtrum-Guide, a five-point Likert scale based on photos displaying different severity levels. Both criteria are crucial to determine the extent of facial dysmorphology and both have to be evaluated independently (Fig. 3.8).

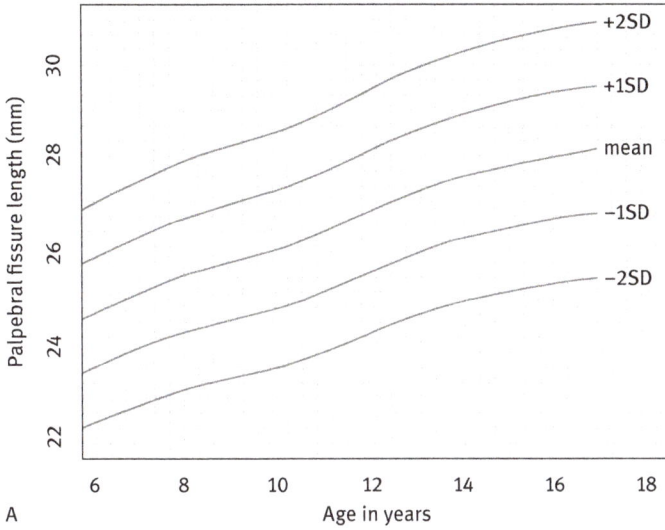

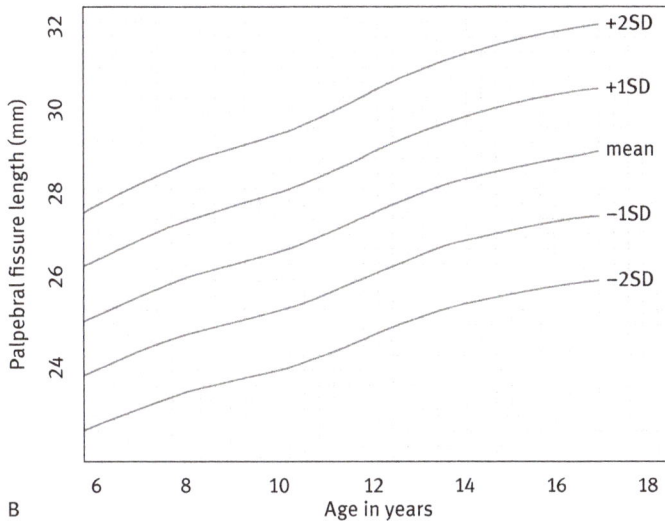

Fig. 3.7: A) Percentile curves for palpebral fissure lengths in girls between the ages of 6 and 18 and B) percentile curves for fissure lengthsin boys between the ages of 6 and 18 [11].

3.3.1 Clinical remarks

In the 4-Digit Diagnostic Code, the extent of the facial dysmorphology is an important difference between FAS and pFAS. If a patient's facial dysmorphology is ranked 3 points on the Likert scale s/he always will receive a diagnosis of partial fetal alcohol syndrome (pFAS), disregarding the severity of impairment in the remaining domains.

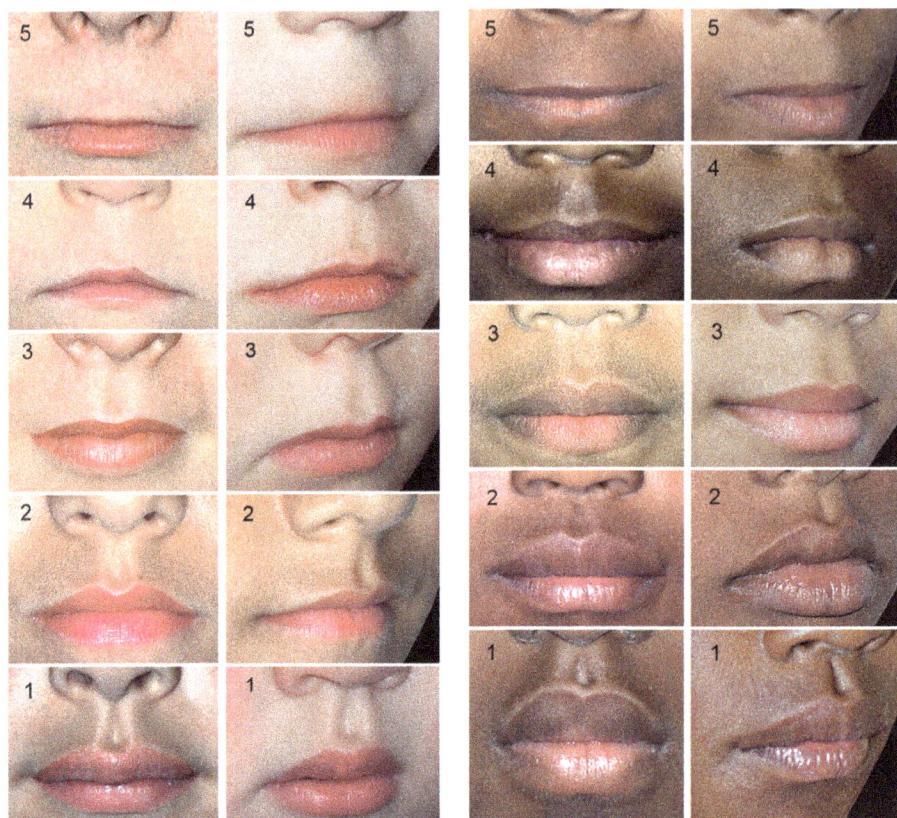

Fig. 3.8: Likert-Scale (Lip-Philtrum Guide), © 2013 Susan Astley PhD, University of Washington.

The precise distinction as to whether a philtrum and upper lip will be ranked 3 or 4 is sometimes a difficult and very subjective clinical decision, and according to the authors' experience, a difficulty in using the 4-Digit Diagnostic Code.

Usually the majority of patients present less marked facial dysmorphic features, therefore it is important to state that pFAS is not simply a benign form of the syndrome, as these patients are often severely affected as well. Nonetheless, a correlation is well known between severity of CNS damage and severity of facial abnormalities.

– Even with extensive familiarity in using the 4-Digit Diagnostic Code, assessment of the facial dysmorphic features is the most difficult part of the diagnosis and requires considerable clinical experience.
– Evaluation of facial dysmorphology in adult patients is particularly difficult, because the characteristic facial features largely diminish over time, and this diagnostic tool only relates to children and adolescents. Therefore, it is necessary to evaluate the severity of facial dysmorphic features in adult patients using photos from their infancy and childhood.

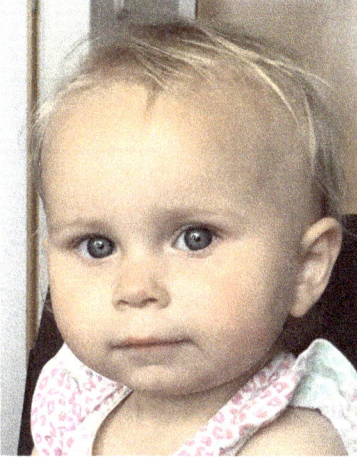

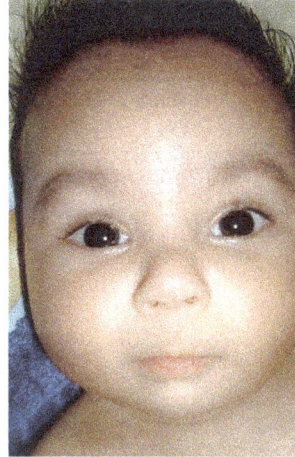

3.4 Central nervous system abnormalities

Alcohol is a teratogen and damages the developing brain irreversibly with various and often-persisting consequences in the form of structural malformations, as well as causing functional brain abnormalities. Postnatal environmental factors may also result in permanent developmental and behavioural impairments without alcohol exposure during pregnancy.

Criteria of the 4-Digit Diagnostic Code ranking damage of the central nervous system portends an increasing probability of functional or structural damage [12].

Current head circumference and data of previous head circumferences are used to identify a possible microcephaly. Functional brain disturbances are examined and analysed with standardised age-adjusted test methods (Chapter 4):

1. intelligence
2. school performance
3. adaptive behavioural skills/social skills
4. executive functioning
5. motor development and sensory processing
6. language development and social communication
7. mental health and
8. general behaviour/attention

Tab. 3.2: Criteria for central nervous system damage in the 4-Digit Diagnostic Code (modified from [3]).

4-Digit-Diagnostic Code (value)	Probability of CNS damage	Evidence
4	Definite	Microcephaly ($\leq$ 3. percentile), pathological MRI findings, prenatal neurological deficits
3	Probable	Significant impairments in 3 or more functional areas (such as cognition, executive functioning, language, memory, concentration)
2	Possible	Signs of functional impairments or developmental delay, which do not meet the criteria of rank 3
1	Unlikely	No evidence for dysfunction or developmental delay, which indicates central nervous system damage.

3.4.1 Clinical remarks

- A correlation between microcephaly and mental retardation has been established in the scientific literature as well as by clinical experience [13, 14].
- Significant structural brain abnormalities may be a consequence of intrauterine alcohol exposure, but might also occur without exposure to alcohol. Due to an increase of clinical MRI-examinations today, these abnormalities are possibly only an incidental finding.
- In general, MRI as a routine method in diagnosing FAS is not useful, because there are no pathognomonic brain abnormalities known, and few experts are able to interpret possible pathological findings. Furthermore, in young children, an MRI examination requires the use of sedatives or even anaesthesia, which would be an additional stress.
- To identify a possible microcephaly measurement of head circumference is a convincing instrument and clinically easy to perform.
- A confirmed microcephaly is rank 4 in the 4-Digit Diagnostic Code; the additional existing functional impairments – even severe – are not separately mentioned.

3.5 Prenatal alcohol exposure

In the majority of cases, a final diagnosis of FAS requires confirmed and significant prenatal alcohol exposure.

Self-report by the birth mother is the preferred information about prenatal alcohol exposure, but determination can also be based on reports of family members and other caregivers who have confirmed information about maternal alcohol consumption during pregnancy or who observed the pregnant birth mother drinking alcohol,

Control animal · Animal with intrauterine alcohol-exposure

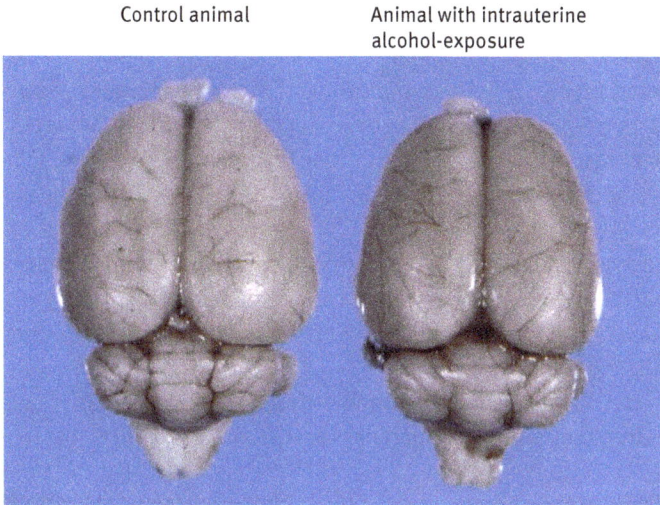

Fig. 3.11: Reduced brain volume in a Wistar rat with intrauterine alcohol exposure compared to a control animal with the same weight (authors' own animal experiment).

and/or information obtained from medical documents or other records. Information obtained by hearsay only or suspected from bad living conditions of the birth mother are insufficient. If available, the amount and types of drinks, drinking patterns, time point and the frequency of alcohol consumption should be recorded.

Furthermore, information about other risk factors during pregnancy should be collected (i.e. additional substance use, illness of the mother, psychosocial risk factors) because they can induce impairment in fetal development as a crucial or an additional factor.

Tab. 3.3: Criteria for prenatal alcohol exposure in the 4-Digit-Diagnostic Code (modified from [3]).

High risk (4)	Alcohol consumption during pregnancy is confirmed as a high risk (i.e. high blood alcohol concentrations at least once a week in early pregnancy).
Medium risk (3)	Alcohol consumption during pregnancy is confirmed and the amount of alcohol is less than described under value 4 or is unknown.
Unknown risk (2)	Alcohol consumption during pregnancy is unknown or denied by the birth mother.
No risk (1)	Alcohol abstinence during pregnancy is confirmed from conception until birth.

3.5.1 Clinical remarks

There are two fundamental problems in the 4-Digit Diagnostic Code documenting alcohol consumption during pregnancy. Firstly, in clinical practice; information on alcohol use during pregnancy may not be available or may be uncertain.

– Birth mothers often underestimate or deny their alcohol consumption during pregnancy.
– In our clinic most affected children are taken into custody due to maternal neglect without noticing that the alcohol abuse is a basic cause of the neglect. Information about the biological family is often underreported or not provided to the foster or adoptive parents due to data privacy.
– Fortunately, Child Services in Berlin, more often evaluate whether a child is suffering from FASD before they allow adoption or placement of the child in a foster family.
– If alcohol consumption during pregnancy remains unknown, the affected child should be transferred for genetic investigation.

Secondly, it is currently impossible to define an amount of alcohol as definitely not being toxic for fetal development and severe alcohol consumption is defined differently:

1. Institute of Medicine (IOM), 1996.
   A pattern of excessive alcohol consumption is characterised by constant and frequent alcohol use or heavy episodic drinking [12].
2. National Institute on Alcohol, Alcoholism and Alcohol Abuse (NIAAA), 2005.
   Heavy alcohol use is defined as the consumption of five or more drinks on occasion at least once a week [15].

3.5.2 Summary and final diagnosis

After the assessment and evaluation of the four diagnostic domains of the 4-Digit Diagnostic Code every domain receives a total score. In theory, a total of 256 separate diagnoses can be given, ranked from 1111 to 4444, which are summarised into the following categories: "fetal alcohol syndrome", "partial fetal alcohol syndrome", as well as the diagnoses: "sentinel physical findings", "static encephalopathy" and "neurobehavioural disorder".

The multitudes of diagnoses presented by the 4-Digit Diagnostic Code are inappropriate in clinical routine, and we only use the following diagnoses: fetal alcohol syndrome (FAS), partial fetal alcohol syndrome (pFAS), and alcohol-related neurodevelopmental disorder (ARND).

Tab. 3.4: Summary of the total scores representing the diagnoses mentioned.

FAS			pFAS					ARND			
2433	3433	4433	1333	1433	2333	3333	4333	1133	1233	2133	2233
2434	3434	4434	1334	1434	2334	3334	4334	1134	1234	2134	2234
2443	3443	4443	1343	1443	2343	3343	4343	1143	1243	2143	2243
2444	3444	4444	1344	1444	2344	3344	4344	1144	1244	2144	2244
2432	3432	4432									
2442	3442	4442									

The complete corresponding scores of the 4-Digit Diagnostic Code are published online [16].

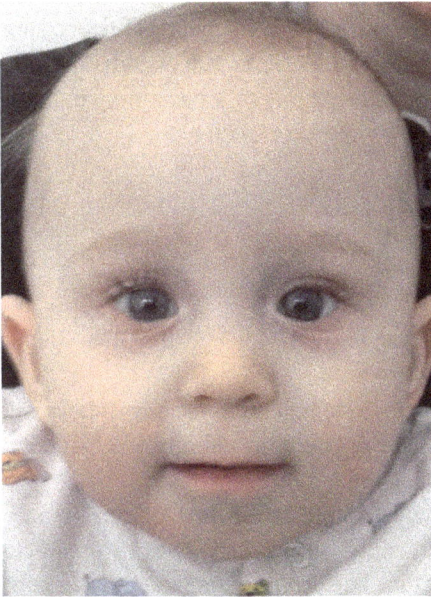

Fig. 3.12: A.S., 9 months old.

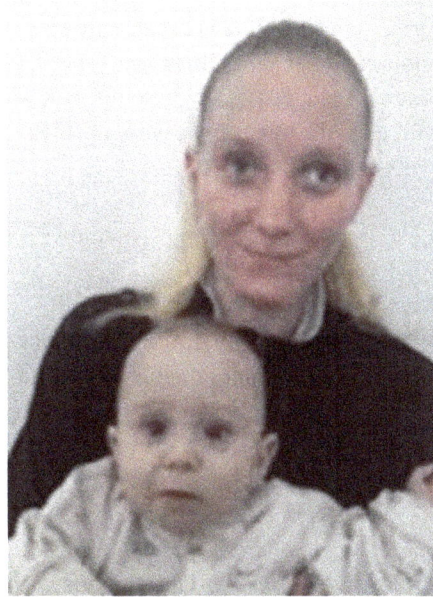

Fig. 3.13: A.S. with her biological mother.

Case report

A.S. born July 2012 (Figs. 3.12, 3.13):

A.S. was a preterm baby diagnosed with intrauterine growth retardation at birth. Postnatally she suffered from a congenital infection and a peripheral pulmonary stenosis.

She was discharged home with the recommendation to consult her paediatrician for controlling weight gain within the next few weeks only.

But the midwife was concerned about her development and suggested further consultation.

At the age of 3 months, she presented with increased neurodevelopmental abnormalities, was examined and finally diagnosed as having "classic" FAS (score 4/4/4/4).

In the medical report of the birth clinic, alcohol abuse of the mother, inpatient alcohol rehabilit-ation in 2008 and distinct facial features were documented. The cooperative mother reported her alcohol abuse during pregnancy, but the possibility of FAS had not been mentioned to her at all.

3.6 Limitation of diagnosing FAS

3.6.1 Diagnostic difficulties

Introduction
The diagnosis of FAS is based only on clinical signs and known medical history. Des-pite diagnostic guidelines i.e., 4-Digit Diagnostic Code, German S3-Guidelines and others, the diagnosis is quite difficult and sometimes limited, especially in patients with partial clinical signs who represent the largest group of patients.

3.6.2 No alcohol consumption during pregnancy

Possible reasons:
- Alcohol exposure during pregnancy is unknown or the biological mother denies alcohol consumption during pregnancy.
- It is important to accept the biological mother's statement, especially if she is still entitled to custody because sometimes she may doubt the validity of a diagnosis of FAS even with help of a lawyer or legal action.
- Women are often unaware of their pregnancies until the second to fourth month or even later. Denying alcohol consumption during pregnancy is not an attempt to justify their behaviour rather they believe that "no alcohol in pregnancy" becomes obligatory after they are aware of the pregnancy. This fact especially holds true for many children exposed to alcohol in early pregnancy.
- Medical awareness is usually focussed on the abuse of illegal drugs during preg-nancy without also taking into account additional alcohol consumption. Treat-ment for drug dependency is well known and easily admitted. Later develop-mental delay or behavioural difficulties of the affected children are often falsely attributed to illegal substance abuse only.
- A recent study from the USA reported that 86% of women suffering from illegal drug abuse additionally consumed alcohol [20]. To date, there is no evidence of long-lasting impairments after intrauterine exposure to illegal drugs (e.g., heroin, cocaine or cannabis).

3.6.3 Microdeletion or microduplication syndromes similar to FAS – "FAS phenocopy"

It rarely occurs that children suffer from growth retardation, facial dysmorphic features, CNS impairment including microcephaly similar to full-blown FAS without intrauterine alcohol exposure. For these particular cases S. Astley (Washington) [2, 11] introduced the term "FAS-phenocopy". Two examples illustrate the increasing differential diagnostic problems of molecular genetic diseasesand the "phenocopy of FAS".

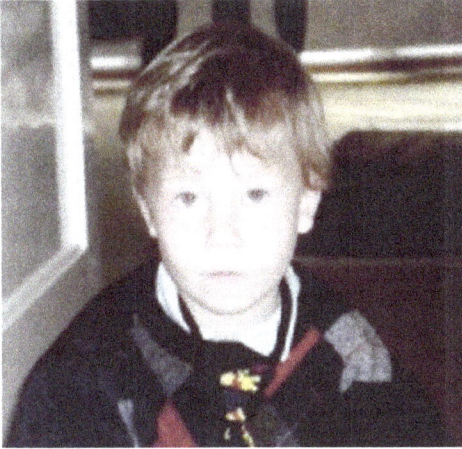

Fig. 3.14: S., born 1996.

Case report I

(16-year-old boy, Fig. 3.14)

S., born in 1996, presented for diagnostic examination at the Charité, Department of Child and Adolescence Psychiatry in November 2012.

Medical history:

- Twin pregnancy, intrauterine fetal death in early pregnancy of the second twin.
  S. was born in the 40th week of pregnancy. Birth weight 2700 g, birth length 47 cm, head circumference 32.5 cm.
- Developmental delay
- epilepsy in infancy and treatment with Valproate until 2010.
- Since the time of school enrolment he had learning difficulties, inattention, hyperactivity and impulsivity.
- Human genetic examination (exclusive of comparative genomic hybridisation) was without any finding in early childhood.
- Recent symptoms: problems in respecting others, accepting and following rules or abiding by an agreement.
- Poor school achievement (school for children with special needs), bad memory, unable to think logically; extremely inattentive.

- Lack of impulse control, violent tantrums with aggressive behaviour.
- Obtrusive behaviour.
- Poor orientation, no sense of time; inability to organise or to structure himself, naïve, suffering from depressive episodes.

Investigation at the age of 16:

- weight: 48 kg (< 3. percentile.), length: 165 cm (3rd to 10th percentile.); microcephaly;
- dysmorphic facial features: short palpebral fissures, epicanthus, smooth and elongated philtrum and thin upper lip (in photographs from early childhood);
- in spite of intensive questioning about alcohol consumption during pregnancy his mother admitted only two or three glasses of white wine and champagne in early pregnancy.

Diagnosis:

According to available guidelines a FAS diagnosis (4-Digit Diagnostic Code 4/4/4/2) was suspected. Because of the credibility of his mother concerning alcohol consumption during pregnancy we initiated a sub-microscopic genetic investigation (Dr. S. Spranger Bremen, Germany)

Based on array comparative genomic hybridisation (aCGH) she diagnosed:

4q22.3q23 (98,548,239–99,919,100)x1 and 6q25.3 (158,392,208–158, 864, 693)x3

The deletion in 4q22.3q23 was interpreted to be pathogenetic but to date there are only some cases with a similar deletion described with clinical findings including developmental delay, "floppy infant", dysmorphic facial features, cognitive deficits and behavioural problems [17].

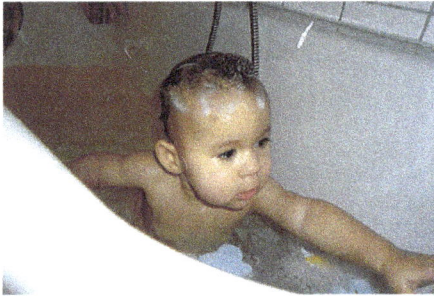

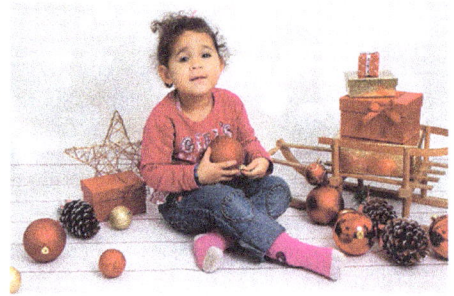

Fig. 3.15: L.-M., born 2011.

Case report II

(4-year-old girl, Fig. 3.15)

Heterozygote duplication in 6q25.3 (the clinical picture is unclear to date).

L.-M., born in 2011

Medical history: Her biological mother as well as her maternal grandmother and some of her siblings are educationally handicapped, her grandfather was of African origin.

The biological mother admitted chronical alcohol consumption also in pregnancy. The biological father also suffered from alcohol dependency and was homeless.

L.-M. lived together with her birth mother in a mother-child-facility for 2 years. Because L.-M. was severely neglected and her mother was pregnant again, she was placed in a foster family in 2013. Now at the age of 4, she suffers from developmental delay, severe behavioural problems, growth disturbance, and microcephaly, as well as dysmorphic facial features.

According to FAS guidelines (4-Digit Diagnostic Code 2/4/4/3) she met the FAS criteria.

Due to a family anamnesis of cognitive impairment we initiated an additional medical genetic investigation. The resulting diagnosis based on aCGH was a micro-duplication 16p11.2. Rare cases are described with developmental delay, slight facial dysmorphic features, underweight, learning disabilities, behavioural problems and autistic symptoms in combination with family history.

3.6.4 Conclusion

It is always important to undertake a medical genetic investigation based on molecular methods if clinical symptoms do not clearly correspond to the diagnostic criteria of FAS or if the history of alcohol abuse in pregnancy is unclear. In recent years, the widespread use of array comparative genomic hybridisation (array CGH) has led to an increased discovery of numerous novel microdeletion and microduplication syndromes. Many phenotypes are still evolving, and it is easily conceivable that the FAS phenocopy is a still unknown microdeletion or microduplication syndrome. The 4-year-old girl suffered from both; a confirmed FAS and a microdeletion syndrome.

Bibliography

[1] Landgraf MN, Notacker M, Heinen F. Diagnosis of fetal alcohol syndrome (FAS): German guideline version 2013. Eur J Paediatr Neurol. 2013, 17(5), 437–446.
[2] Astley SJ, Clarren SK. Diagnosing the full spectrum of alcohol exposed individuals: Introducing the 4-Digit Diagnostic Code. Alcohol & Alcoholism 2000, 35(4), 400–410.
[3] Astley SJ. Diagnostic guide for Fetal Alcohol Spectrum Disorders: The 4-Digit Diagnostic Code. 3rd edn. University of Washington Publication Services, Seattle WA 2004.
[4] Clarren SK, Smith DW. The Fetal alcohol syndrome. New Engl J Med 1978, 298, 1063–1067.
[5] Castells S, Mark E, Abaci F, Schwartz E. Growth Retardation in Fetal Alcohol Syndrome. Unresponsiveness to Growth-Promoting Hormones. Dev Pharmacol Ther 1981, 3, 232–241.
[6] Smith DW. Fetal alcohol syndrome and fetal alcohol effects. Neurobehavioral Toxiology and Teratology 1981, 3, 127.

[7]   Astley SJ. Profile of the first 1400 patients receiving diagnostic evaluation for the fetal alcohol spectrum disorder at the Washington State. Fetal Alcohol Syndrome Diagnostic & Prevention Network. Can J Clin Pharmacol 2010, 17(1), e132–164.

[8]   Streissguth AP, Clarren KS, Jones KL. Natural History of the Fetal Alcohol Syndrome: A 10-year-Follow-up of eleven Patients. Lancet 1985, 2(8446), 85–91.

[9]   Astley SJ, Stachowiak J, Clarren SK, Clausen C. Application of the fetal alcohol syndrome facial photographic screening tool in a foster care population. J Pediatrics 2002, 141 (5), 712–717.

[10] Hall JG, Froster-Iskenius UG, Allanson JE. Handbook of Normal Physical Measurements. Oxford University Press, New York 1989.

[11] Clarren SK, Chudley AE, Wong L, Friesen J, Brant R. Normal distribution of palpebral fissure length in Canadian school age children. Can J Clin Pharmacol 2010, 17(1), e67–78.

[12] Institute of Medicine (IOM), Stratton KR, Howe CJ, Battaglia FC (eds). Fetal alcohol Syndrome: Diagnosis, Epidemiology, Prevention, and Treatment. National Academy Press, Washington, D.C. 1996.

[13] Chudley AE, Conry J, Cook JL, Cook C, Rosales T, LeBlanc N. Fetal alcohol spectrum disorder: Canadian guidelines for diagnosis. CMAJ 2005, 172(5suppl), S1–S21.

[14] Dolk H. The predictive value of microcephaly during the first year of life for mental retardation at seven years. Developmental Medicine and Child Neurology 1991, 33, 974–983.

[15] Epidemiology of Alcohol Problems in the United States; National Institute on Alcohol, Alcohol Abuse and Alcoholism (NIAAA),2005; https://pubs.niaaa.nih.gov/index.html.

[16] http://depts.washington.edu/fasdpn/htmls/4-digit-code.htm.

[17] 4q deletions: various between 4q21 and 4q31: http://www.rarechromo.org.

[18] Hempel M, Brugues N, Lederer G et al. Microdeletion syndrome 16p11.2: clinical and molecular characterization. Am J Med Genet A 2009, 10, 2106–12.

[19] Coles CD, Gailey AR, Mulle JG, Kable JA, Lynch ME, Jones KL. A Comparison Among 5 Methods for the Clinical Diagnosis of Fetal Alcohol Spectrum Disorders. Alcohol Clin Exp Res 2016, 40(5), 1000–1009 doi: 10.1111/acer.13032.

[20] Singer LT, Nelson S, Short E, Min NO, Levis B, Russ S, Minnes S. Prenatal cocain exposure: Drug and environmental effects at 9 years. J Peditr 2008, 153(1), 105–111.

4 Neuropsychological aspects of fetal alcohol syndrome

Betteke Maria van Noort

4.1 Introduction

Besides physically visible characteristics, such as craniofacial abnormalities, growth deficiency and microcephaly, fetal alcohol syndrome is characterised by damage to the central nervous system resulting in functional disruptions in executive functioning (see Chapter 3). *Executive functions* encompass those cognitive abilities that allow us to adapt our behaviour to our continuously changing environment. These cognitive functions enable us to focus our attention consciously on a task or object, to set goals, to plan actions or to control our impulses [1].

Executive functions and other cognitive functions such as intelligence, language or memory can be evaluated via neuropsychological tests. *Neuropsychology* aims to find correlations between physiological factors and human behaviour and evaluate the effects of impairments and damage to the brain [1].

In fetal alcohol syndrome, the brainhas been damaged during its prenatal development due to the toxic effects of alcohol exposure. Prenatal alcohol exposure may have different effects on cognition, depending on the dosage and duration of exposure. *Neuropsychological evaluations* allow us to identify the exact cognitive deficits resulting from the prenatal brain damage, as well as to assess their severity. The known biological and physiological effects of prenatal alcohol exposure are described in more detail in Chapter 11. Overall, many different areas of the brain seem to be affected, including the pre-frontal cortex, corpus callosum, hippocampus, basal ganglia, cerebellum and thalamus [2, 3]. Figure 4.1 shows a simplified presentation of the affected areas of the brain and the associated cognitive abilities.

4.2 Neuropsychological evaluation

According to the 4-Digit Diagnostic Code, damage to the central nervous system may lead to impairments in the following cognitive domains in FAS: general cognitive performance, attention, planning, memory, visual–spatial perception, social ability, language and motor ability. Cognitive impairments differ individually, depending on factors such as genetic predisposition, dosage or duration of the alcohol exposure. In other words, not every person experiencing prenatal alcohol exposure will present with the same cognitive impairments [4, 5]. Therefore, it is highly recommended that

https://doi.org/10.1515/9783110436563-004

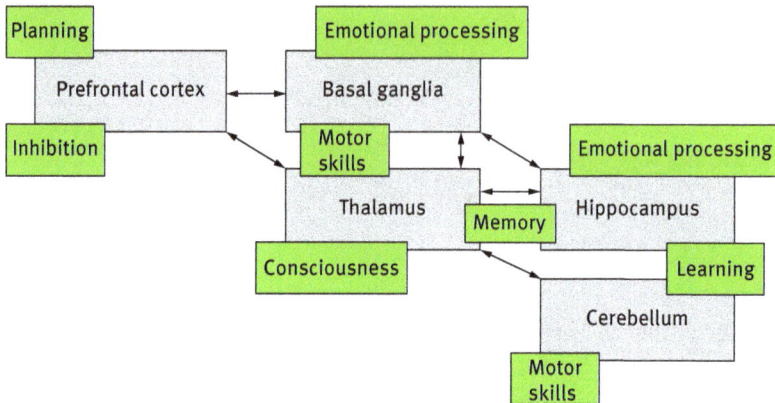

Fig. 4.1: Simplified illustration of individual brain areas (grey) and cognitive functions (green).

an extensive neuropsychological examination be conducted for every patient to determine personal cognitive strengths and weaknesses.

The duration of the neuropsychological evaluation should be tailored to the typical low attention span of patients and to the often existing behavioural difficulties. It is, therefore, recommended that a pre-selection of neuropsychological tests be made. As a guide for the test selection, the 4-Digit Diagnostic Code suggests a short interview (see Table 4.1) with the parents or legal guardians to assess the severity of the problem and the level of cognitive impairment. Table 4.2 shows an example of different neuropsychological tests selected for an 8 year-old patient with FAS. The total test duration is about 160 minutes.

During neuropsychological assessments, there is a constant struggle between the aim to examine as many cognitive areas as possible and, on the other hand, not to exhaust the participant. It is, therefore, important to offer short breaks frequently, to assess the patient's well-being regularly, to document the test order, to discontinue a test when necessary or even to interrupt the entire assessment and continue at a later time and/or day.

4.3 Cognitive deficits in children and adolescents with FAS

Neuropsychological studieshave found that children and adolescents with FAS show problems, particularly in processing and integrating new information. Furthermore, they often present with impairments in cognitive areas such as intelligence, learning, memory, language, flexibility, emotional processing and motor skills [7, 8]. Deficit severity increases simultaneously with an increase in task complexity. Moreover, cognitive deficits reinforce one another; impaired attention, for example, makes it complicated to develop adequate language skills, which in turn can hinder the develop-

Tab. 4.1: Cognitive abilitiesof the patient from a caregiver's perspective (modified according to [6]).

Ability	Delay/Impairment	Severity
Planning	Needs help planning and organising everyday tasks	0 – 1 – 2 – 3
	Doesn't understand concept of 'time'	0 – 1 – 2 – 3
	Experiences difficulties during multi-step tasks	0 – 1 – 2 – 3
Behavioural regulation	Finds it difficult to regulate anger	0 – 1 – 2 – 3
	Experiences mood swings	0 – 1 – 2 – 3
	Impulsiveness	0 – 1 – 2 – 3
	Inattentiveness	0 – 1 – 2 – 3
	Shows unusual activity levels (either high or low)	0 – 1 – 2 – 3
	Lies and/or steals	0 – 1 – 2 – 3
Abstract thinking	Poor judgement	0 – 1 – 2 – 3
	Unable to think in abstract terms/concepts	0 – 1 – 2 – 3
	Cannot be left alone	0 – 1 – 2 – 3
Memory and learning	Poor recall of learned information	0 – 1 – 2 – 3
	Slow in learning new skills	0 – 1 – 2 – 3
	Not able to learn from previous experiences	0 – 1 – 2 – 3
	Finds it difficult to recognise consequences from own actions	0 – 1 – 2 – 3
	Experiences difficulty/is slow in information processing	0 – 1 – 2 – 3
Spatial skills	Gets lost	0 – 1 – 2 – 3
	Navigation difficulties	0 – 1 – 2 – 3
Social skills	Clearly behaves younger than chronological age	0 – 1 – 2 – 3
	Poor social skills	0 – 1 – 2 – 3
Motor skills	Poor or delayed development of motor skills	0 – 1 – 2 – 3
	Poor balance	0 – 1 – 2 – 3

ment of social skills [4, 9]. In the following section, current research results in children and adolescents with FASD are summarised for the most significant cognitive areas.

Intelligence: the cognitive domain that is studied the most in children and adolescents with FAS is intelligence. A standardised intelligence test can be used to determine an intelligence quotient (IQ) for each person. The IQ of children with prenatal alcohol exposure can vary greatly, from mental retardation (IQ < 60), to average intelligence (IQ = 85–115) or even above average intelligence (IQ = 115–125), as seen in a small set of children [10]. Although FAS is one of the most common causes for mental retardation [11], not every patient with FAS suffers from it [8]. On average, children with FAS have an IQ of about 70, which is considered to be a below average intelligence level [12]. Prenatal alcohol exposure causes a significantly greater reduction in IQ scores compared to prenatal psychotropic drugs exposure [13]. Long-term studies show that these low intelligence levels remain stable over time [14, 15] and have a negative influence on the educational level of the patient, his psychiatric condition and his overall quality of life [16]. These long-term negative effects of prenatal alcohol exposure emphasise the need for adequate prevention. Even the relatively moderate

Tab. 4.2: Selection of neuropsychological tests for an 8-year-old patient; total duration around 160 minutes.

Domain	Neuropsychological test	Duration
Intelligence	Wechsler Intelligence Scale for Children – 4th Edition (WISC-IV)	90 min.
Language	Subtest "Vocabulary" of the WISC-IV	–
	Subtest "Comprehension" of the WISC-IV	–
Visual-spatial skills	Rey Complex Fig. Test and Recognition (RCFT)	15 min.
	Subtest "Matrix Reasoning" of the WISC-IV	–
Memory	Subtest "Working Memory" of the WISC-IV	–
Executive functions	Test of Attentional Performance (TAP)	30 min.
Attention	Test of Attentional Performance (TAP)	–
Fine motor skills	Movement Assessment Battery for Children (M-ABC-2)	25 min.
Social abilities and behaviour	Child-Behavior-Checklist (CBCL) filled out by care giver	–
	Strengths and Difficulties Questionnaire (SDQ) filled out by care giver	–

consumption of two alcoholic units a day during pregnancy is associated with reduced intelligence levels in the child [17]. According to May et al. (2013), the child's intelligence is particularly at risk when the prenatal alcohol exposure takes place during the first or second trimester [18].

Language: Children with FASD show speech difficulties and problems in verbal communication, for example problems with comprehension, object naming and semantics in general [8, 19, 20]. Adequate language skills are essential for social interaction with peers and the development of general knowledge. Several studies have tried to identify the exact mechanisms causing language deficits in FASD. Some results suggest that the more basic language processes are affected, because children with FASD show impairments in phonological skills (i.e. auditory processing skills) [21]. Other results suggest that more complex language difficulties, such as an articulation disorder or loss of hearing hinder adequate language development [8, 10]. An alternative hypothesis is that the language difficulties are caused by the mental retardation seen in some of the patients [22]. It is clear however, that these verbal impairments lead to social, academic and general behavioural difficulties. In contrast to the findings for intelligence, language abilities do not seem highly affected by moderate alcohol exposure. However, language development is (similarly) very vulnerable during the second trimester [23].

Memory and learning: Our memory consists of different processes including learning of new information, information storage and retrieval of stored information (see Fig. 4.2). When a memory system is intact it receives input from the external environment, which resides in our sensory memory. Using selective attention, specific inform-

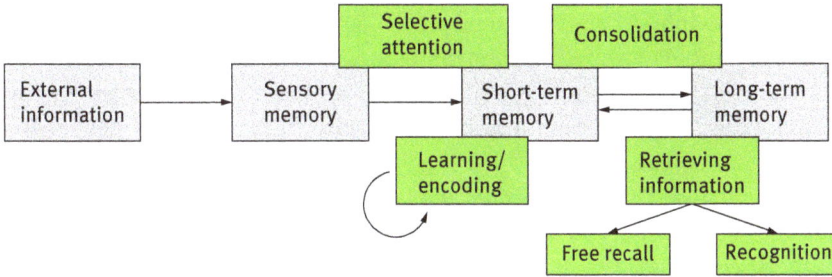

Fig. 4.2: Memory processes in unaffected individuals.

ation is then selected for the short-term memory (a very quick and subconscious process). In our short-term memory, information is learned (encoded), and this learned information can then be stored in the long-term memory (consolidation). The processes of free recall or recognition allow us to remember learned and stored information, which then shifts from the long-term memory back into the short-term memory.

Children and adolescents with FAS show, analogous to their language difficulties, weaknesses in verbal memory [19, 24, 25]. Moreover, the non-verbal memory, in particular the spatial memory, seems to be impaired as well, despite the fact that there are some inconsistent findings [25, 26]. In a review article, Glass et al. (2014) conclude that the process of storing information is not affected by FASD [10]. However, children and adolescents with FASD show clear difficulties in learning information and in retrieving information from long-term memory [26, 27]. Moreover, imaging studies have shown that neurophysiological brain processes taking place during recognition are different in children with FASD compared to healthy children [28]. Taken together, the majority of the memory system seems to be affected by prenatal alcohol exposure.

Flexibility and inhibition: Cognitive abilities are divided into basic and higher-level skills. Higher cognitive processes are necessary in order to adapt our behaviour in a targeted manner according to our ever-changing environment, i.e. *cognitive control*. Basic cognitive processes are essential to higher cognitive processes. When basic cognitive skillsare impaired, more complex skills such as flexibility or inhibition are negatively affected. General processing speed is, indeed, a basic process that is clearly impaired in patients with FAS [7]. A recent diffusion tensor imaging (DTI) study, which is a technique allowing the depiction of neural tracts, was able to show that the network connections of children and adolescents with FASD are significantly longer and more inefficient than the network connections of healthy controls [29]. These longer and more inefficient network connections can account for the slow processing speed seen in FAS.

Problems with flexibility, however, also arise irrespective of problems with processing speed. Several studies show that children with FAS have deficits in flexible and abstract thinking, as well as deficits in switching flexibly between different tasks or concepts [9, 19, 30]. The ability to switch back and forth seamlessly between tasks requires the ability to inhibit competing thoughts or impulses at the same time. Children and adolescents with FAS show impaired inhibition, both during verbal tasks [19, 30] and motor tasks [31]. These deficits in higher cognitive skills, i.e. flexibility and inhibition, are associated with behavioural problems, impulsivity during social interactions and adjustment problems [32–34].

Social cognition and emotional processing: The ability to put one's self in another person's shoes and understand their emotional state and motives is called *theory of mind* or social cognition. The development of social cognition is disrupted in children with FAS [34]. Both behavioural experiments and observations of caretakers and teachers confirm that children with FAS experience great difficulties with recognition of emotions [35, 36]. Emotion recognitioncombines information taken from body language, intonation and facial expressions. Kerns et al. (2015) highlight the importance of this ability for the development of social skills [35]. Examinations with the *Social Skills Rating System* show that deficits in social cognition and emotion recognition are associated with a reduced sense of responsibility, hyperactivity, internalisation of emotions and problems with social skills in general [37]. Subsequently, children with FAS are not able to solve problems in social situations correctly and quickly [38]. Taken together, these social deficits lead to restlessness in school settings, unstable behaviour and limited social contact with peers [39].

Motor: Motor skills encompass all actions coming from the muscular system of a human being. When talking about motor development, a distinction is made between fine and gross motor skills. Children with FAS show impairments in both their fine motor skills, as well as in their gross motor skills. Nonetheless, fine motor skills are affected by FAS more often and more severely [46]. Deficits in fine motor skills lead to reduced movement speed, coordination errors and delayed response times [40–42]. Impairments of gross motor skills include an unusual gait, imbalance, instable posture, weak grip, problems with goal-oriented movements and reduced hand–eye coordination [43–45].

Besides fine and gross motor skills, some researchers are specifically interested in the oculomotor abilities of patients with FAS. They have shown that children with FAS have reduced control of eye movement compared to healthy children, which leads to more errors on visual tasks [40, 47]. Moreover, these oculomotor problems are found to be associated with reduced cognitive performance [47].

Severity of cognitive deficits: Some findings suggest that the degree of facial dysmorphia is directly related to the severity of cognitive deficits. More specifically, FASD patients with more distinct craniofacial abnormalities show more severe cognitive impairments [48]. However, other findings suggest that the severity of cognitive deficits is related to the level of growth deficiency rather than facial dysmorphia [49]. What can be said for certain is that a simultaneous manifestation of craniofacial abnormalities and growth deficiency is clearly associated with severe cognitive deficits [49, 50]. Chasnoff et al. (2010) compared cognitive performance of children with either FAS, pFAS or ARND. Firstly, children with FAS show significantly lower intelligence and have significantly more memory problems than children with ARND. In addition, children with FAS have significantly more communication difficulties and motor disorders than children with pFAS. Moreover, cognitive flexibility is significantly weaker in children with FAS compared to both children with pFAS or ARND. Taken together, in this study, children with FAS have more cognitive problems than children with pFAS or ARND [13, 46, 49].

4.4 Cognitive deficits in adults with FAS

Effects of fetal alcohol syndrome on cognition in adulthood have been examined considerably less often than effects on cognition in childhood and adolescence. Chapter 13 of this book provides a detailed description of the currently known information about adults with FAS. As mentioned earlier in the current chapter, cognitive deficits have far-reaching consequences for the social and academic development of FAS patients [12, 16]. Therefore, for adult patients it is also recommended that an extensive neuropsychological examination be performed. A neuropsychological assessment can aid and guide the patient's professional orientation when necessary.

Despite relatively few studies, findings so far suggest that the level of intelligence in adult patients remains low, in accordance with the findings in children and adolescents with FAS [15]. Similarly, fine motor skills and balance remain affected by FASD in adulthood [51]; flexibility, attention, visuospatial skills, memory, learning, planning and language continue to be impaired [52–54]; and social skills of adult patients show clear developmental delay [12]. Adults with FAS possess fewer everyday life skills, even when compared to a control group with a similar low intelligence level [55]. Results of imaging studies are in line with the findings described in this paragraph, i.e. they suggest that brain structures of adult patients show irregularities and that their brain connectivity is different in comparison to healthy adults [56, 57].

Overall, the cognitive deficits caused by prenatal alcohol exposure do not seem to improve going into adulthood. As a result, besides preventative measures, there is a high need for an early identification and potential treatment of these cognitive impairments, so as to reduce the negative long-term consequences for patients, parents and caregivers as much as possible.

4.5 Treatment of cognitive deficits in FAS

Cognitive impairments have clear consequences for the everyday lives of patients with FASD, in terms of social interactions with other people, academic performance and their professional lives. A more detailed description of the everyday difficulties encountered by patients with FAS can be found in Chapter 5. Of great interest for the patients and their families is the question of whether these cognitive deficits can be treated and thus both acute and long-term consequences reduced. Because the cognitive problems encountered by patients with FAS are so versatile, there are several training approaches focussing on different target areas [58, 59].

So far, current therapeutic approaches target single cognitive domains, such as language, attention, memory or social skills. Wells et al. (2012) and Nash et al. (2015) evaluated the effectiveness of the "Alert Program" in children with FAS [60, 61]. This intervention program targets *self-regulation*, which is the mental ability that allows us to deal with emotions adequately, lets us act in a goal/target-oriented manner, and directs our attention and impulses. Self-regulation requires cognitive abilities that function properly and is, therefore, impaired in patients with FAS. The first randomised controlled trials by Wells et al. and Nash et al. were able to achieve promising preliminary results: both behavioural and emotional regulation of children with FAS seems improved directly after the intervention according to observer ratings [60, 61]. An attention training program [62], language skills training [63], memory training program [64] and maths training program [65] were all able to achieve equally positive effects in their respective cognitive areas. Furthermore, children with FAS seem to benefit from social skills training. The benefits are, however, primarily visible at home in familial situations and not in school environments [66].

The current therapeutic approaches have in common that they are predominantly focused on children and adolescents. Furthermore, the actual efficacy is not yet confirmed for any of the approaches available. The effectiveness of a therapeutic approach needs to be examined via a *randomised controlled trial* (RCT) with a large sample size. So far, there are few randomised controlled trials in the field of FAS. Recently however, a few RCTs were started in South Africa, Canada and the United States [67]. The evaluation of long-term benefits (adulthood) of the various therapeutic approaches is pending.

Taken together, these first achievements by the various training approaches seem to be positive. It should be noted, however, that it remains unclear how long these benefits will remain and whether they can be transferred to other domains, e.g. academic performance. Moreover, it is unclear which patients will benefit from which interventions. Because the cognitive profile of patients with FAS is highly heterogeneous and cognitive abilities very limited in some patients, future studies should continue to examine which interventions are appropriate for each patient, with which frequency and of which duration. It is recommend that an intensive, individually tailored treatment program, targeting all affected cognitive domains be offered. In addition, regular progress evaluations should be implemented [68].

Bibliography

[1]   Lezak MD, Howieson DB, Bigler ED, Tranel D. Neuropsychological Assessment. 5th edn. Oxford University Press, Inc, New York 2012.

[2]   Donald KA et al., Neuroimaging effects of prenatal alcohol exposure on the developing human brain: a magnetic resonance imaging review. Acta Neuropsychiatr 2015, (5), 1–19.

[3]   Mattson SN et al. A decrease in the size of the basal ganglia in children with fetal alcohol syndrome. Alcohol Clin Exp Res 1996, 20(6), 1088–93.

[4]   Roszel EL. Central nervous system deficits in fetal alcohol spectrum disorder. Nurse Pract 2015, 40(4), 24–33.

[5]   Reynolds JN et al. Fetal alcohol spectrum disorders: gene-environment interactions, predictive biomarkers, and the relationship between structural alterations in the brain and functional outcomes. Semin Pediatr Neurol 2011, 18(1), 49–55.

[6]   Astley SJ. Diagnostic guide for Fetal Alcohol Spectrum Disorders: The 4-Digit Diagnostic Code. 3rd edn. University of Washington Publication Services, Seattle WA 2004.

[7]   Kodituwakku PW. Neurocognitive profile in children with fetal alcohol spectrum disorders. Dev Disabil Res Rev 2009, 15(3), 218–24.

[8]   Mattson SN, Crocker N, Nguyen TT. Fetal alcohol spectrum disorders: neuropsychological and behavioral features. Neuropsychol Rev 2011, 21(2), 81–101.

[9]   Vaurio L, Riley EP, Mattson SN. Neuropsychological comparison of children with heavy prenatal alcohol exposure and an IQ-matched comparison group. J Int Neuropsychol Soc 2011, 17(3), 463–73.

[10] Glass L, Ware AL, Mattson SN. Neurobehavioral, neurologic, and neuroimaging characteristics of fetal alcohol spectrum disorders. Handb Clin Neurol 2014, 125, 435–62.

[11] Abel EL, Sokol RJ. Fetal alcohol syndrome is now leading cause of mental retardation. Lancet 1986, 2(8517), 1222.

[12] Streissguth AP et al. Fetal alcohol syndrome in adolescents and adults. JAMA 1991, 265(15), 1961–7.

[13] Dalen K et al. Cognitive functioning in children prenatally exposed to alcohol and psychotropic drugs. Neuropediatrics 2009, 40(4), 162–7.

[14] Streissguth AP, Randels SP, Smith DF. A test-retest study of intelligence in patients with fetal alcohol syndrome: implications for care. J Am Acad Child Adolesc Psychiatry 1991, 30(4), 584–7.

[15] Spohr HL, Willms J, Steinhausen HC. Prenatal alcohol exposure and long-term developmental consequences. Lancet 1993, 341(8850), 907–10.

[16] Steinhausen HC, Spohr HL. Long-term outcome of children with fetal alcohol syndrome: psychopathology, behavior, and intelligence. Alcohol Clin Exp Res 1998, 22(2), 334–8.

[17] Streissguth AP, Barr HM, Sampson PD. Moderate prenatal alcohol exposure: effects on child IQ and learning problems at age 7 1/2 years. Alcohol Clin Exp Res 1990, 14(5), 662–9.

[18] May PA et al. Maternal alcohol consumption producing fetal alcohol spectrum disorders(FASD): quantity, frequency, and timing of drinking. Drug Alcohol Depend 2013, 133(2), 502–12.

[19] Rasmussen C et al. Neuropsychological impairments on the NEPSY-II among children with FASD. Child Neuropsychol 2013, 19(4), 337–49.

[20] Wyper KR, Rasmussen CR. Language impairments in children with fetal alcohol spectrum disorders. J Popul Ther Clin Pharmacol 2011, 18(2), e364–76.

[21] Streissguth AP et al. Drinking during pregnancy decreases word attack and arithmetic scores on standardized tests: adolescent data from a population-based prospective study. Alcohol Clin Exp Res 1994, 18(2), 248–54.

[22] McGee CL et al. Impaired language performance in young children with heavy prenatal alcohol exposure. Neurotoxicol Teratol 2009, 31(2), 71–5.

[23] O'Leary C et al. Prenatal alcohol exposure and language delay in 2-year-old children: the importance of dose and timing on risk. Pediatrics 2009, 123(2), 547–54.

[24] Lewis CE et al. Verbal learning and memory impairment in children with fetal alcohol spectrum disorders. Alcohol Clin Exp Res 2015, 39(4), 724–32.

[25] Mattson SN, Roebuck TM. Acquisition and retention of verbal and nonverbal information in children with heavy prenatal alcohol exposure. Alcohol Clin Exp Res 2002, 26(6), 875–82.

[26] Pei J et al. Executive function and memory in children with Fetal Alcohol Spectrum Disorder. Child Neuropsychol 2011, 17(3), 290–309.

[27] Crocker N et al. Comparison of verbal learning and memory in children with heavy prenatal alcohol exposure or attention-deficit/hyperactivity disorder. Alcohol Clin Exp Res 2011, 35(6), 1114–21.

[28] Burden MJ et al. The effects of maternal binge drinking during pregnancy on neural correlates of response inhibition and memory in childhood. Alcohol Clin Exp Res 2011, 35(1), 69–82.

[29] Wozniak JR et al. Global functional connectivity abnormalities in children with fetal alcohol spectrum disorders. Alcohol Clin Exp Res 2013, 37(5), 748–56.

[30] Rasmussen C, Bisanz J. Executive functioning in children with Fetal Alcohol Spectrum Disorders: profiles and age-related differences. Child Neuropsychol 2009, 15(3), 201–15.

[31] Noland JS et al. Executive functioning in preschool-age children prenatally exposed to alcohol, cocaine, and marijuana. Alcohol Clin Exp Res 2003, 27(4), 647–56.

[32] Ware AL et al. Executive function predicts adaptive behavior in children with histories of heavy prenatal alcohol exposure and attention-deficit/hyperactivity disorder. Alcohol Clin Exp Res 2012, 36(8), 1431–41.

[33] McGee CL et al. Deficits in social problem solving in adolescents with prenatal exposure to alcohol. Am J Drug Alcohol Abuse 2008, 34(4), 423–31.

[34] Rasmussen C, Wyper K, Talwar V. The relation between theory of mind and executive functions in children with fetal alcohol spectrum disorders. Can J Clin Pharmacol 2009, 16(2), e370–80.

[35] Kerns KA et al. Emotion recognition in children with Fetal Alcohol Spectrum Disorders. Child Neuropsychol 2015, (3), 1–21.

[36] Greenbaum RL et al. Social cognitive and emotion processing abilities of children with fetal alcohol spectrum disorders: a comparison with attention deficit hyperactivity disorder. Alcohol Clin Exp Res 2009, 33(10), 1656–70.

[37] Rasmussen C et al. An evaluation of social skills in children with and without prenatal alcohol exposure. Child Care Health Dev 2011, 37(5), 711–8.

[38] Stevens SA et al. Social problem solving in children with fetal alcohol spectrum disorders. J Popul Ther Clin Pharmacol 2012, 19(1), e99–110.

[39] Kjellmer L, Olswang LB. Variability in classroom social communication: performance of children with fetal alcohol spectrum disorders and typically developing peers. J Speech Lang Hear Res 2013, 56(3), 982–93.

[40] Green CR et al. Oculomotor control in children with fetal alcohol spectrum disorders assessed using a mobile eye-tracking laboratory. Eur J Neurosci 2009, 29(6), 1302–9.

[41] Jirikowic T, Olson HC, Kartin D. Sensory processing, school performance, and adaptive behavior of young school-age children with fetal alcohol spectrum disorders. Phys Occup Ther Pediatr 2008, 28(2), 117–36.

[42] Simmons RW et al. Motor response selection in children with fetal alcohol spectrum disorders. Neurotoxicol Teratol 2006, 28(2), 278–85.

[43] Simmons RW et al. Children with heavy prenatal alcohol exposure exhibit deficits when regulating isometric force. Alcohol Clin Exp Res 2012, 36(2), 302–9.

[44] Roebuck TM et al. Prenatal exposure to alcohol affects the ability to maintain postural balance. Alcohol Clin Exp Res 1998, 22(1), 252–8.

[45] Domellof E et al. Goal-directed arm movements in children with fetal alcohol syndrome: a kinematic approach. Eur J Neurol 2011, 18(2), 312–20.

[46] Kalberg WO et al. Comparison of motor delays in young children with fetal alcohol syndrome to those with prenatal alcohol exposure and with no prenatal alcohol exposure. Alcohol Clin Exp Res 2006, 30(12), 2037–45.

[47] Paolozza A et al. Working memory and visuospatial deficits correlate with oculomotor control in children with fetal alcohol spectrum disorder. Behav Brain Res 2014, 263, 70–9.

[48] Astley SJ, Clarren SK. Measuring the facial phenotype of individuals with prenatal alcohol exposure: correlations with brain dysfunction. Alcohol 2001, 36(2), 147–59.

[49] Chasnoff IJ et al. Neurodevelopmental functioning in children with FAS, pFAS, and ARND. J Dev Behav Pediatr 2010, 31(3), 192–201.

[50] Ervalahti N et al. Relationship between dysmorphic features and general cognitive function in children with fetal alcohol spectrum disorders. Am J Med Genet A 2007, 143A(24), 2916–23.

[51] Connor PD et al. Effects of prenatal alcohol exposure on fine motor coordination and balance: A study of two adult samples. Neuropsychologia 2006, 44(5), 744–51.

[52] Connor PD et al. Direct and indirect effects of prenatal alcohol damage on executive function. Dev Neuropsychol 2000, 18(3), 331–54.

[53] Kerns KA et al. Cognitive deficits in nonretarded adults with fetal alcohol syndrome. J Learn Disabil 1997, 30(6), 685–93.

[54] Monnot M et al. Neurological basis of deficits in affective prosody comprehension among alcoholics and fetal alcohol-exposed adults. J Neuropsychiatry Clin Neurosci 2002, 14(3), 321–8.

[55] Temple V et al. Comparing Daily Living Skills in Adults with Fetal Alcohol Spectrum Disorder (FASD) To An IQ Matched Clinical Sample. J Popul Ther Clin Pharmacol 2011, 18(2), e397–e402.

[56] Bookstein FL et al. Corpus callosum shape and neuropsychological deficits in adult males with heavy fetal alcohol exposure. Neuroimage 2002, 15(1), 233–51.

[57] Ma X et al. Evaluation of corpus callosum anisotropy in young adults with fetal alcohol syndrome according to diffusion tensor imaging. Alcohol Clin Exp Res 2005, 29(7), 1214–22.

[58] Peadon E et al. Systematic review of interventions for children with Fetal Alcohol Spectrum Disorders. BMC Pediatr 2009, 9, 35.

[59] Bertrand J. Interventions for children with fetal alcohol spectrum disorders (FASDs): overview of findings for five innovative research projects. Res Dev Disabil 2009, 30(5), 986–1006.

[60] Wells AM et al. Neurocognitive habilitation therapy for children with fetal alcohol spectrum disorders: an adaptation of the Alert Program(R). Am J Occup Ther 2012, 66(1), 24–34.

[61] Nash K et al. Improving executive functioning in children with fetal alcohol spectrum disorders. Child Neuropsychol 2015, 21(2), 191–209.

[62] Kerns KA et al. Investigating the efficacy of an attention training programme in children with foetal alcohol spectrum disorder. Dev Neurorehabil 2010, 13(6), 413–22.

[63] Adnams CM et al. Language and literacy outcomes from a pilot intervention study for children with fetal alcohol spectrum disorders in South Africa. Alcohol 2007, 41(6), 403–14.

[64] Loomes C et al. The effect of rehearsal training on working memory span of children with fetal alcohol spectrum disorder. Res Dev Disabil 2008, 29(2), 113–24.

[65] Kable JA, Coles CD, Taddeo E. Socio-cognitive habilitation using the math interactive learning experience program for alcohol-affected children. Alcohol Clin Exp Res 2007, 31(8), 1425–34.

[66] O'Connor MJ et al. A controlled social skills training for children with fetal alcohol spectrum disorders. J Consult Clin Psychol 2006, 74(4), 639–48.

[67] Paley B, O'Connor MJ. Intervention for individuals with fetal alcohol spectrum disorders: treatment approaches and case management. Dev Disabil Res Rev 2009, 15(3), 258–67.

[68] Kodituwakku PW, Kodituwakku EL. From research to practice: an integrative framework for the development of interventions for children with fetal alcohol spectrum disorders. Neuropsychol Rev 2011, 21(2), 204–23.

5 Diagnostic characteristics across lifespan

FAS is a lifelong disorder, and the cluster of symptoms differ in each developmental stage along the lifespan.

Apart from in exceptional cases FAS is not diagnosed at birth and, therefore, potential foster or adoptive parents usually take care of a newborn or a neonate without any clinical diagnosis. Relevant information about potential alcohol and drug abuse in the biological family, even if known by child services, are usually not communicated to adoptive or foster parents.

With increasing awareness of FAS in the recent past, the situation has improved considerably, but as long as these children are discharged from maternity clinics without a precise diagnosis, child services typically only speak about difficult conditions and neglect as a compelling reason for removal of children from their biological family.

The general information that the child has "only" been neglected, reinforces the desire of caregivers to provide a better education in order to offer a brighter future to these children.

Children with alcohol damage are, however, "different" and often have numerous and severe developmental problems and behavioural abnormalities, which quickly become a major challenge for the "new parents". Despite extensive effort and support, only limited educational improvements can be attained. If foster or adoptive parents had been informed of the diagnosis of FAS, implicating that the child is likely to be impaired for life, they would have had the individual choice whether or not to take a disabled child into their family (see Fig. 5.1).

> "FASD also affects all other members of the immediate family, including siblings and the extended family. Emotional, financial and social burdens can be considerable. Indeed, the stress of living with a child affected with FASD may result in family discord or breakup. Adoptive and foster families confront similar issues in dealing with the needs of affected children. Again proper supports are essential."
>
> Ipsiroglu (2012; [2]), FASD und sleep researcher (Vancouver)

5.1 Infancy

Common morphological signs and clinical abnormalities associated with FAS directly after birth (Figs. 5.2–5.5)
- premature birth (small for date);
- small head circumference (microcephaly);
- lack of weight gain (dystrophy);
- growth deficiency;

https://doi.org/10.1515/9783110436563-005

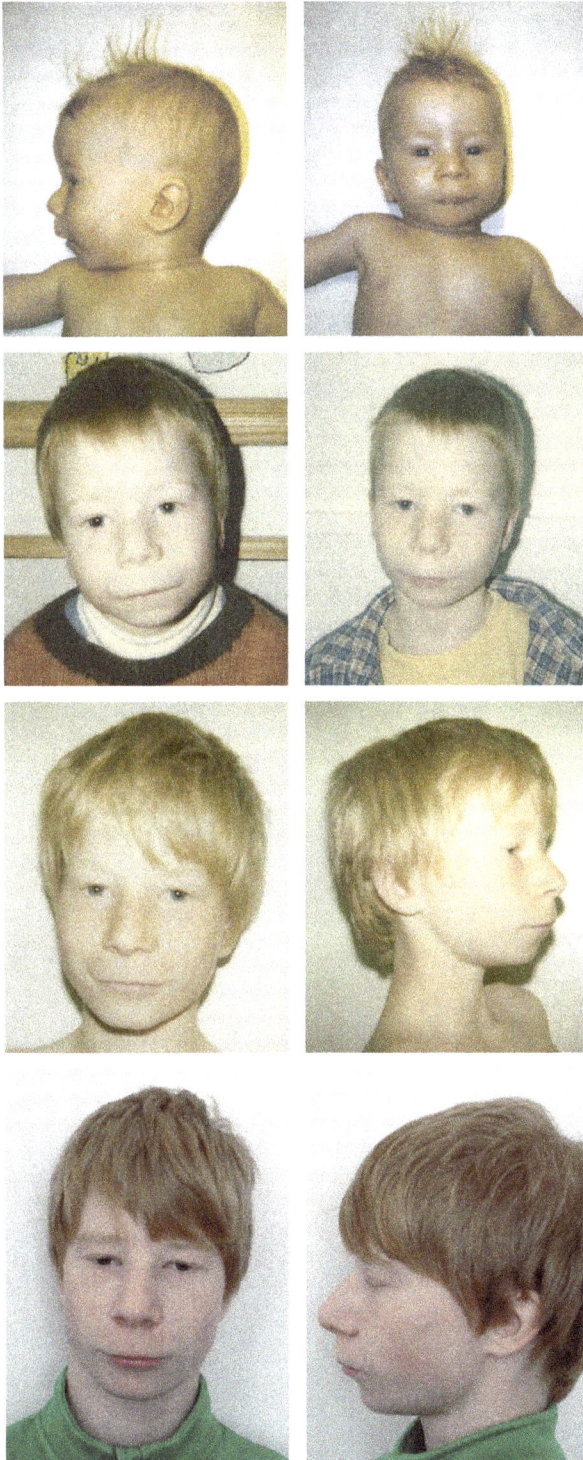

Fig. 5.1: Patient with FAS at different ages: first row at 8 months old, second row at 4 and 8 years old, third row at 11 years old, and fourth row at 16 years old.

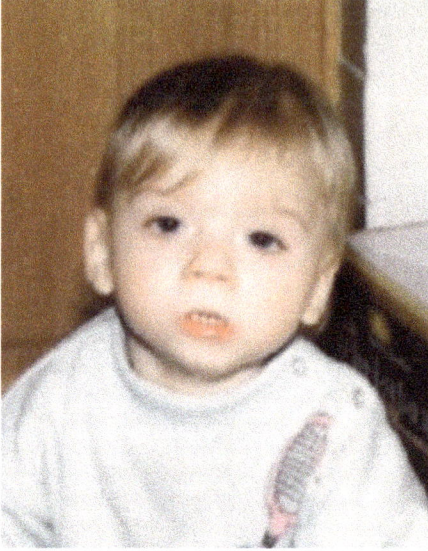

Fig. 5.2: FAS, 13-month-old boy.

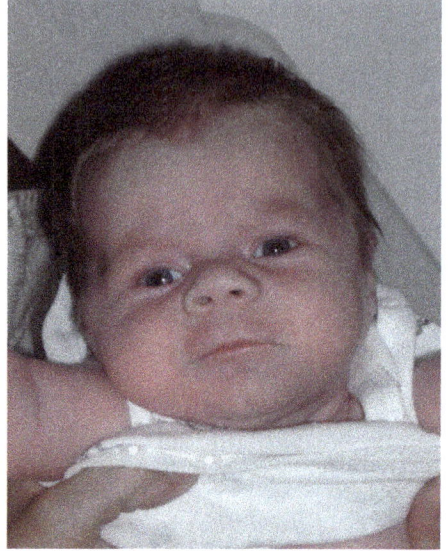

Fig. 5.3: FAS, 3-month-old boy.

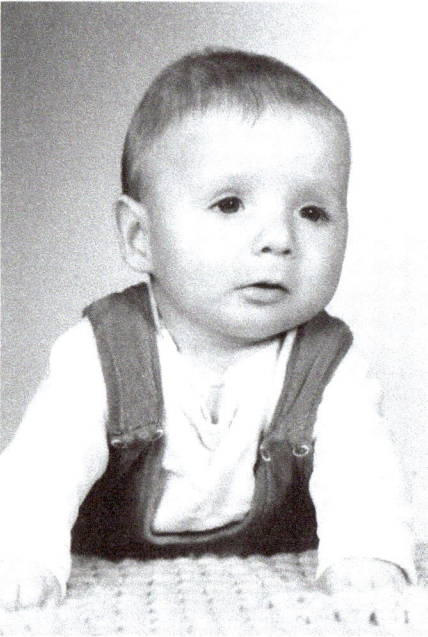

Fig. 5.4: FAS, 8-month-old boy.

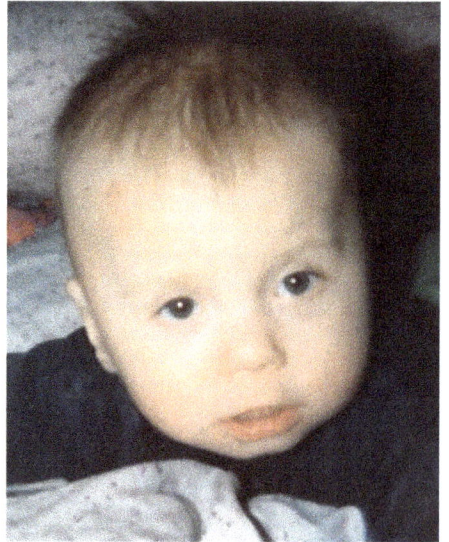

Fig. 5.5: FAS, 9-month-old boy.

- characteristic facies with small eyes, low nose bridge, short, upturned nose, and backwardly rotated ears (less pronounced in infancy);
- major malformations (i.e. heart, renal, skeletal, cleft palate), with congenital heart anomalies the most frequent, such as ventricular septal defect (VSD) or atrial septal defect (ASD).

Common signs in infancy are
- symptoms of alcohol and drug withdrawal (i.e. restlessness, irritability, perspiration, trembling);
- often long lasting sleep problems;
- feeding and swallowing problems (dysphagia, weak sucking reflex);
- increased susceptibility to infections;
- general muscle hypotonia.

5.1.1 Irritability and alcohol withdrawal symptoms

It is well known that women abusing alcohol are often additionally not only nicotine dependent, but also tend to consume illegal substances.

In everyday life, however, symptoms of illegal drug abuse are clinically more obvious and more frequently admitted by women, and due to the severity of symptoms, treatment is often focused on drug abuse only. The additional alcohol consumption in drug dependent women, which is as high as 86% of women according to a study by Singer et al. [3], often remains unnoticed.

These newborns often suffer from neonatal withdrawal syndrome. The clinical symptoms of intrauterine alcohol exposure may be noticed not before the reduction of acute withdrawal symptoms, and when dystrophy, growth deficiency, microcephaly, feeding and sleeping disorders and general developmental delay become apparent.

5.1.2 Sleep disorders

Many patients suffer from severe sleep problems postnatally and in early infancy, especially after long hospitalisation or when the newborn was living under difficult and neglectful conditions with their biological parents before being removed from the family (see Section 6.1).

Overall, sleep disorders often stress the whole family, and in some cases remain a problem for years.

Case report

Our infant suffered from developmental delay and from severe sleep disorders right from the very beginning. He was hardly able to fall asleep, waking up regularly at night to make sure that his foster parents were still present. Sleep disturbances lasted for many months and improved only when, fortunately, he was treated with melatonin for a period of time.

5.1.3 Feeding and regulation disorders

Even in healthy newborns, infants or small children, feedingproblems and regulation disorders such as excessive clinging to parents, and aggressive or oppositional behaviour often occur for a certain period of time [4].

Early-onset regulation disorders include an inability to regulate behaviour appropriately, i.e. excessive crying, inappropriate aggressive behaviour, sleep or feeding disorders. Chronic exhaustion of both parents and the child burdens the relationship.

Many infants with FAS are often irritable, anxious and cry for hours. Despite medical and psychological assistance these symptoms can persist over a period of many months.

Problems with sucking and swallowing are often responsible for difficulties in feeding, possibly because of the delayed neurological maturation of the swallowing reflex. Infants frequently spit, vomit or refuse food completely and are only able to drink small amounts at a time, resulting in additional stress and burden for caretakers, and necessitating feeding the child almost hourly.

Many children hardly gain any weight despite sufficient food intake and they remain underweight and growth delayed throughout childhood.

Consequently, foster parents try even harder to increase weight in their children, but mostly without any success. This understandable desire to help their children grow is regrettably often a futile effort. Fortunately, not a single child with FAS among the many diagnosed children ever had a serious or acute danger for their life due to their low weight.

In adulthood, female FAS patients often become significantly obese, until now there is no sufficient endocrinological explanation for this phenomenon.

Report of a foster mother

"... After the first 3 days, I slept nearly 2 hours on average at night because of my foster daughter's feeding problems. She was only able to drink 40–50 ml per meal. I started to feed her almost every hour because I was worried that otherwise she would starve. Each meal was like a battle and out of 10 meals I lost 4 of them because if I tried to give her 60 ml milk per meal instead of 50 ml she vomited out the whole meal. Afterwards it took almost 20 minutes until she was able to take some food again, and everything started all over again. If a healthy child of the same age needs about

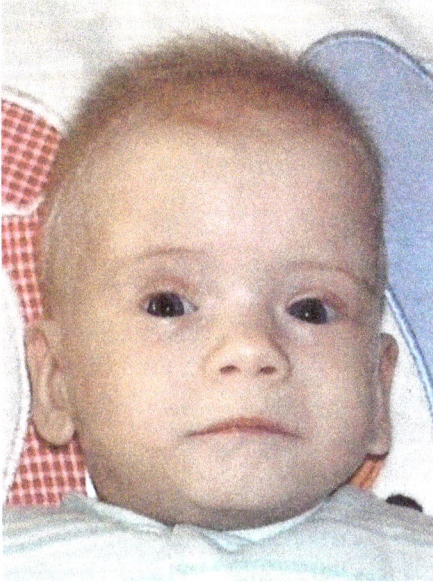

Fig. 5.6: FAS, 5-month-old girl.

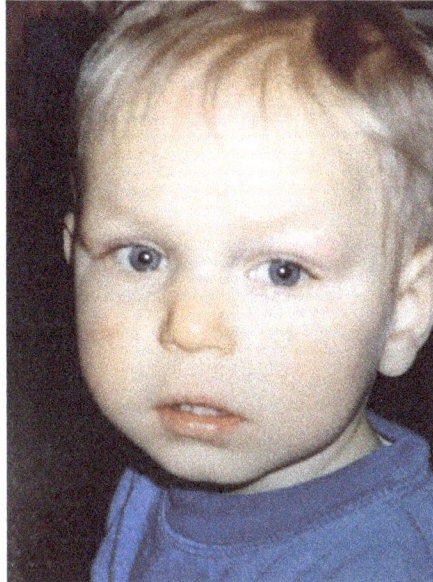

Fig. 5.7: FAS, 2-year-old boy.

1000 ml per day, this little child was surviving with only 500 ml. These feeding problems even at night caused permanent sleep deprivation. Therefore, my husband and I took turns feeding her at night, so that one of us could sleep while the other tried to feed and calm down our frequently crying child."

5.1.4 Susceptibility to infections

Many young patients with FAS additionally suffer from an increased susceptibility to infections, particularly of the upper respiratory tract, the middle ear or tympanic inflammation and sinusitis. This could be due to their former suboptimal living conditions in their biological family but could also be due to "midface hypoplasia", leading to insufficient ventilation of sinuses and the middle ear, and even in a stable living environment these children may suffer from frequent infections. With increasing age, these problems tend to ameliorate.

5.1.5 Congenital heart defects

The majority of patients suffer from ventricular septal defect (VSD) or atrial septal defect (ASD), which only require surgical repair in rare cases. Generally, a paediatric cardiologist will follow them, and most children are not severely affected. With increasing age, the cardiac wall closes and does not require further treatment or monitoring (see also Section 6.2).

5.2 Early childhood (preschool)

In early childhood, FAS is diagnosed most commonly because of the more pronounced morphological signs and symptoms, cognitive deficits and behavioural difficulties. In kindergarten and preschool, behavioural difficulties and impairments usually become clearly apparent. Children are no longer only at home and thus they are compared to peers, revealing their significant developmental delay (i.e. motor, language, speech, cognition, emotional-social abilities and behaviour).

Language delay includes both expressive and receptive speech, which means that they are often unable to talk like their peers and especially that their ability to understand what is being said is limited and not always immediately recognisable.

The most common morphological signs and clinical abnormalities associated with FAS in early childhood (preschool) are:
- lack of weight gain (dystrophy)
- growth deficiency
- small head (microcephaly)
- developmental delays in:
  gross and fine motor skills; perception; speech
- cognitive disorders
- abnormal social interaction and communication
- hyperactivity, impulsivity and attention deficits

5.2.1 Growth deficiency, dystrophy and craniofacial dysmorphia

Growth deficiency becomes noticeable at the latest during preschool age, also in affected children without any typical craniofacial dysmorphic features. Weight, height and head circumference are often documented to be below average, i.e. 3rd–10th percentile, meaning that those children are clearly smaller than their peers. Reflective of the very small head circumference, mothers sometimes report that the child is still wearing a baby cap.

Because most children are smaller than their peers, they may be mistaken to be of much younger age, and their behaviour and development erroneously presumed to be age appropriate.

Severely affected children have typical facial features (i.e. small palpebral fissures, short and upturned nose, thin upper lip and a flat and smooth philtrum).

Often, these children may present with additional facial features such as a flattened midface (midface hypoplasia) and dysmorphic and backwardly rotated ears.

All of these characteristics and anomalies may be present in varying degrees of severity, and in cases of less marked facial features are sometimes only recognisable by specialists.

5.2.2 Developmental delay of motor abilities

Most affected children suffer from developmental delays and in infancy they are particularly focused on difficulties in motor skills. Gross motor skills are normally less affected but due to poor perception, fine motor skill deficiencies are often evident with problems in hand–eye coordination; these children are clumsy and unable to play football, cycle or ride scooters, and they have difficulties in painting or writing.

Due to hyperactivity and lack of concentration combined with difficulties in recognising danger, these children very often are at increased risk of accidents and injury whilst playing or climbing.

Report of a foster mother

After suffering initially from developmental delay and little motor skills, he learned to walk freely at the age of 20 months after physiotherapy treatment. For a long time, he was rather unsteady on his feet and he regularly stumbled against everything. Now he is very hyperactive, is unaware of any danger and unable to assess dangerous situations properly.

Furthermore, he behaves obtrusively without accepting personal limits and he talks a lot but it often remains unintelligible. He cannot concentrate and is oblivious to daily life routine. He is not able to learn to tell time, handle money or deal with daily structure. During infancy, he was insensitive to heat or cold and to pain.

5.2.3 Language developmental disorders

Expressive and receptive speech and language development is often delayed. Compared to peers, the language of children with FAS still seems very superficial and childlike; in some cases, these children only use single words or half-sentences and they tend to answer with stereotypies instead of meaningful and appropriate responses. They may give the impression that their language skills are quite normal, but listening more carefully, there is a lack of any sense.

Speech is not an element of communication for them; rather they talk without any interest in their conversational partner. They frequently talk without interruption and are very focused on their own talking, not realising that they annoy others. Foster and adoptive parents often report that they desperately want to find a way to stop their disturbing chatter.

In contrast, several FAS children have very good language abilities and use them to cover up many of their other social problems. Foster or adoptive parents report that the children show great imagination in creating stories and talking about fictional experiences.

Case report

The foster parents report that their son has great adaptation difficulties. He has suffered from severe sleep problems. In addition to his constant restlessness and fidgeting, he started having strong concentration problems. He talks all day incessantly and interrupts and prevents others from speaking. The content of what he is talking about is often incomprehensible for others, and he senselessly repeats himself. On the other hand, he has good speech comprehension, likes to sing and is able to memorise melodies quickly.

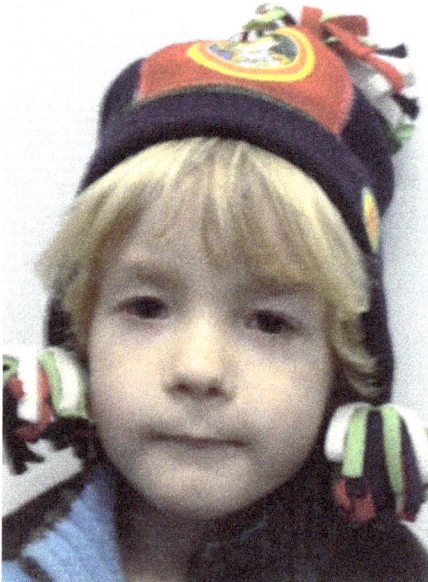

Fig. 5.8: FAS, 4-year-old boy.

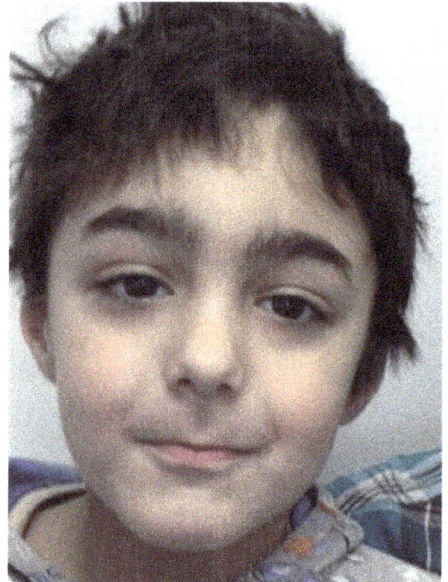

Fig. 5.9: FAS, 5-year-old boy.

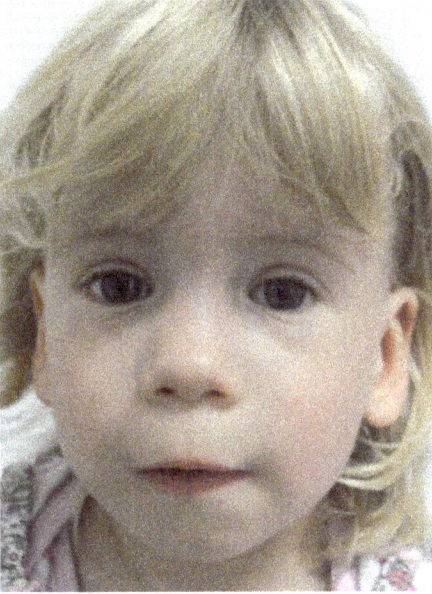

Fig. 5.10: FAS, 28-month-old girl.   Fig. 5.11: FAS, 24-month-old girl.

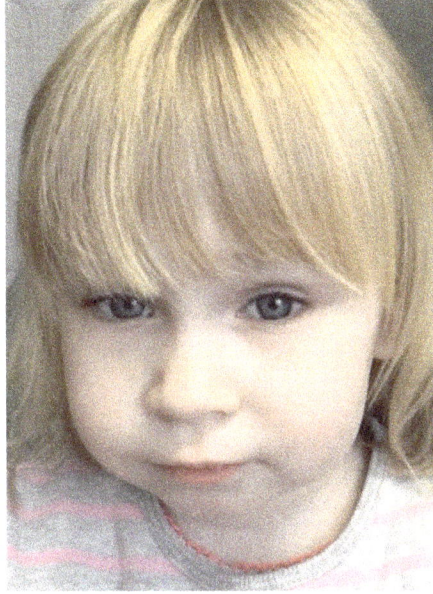

Cognitive abnormalities and perception disturbance

Although these children practise daily routines extensively, i.e. how to get dressed and undressed, how to perform personal hygiene, wash and brush teeth, or how to perform family rituals like setting the table, etc., the children forget basic rules and routines, even when they are repeated regularly due to persisting memory deficits. They always need to be encouraged and motivated for daily routine activities because they are completely unresourceful.

All of the rules need to be re-taught every day, need to be repeated constantly and practised repetitively. A particular problem is the inability of these children to understand the cause and effect of their actions.

Neither the educators in kindergarten, nor neighbours, friends or physicians unfamiliar with FAS syndrome are able to understand this forgetfulness and slow-wittedness properly and are easily convinced that these children are just unwilling or badly raised.

Due to their problems in social perception, children with FAS discern their social environment differently. They behave obtrusively and are obviously unable to apprehend the needs of other persons; as a consequence, they do not understand other people's reactions properly. Furthermore, many of them have limited impulse control, are dominant, particularly towards other children, and quickly become encroaching without accepting personal limits. Due to this behaviour, they become socially isolated.

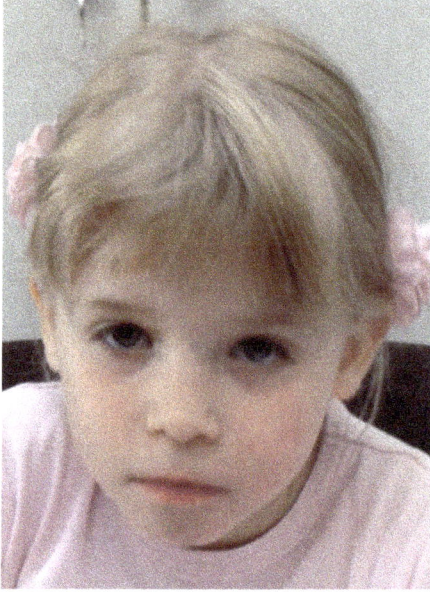

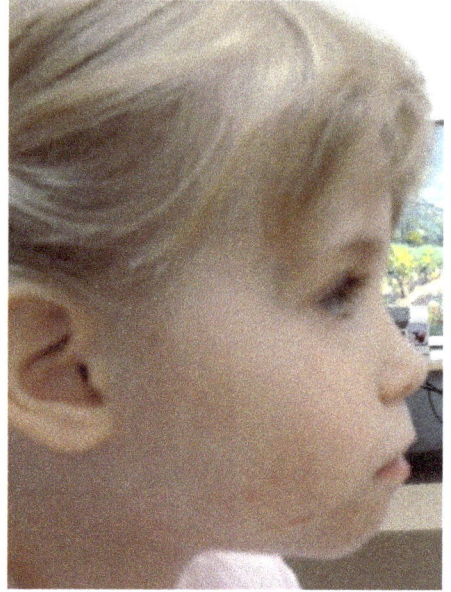

Fig. 5.12: FAS, 5-year-old girl.

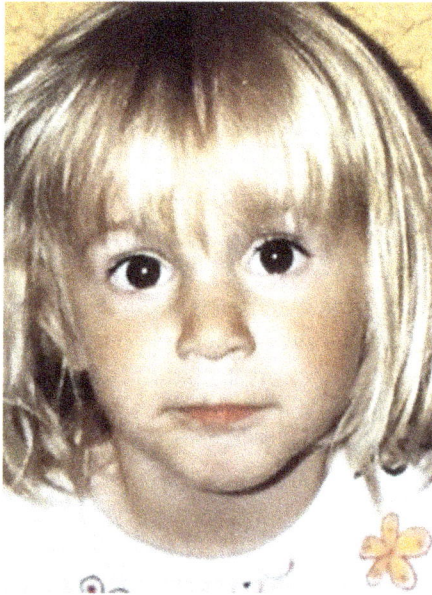

Fig. 5.13: FAS, 3-year-old girl.

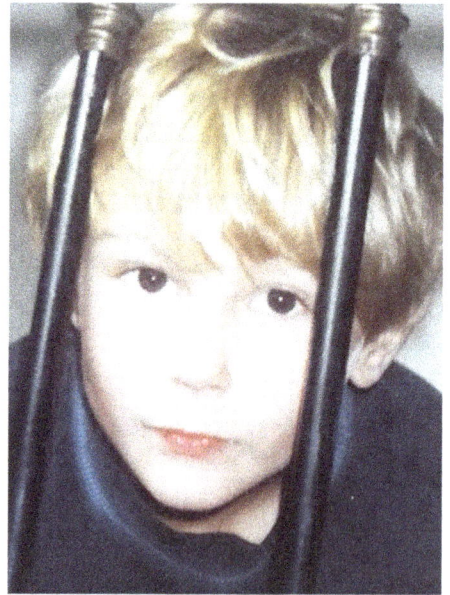

Fig. 5.14: FAS, 5-year-old boy.

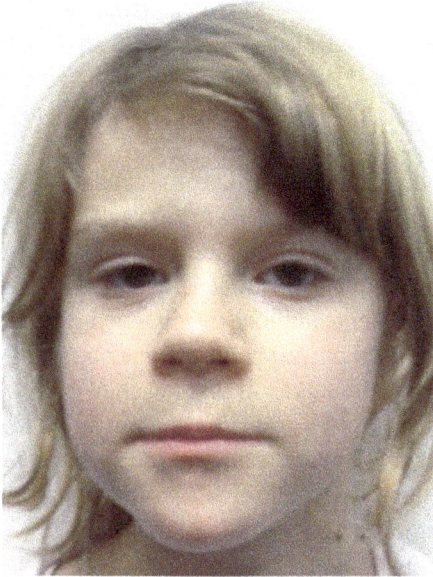

Fig. 5.15: FAS, 5-year-old girl.

Moreover, children with FAS do not understand the concept of friendship.They are unable to be in a constant and close relationship, but they quickly call anyone a friend, even if it is only a casual acquaintance. When asked, they usually report that they have many friends, but parents report that none of these so-called friends ever come to see them at home. When playing with others, the inability to control their impulses and to estimate the impact of their actions leads to acute danger for themselves and other children.

Some children with FAS develop sexualised behaviour already in early childhood. They often have been seriously neglected and sometimes have experienced physical and sexual abuse in their biological families.

Due to their encroaching behaviour and inability to detect any possible dangers, they walk out and even go along with strangers who behave in a friendly manner towards them, without regarding the often-repeated warnings of their parents.

Derived from these facts there is an essential need for a protective home environment with stable caretakers, strict rules, a structured and regular daily routine and an unexciting, i.e. stimulus free, living environment in order to support these children.

5.2.4 Social problems, hyperactivity, ADHD

Even the very young children are soon perceived as being different from their peers. They are either completely distraught and, for example, refuse to go to kindergarten or they clown around, spreading chaos and trouble. Due to their low impulse control, they often respond with destructive and aggressive behaviour. They often have tantrums ("explosive episodes") for the slightest reasons and thereby frighten other children. As a result, they usually become socially isolated very quickly without understanding the nature and cause of the rejection.

In addition, many affected children are hyperactive with further and clear symptoms of ADHD already in early childhood.

If a child is very hyperactive, parents should carefully structure and adapt daily activities, i.e. put a limit on watching television, reduce exposure to loud and aggressive music, and protect the child from overstimulation by light, movements, sounds, toys, noise, colour, activities, and large groups of people. Moreover, sport activities are helpful for many children with FAS, also in order to improve their low self-esteem.

Symptoms of ADHD (hyperactivity, impulsivity, attention deficits) may be so distinctive sometimes even in early childhood that parents report that the child is buzzing around the entire day unable to concentrate and play normally. One way to reduce child's tension is, for instance, playing in the garden or at the playground so that s/he is exhausted and falls asleep easily at night, but the next morning the same problems start again. In these cases, treatment with stimulants is reasonable, even in early childhood (see Section 6.5).

Report of an adoptive mother

"Imagine a child that is moving around on the floor like a never-ceasing humming top. Imagine this child is squeaking continuously, talking loudly and with a shrill voice. Imagine that the child is attacking you with questions continously, but is hardly interested in any answers. Just imagine a very loud, hyperactive, four-and-a-half-year-old girl who seems to be like a two-year-old, running around with agitated movements, talking incessantly in order to make contact with anybody without the slightest idea of closeness or distance. If you imagine all that, you have a good idea of my daughter N. ..."

5.3 School age

At this age, the problems at school lead to increasing diagnostic examinations and therapeutic measures.

The most frequent problems are restlessness, attention deficits, impulsivity, memory disorders, and developmental problems in language and mathematics.

The children can only concentrate for short periods of time; they are easily distracted, and tend to disrupt the class. Despite extensive parental support during homework, they are often unable to understand the context and always forget what they had already learned. Hence, they often react with aggressivetantrums for no reason and become outsiders at school. Some of these children react with withdrawing, are shy, anxious, or depressed.

Examinations should be initiated at the latest at this age if intrauterine alcohol exposure is suspected because children have to attend school, and the parents are no longer able to protect them intensively.

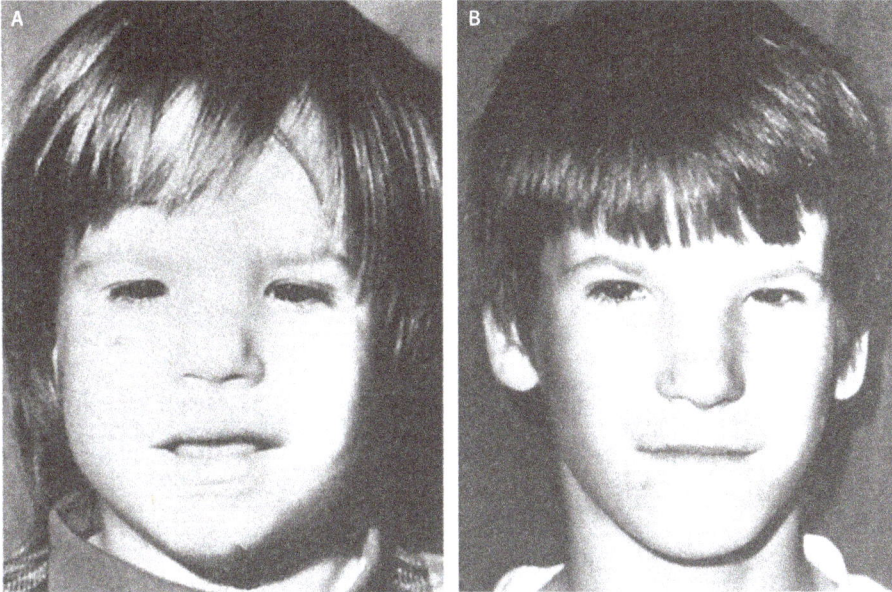

Fig. 5.16: Patient from the first description of FAS by Jones and Smith (1973). A) 2-year-old, B) 12-year-old [5].

The most common morphological signs and clinical abnormalities associated with FAS at school age are:
- dysmorphic features
- significant developmental deficiencies
- learning difficulties
- no sense of space and time
- social difficulties (conflicts, bullying at school, inappropriate friends)
- executive functioning disorder
- conflicts with adoptive/foster parents
- attention disorder
- impulsive behaviour
- forgetfulness

5.3.1 Significant developmental disorders and dysmorphic features

At school age, affected children are suffering even more from their short stature and low weight compared to their peers. They are slender, hyperactive, love sports and playing around. They suffer from delays in motor, language and emotional development and often display a dominant behaviour. They prefer to play with younger children because peers often do not accept them.

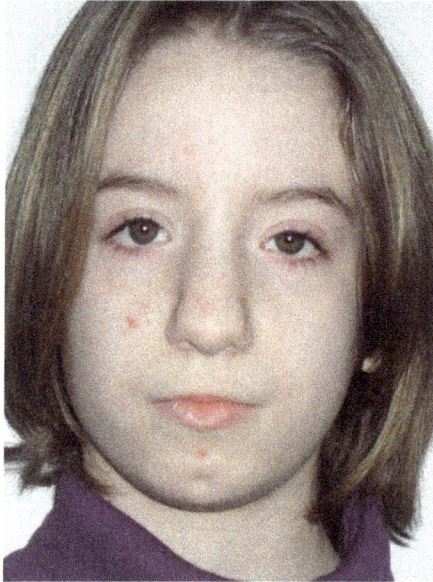

Fig. 5.17: FAS, 12-year-old girl.

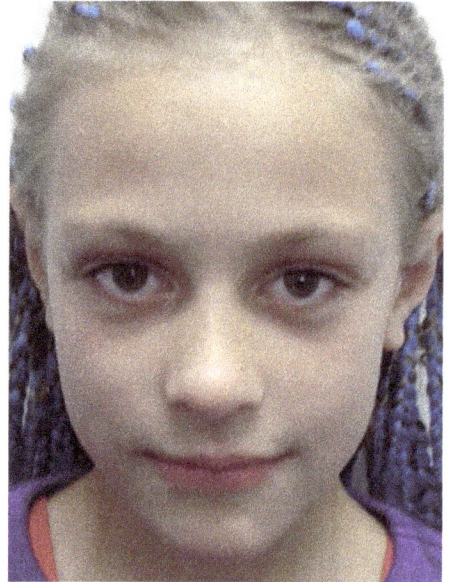

Fig. 5.18: pFAS, 10-year-old girl.

The typical craniofacial dysmorphic features are usually visible at this age: small palpebral fissures, thin upper lip, and a smooth philtrum in combination with microcephaly, giving them a characteristic facial expression. In the majority of children the facial features are less obvious and a diagnosis is more difficult to ascertain and must be evaluated using, for example, the 4-Digit Diagnostic Code.

5.3.2 Learning and social difficulties

Due to their developmental delay and short stature, most children with fetal alcohol syndrome, whether diagnosed or not, start school at the earliest age of 7 years. Starting school earlier may be stressful for parents or caregivers of children with FAS and increases the risk of an early school failure, especially in the absence of a diagnosis.

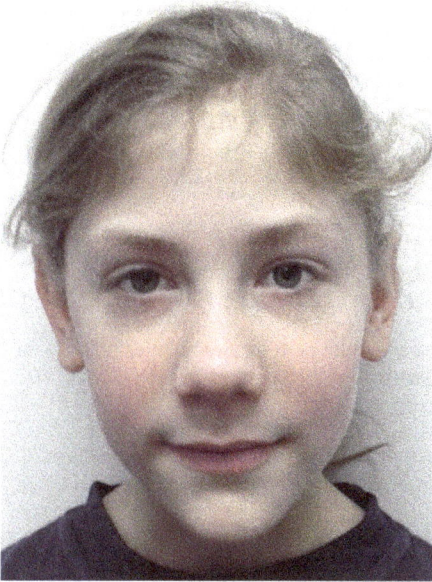

Fig. 5.19: pFAS, 11-year-old girl.

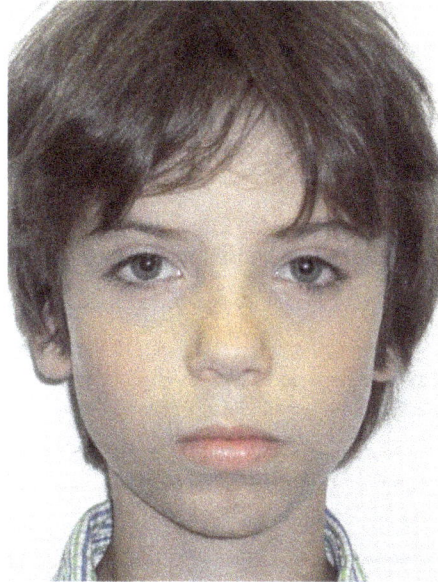

Fig. 5.20: FAS, 10-year-old boy.

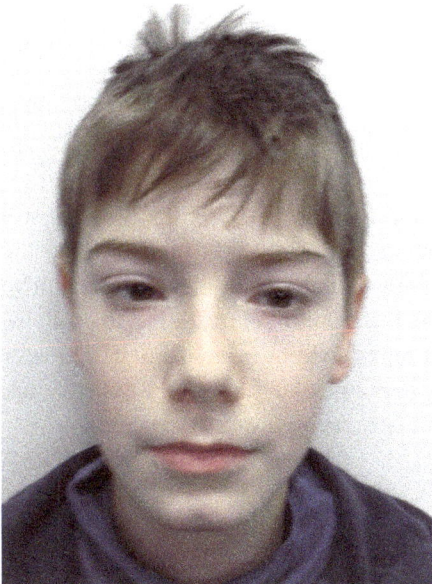

Fig. 5.21: FAS, 13-year-old boy.

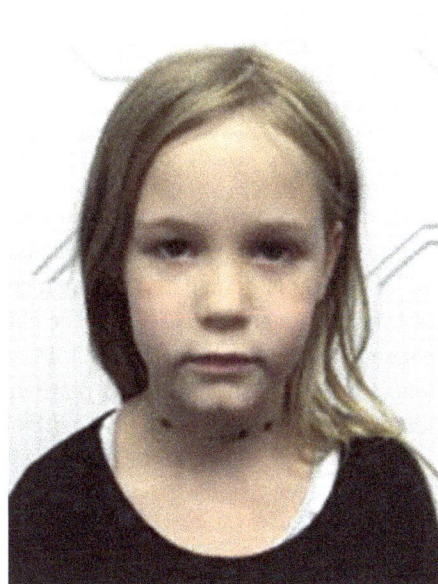

Fig. 5.22: FAS, 6-year-old girl.

In some children, cognitive developmental delay has been recognised since early childhood. Severe developmental deficiencies in language, inability to understand even simple everyday routines, and difficulty in learning and remembering them, as well as working memory deficits, and sometimes severe attention difficulties, and restlessness together with social problems, often results in their inability to attend a regular school.

Report from a foster mother

"Her developmental delay raised the question of what might be the best time for school enrolment.

A neuropsychological test conducted to determine her current performance abilities, taking into account her hearing and speech disorder, revealed an IQ of 74. She clearly had learning disabilities and she started school at a special-needs school at the age of 7.

To her, going to school was an arduous path, and mathematics was a major difficulty; on the other hand, she was good at reading and copying. However, since she started attending school, she reached her physical limits more often.

Her everyday life activities were only manageable with a lot of family support 24 hours a day. She was unable to grasp the sense of time, date, and the four seasons, and she was unable to remember them.

She is easily fooled into doing anything stupid without being able to realise the dangers or consequences of her irresponsible behaviour.

... She is now in the fifth grade at a school for children with special needs. She is able to read and copy but without understanding the sense of it. She is only able to calculate numbers up to 10 by using her fingers and she is only able to solve all other tasks with difficulty and with a lot of support. We decided to transfer her to a school for children with a mental disability. At this school she feels accepted and learns, according to her abilities, everyday practical skills. She will never receive a high school diploma, but that is not so important for us."

If the cognitive deficits of the affected children are not very striking, they are still able to start and participate in a regular school during the first grades, when the subject matter is trained and repeated constantly at home. With increasing cognitive demands, teachers realise that these children lag behind their classmates. Initially, teachers often presume that these children are only unwilling to learn. But with greater demands for straight reasoning, particularly in mathematics, despite extensive support and great effort, their learning difficulties become more and more apparent.

5.3.3 No sense of time

The affected children do not develop an age-appropriate sense of time either and often they are unable to tell time. Most children use a digital watch but, nonetheless, the sense of time remains difficult even in recurring daily routines.

5.3.4 Spatial orientation

Outside their home environment these children often get lost, but sometimes it is possible for them to learn and to know routine routes after a long time of guided practice (i.e. the way to school).

Details from a report of a foster mother

"… Since 3 years our daughter has been using an alarm clock that helps her to get up in the morning by herself and a list with an exact time schedule to get the school bus on time. One morning I got up and saw her sitting at the kitchen table. I asked her why she wasn't eating breakfast. She answered that it wasn't 5.40 am yet. When she gets up earlier, the entire list needs to be adapted as well.…"

"… F., now 14 years old, ought to manage the route to her weekly psychotherapy session independently. Because we live in a small village, F. is used to take public transportation to get to school, but for therapy sessions – located in another town- the way is different. Hence, she had to learn to connect different stages and, therefore, we presented her a second list. Initially, we taught her the first step, going from school into town by train. This presented a lot of difficulties; it was a Tuesday and her school bus left 1 hour later. Therefore, F. concluded that the train to therapy session would also be 1 hour later. After 3 weeks she understood that she has to follow the exact dates on her list. So, she had learned the first step.

Then she had to find the right tramline to the correct direction. It also took several weeks until she was at least able to do it correctly. Taken all together, our training continued from the end of August until December when she finally was able to manage the entire route by herself without contacting us for questions… "

5.3.5 Conflicts, bullying in school, inappropriate friends

Persistent problems with social interaction lead to isolation, in school and at home, and sometimes start as early as in kindergarten. These children are disliked; they often are friendless and without playmates. Because they are unable to recognise and respond appropriately to the needs of other children, they experience social rejection more and more without being able to interpret and understand the reactions of peers.

They are "different", and because of their inability to respond age-appropriately they easily become a target for bullying. They have a strong wish to make friends and they often try to please others by giving presents. In order to buy them, they even steal money from their parents. They desperately want these "false friends" to like them, not realising that they are being exploited.

5.3.6 Executive functioning disorders

Many patients damaged by alcohol exposure during pregnancy have deficits in executive functioning. One of the functions is the control of non-automated behaviour in everyday life (see Chapter 4).

Even with an IQ in a normal range, children with an executive dysfunction are unable to focus attention on relevant and important information while disregarding irrelevant, and unimportant information, i.e. to distinguish between important and unimportant things in everyday life. Because deficits in executive function are independent of intelligence, and also occur in children with normal intelligence, teachers and educators often wrongly assess that normal intelligent children cannot suffer from fetal alcohol syndrome.

These children have difficulties in handling daily routines, due to their poor working memory abilities, as they are unable to memorise lessons learned, and thus, always make the same mistakes. Consequently, daily tasks such as getting dressed, washing, brushing teeth, and setting the table must be repeated often and constantly. Children often react with tantrums because they do not understand what they are supposed to do.

Case report

C., a 16-year-old lovely girl, presented for diagnosis of FAS by her foster parents. She finished school but without school-learning graduation despite great efforts and intensive support.

Currently she is working in the kitchen of a hotel: she reported with joy that she really likes her job. Among other duties in the kitchen, she has for example, to wash the vegetables, or to peel potatoes under the guidance of the kitchen chef. She reported to be very good at it and likes to go there every day. The day before yesterday she had peeled cucumbers with zeal the whole day. In the evening, the kitchen chef had told her that carrots had to be peeled the next day. Her foster father added that the next day the kitchen chef said to C.: "Before you start with the carrots, please finish the last 20 cucumbers that weren't peeled yesterday." He had given the peeling knife to her and pointed to the cucumbers, but C. was completely at a loss because she couldn't remember what to do with the cucumber. With tears in her eyes she had to admit that she doesn't know how to peel cucumbers anymore!

5.3.7 Conflicts with adoptive or foster parents

With increasing age, children often strive for more independence, although they are incapable handling the requirements of daily life. The resulting conflicts with their parents are more difficult to control and become an added burden.

Conflicts with their parents, rejection by peers, and learning difficulties at school often result in a depressed mood, anxieties, skipping school, and aggressive behaviour. Lying and stealing are daily fare and stress their family relationships.

On the other hand, the affected children have many good character attributes; they are often very loving and willing to help, gifted in music, talkative and charming, deal well with younger siblings, lovingly take care of pets, and their childlike affection for their parents is special.

5.4 Late childhood and adolescence

At this age, severe behavioural problems and learning difficulties are rarely considered to be the result of intrauterine exposure to alcohol. Patients often have already received a variety of psychiatric diagnoses and several treatments have been started, but mostly without any improvement. Foster and adoptive parents often have given up hope and come to terms with the deficits and difficulties of their children, whilst the treating physicians do not know how to manage these persistent symptoms. Affected adolescents are usually isolated from their peers and increasingly refuse help and support.

The most common morphological signs and clinical abnormalities associated with FAS in late childhood and adolescence are:
- dysmorphic facial features
- weight gain
- learning difficulties school failure

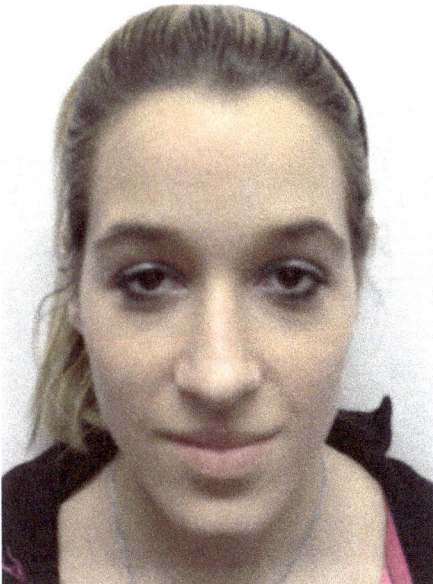

Fig. 5.23: FAS, 17-year-old girl.

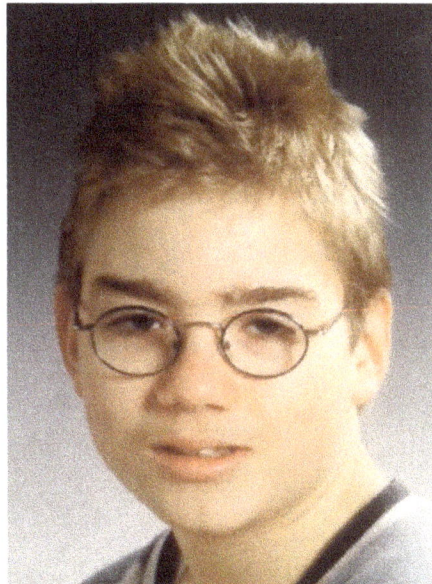

Fig. 5.24: FAS, 14-year-old boy.

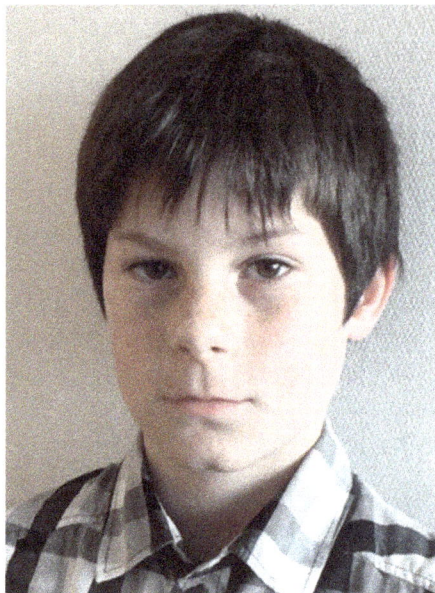

Fig. 5.25: FAS, 11-year-old boy.

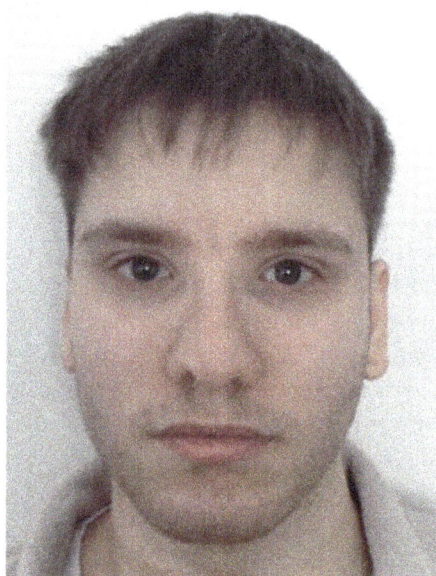

Fig. 5.26: FAS, 17-year-old boy.

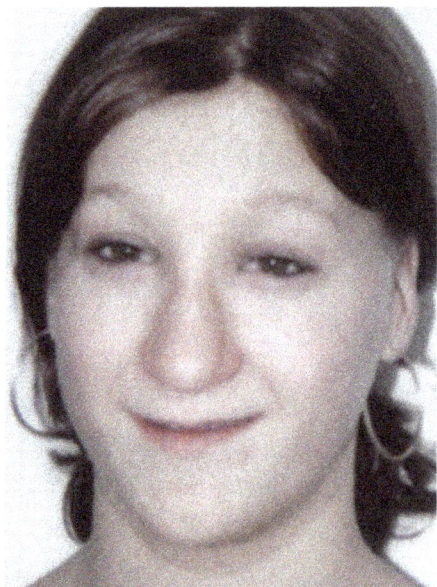

Fig. 5.27: FAS, 18-year-old girl.

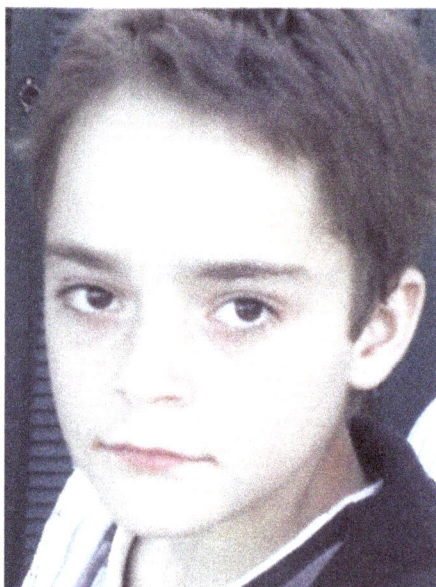

Fig. 5.28: pFAS, 13-year-old boy.

- vocational training problems
- inappropriate sexual behaviour
- criminal behaviour/problems with the law
- mental health problems, primarily ADHD and depression
- lacking independence
- limited contractual capability

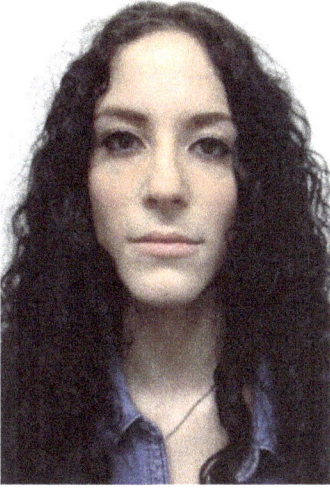

Fig. 5.29: pFAS, 17-year-old girl.

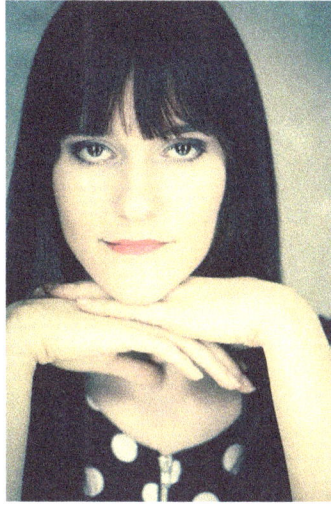

Fig. 5.30: FAS,16-year-old girl.

5.4.1 Late or missing diagnosis

With increasing awareness of the risk of FAS after intrauterine alcohol exposure today more adolescents come to our specialised FAS centre. They have been suffering for years from numerous behavioural, cognitive, social, and emotional problems without identified reasons before they ascertain the alcohol abuse of their biological mother during pregnancy.

In general, it is difficult to obtain conclusive information about potential alcohol consumption in a pregnancy years ago, in particular as the information is often not passed on to foster or adoptive parents or it is not available because children often came from disorganised and neglectful families lost to further contact.

Nevertheless, it is absolutely essential for an accurate diagnosis to acquire knowledge about possible maternal alcohol consumption during pregnancy by gathering information in any and every possible way.

Case report

J. came to our specialised centre at the age of 17 accompanied by his adoptive father. He had read about FAS on the Internet and recognised striking similarities with many thoughts and feelings described by young affected patients. He now wanted to know whether he probably was suffering from this syndrome. He was tall, did not show any facial abnormalities, but had a lot of social problems and was bullied extensively at school and, therefore, left school early. He was adopted right after birth, and his adoptive parents had neither information about his biological family nor knowledge about any maternal alcohol consumption during pregnancy.

When asked about siblings, his father remembered that J. had an older biological sister, but they were not in contact.

Father and son were sent home without a diagnosis, but with the advice to find the sister in order to get information about whether their biological mother had drunk alcohol while pregnant with him.

After 6 weeks they returned, and J. reported that they had found his 9 years older sister who had answered straight away: "Didn't you know that our mother was an alcoholic? She drank heavily while being pregnant with you!"

Note: Due to this information, we were able to diagnose FAS. In a trial years later, he was accused of burglary but because of his diagnosis he was acquitted.

5.4.2 Dysmorphic features

Dysmorphic features are still present in adolescence but might be a little less pronounced. The previous small, short and upturned nose the "nez en trompette", as the French named this characteristic short nose, often becomes large with a broad nasal bridge, which is medically unclear to date (see Figs. 5.20, 5.22, 5.23). Furthermore, the majority of patients still has a small head, a reduced height, and are underweight. The thin upper lip, the smooth philtrum, and particularly the small palpebral fissures, often remain clearly visible. Postpubertal girls tend to become overweight, sometimes even obese.

5.4.3 Learning difficulties, school failure, problems with vocational training

Often, severe social difficulties may continue into adulthood, and further academic failure leads to intensive diagnostic procedures, sometimes resulting in the diagnosis of FAS.

In some circumstances, affected children are able to pass the first 1–2 years of primary school without great difficulties, although almost uniformly extensive support and help by the parents is necessary. Children often receive a special needs-status and following that, the goodwill of their teachers. But later on, learning difficulties and social problems become so serious as to require a change of school, i.e. a special-needs school with smaller classes, with regard to their school performance is a useful and recommendable measure.

If FAS is still not diagnosed by the time of adolescence, difficulties may become increasingly serious with many of the affected people not being able to graduate from school or to complete professional training later on.

If they already had received a diagnosis of FAS, they are clearly classified as being mentally and physically handicapped and thereby entitled to help and support, i.e. special school projects in order to finish school successfully or special education programmes of the Federal Employment Agency.

Case report

The psychiatric diagnoses of this adolescent were: depression in combination with the development of an emotionally unstable personality disorder, substance abuse disorder, and conduct disorder. According to the adoptive father, his son is not an "easy person" and is very sensitive and quick-tempered. Because he was different from the others he was harassed in school for many years and despite help and support of his parents he skipped school for fear of his schoolmates. Finally, he refused to go to school at all; and only his father's support prevented him from being expelled from school.

5.4.4 Adolescence and sexual problems, delinquency, and comorbidity

Adolescents withdraw more and more out of control of their parents and caregivers. They withdraw from family life and partially act like other teenagers; they desire more independence and refuse well-intentioned advice from their parents. Conflicts with parents increase in frequency and severity, and parents sometimes are even attacked physically by their children, with possibly far-reaching consequences.

If the living conditions become unbearable because family members are unable to cope with the aggressive and impulsive behaviour any longer, sometimes placement in an institution becomes necessary.

Case report

Her foster son, now 12-years old, became more and more aggressive, and for quite some time his foster mother had become increasingly scared of him. One day, he was beside himself with rage and assaulted her physically; his foster father had to hold him back in order to break up this fight, and the critical situation ended. The next day, however, the boy went to the child protective services to report that his parents had hit and mistreated him. Without any consultation of the foster parents he was referred to a protectory. Soon he became homesick, but it was only after 14 days that he was allowed to return home and this only with legal support. Now his foster parents are under threat of a charge based on child abuse.

Foster parents often report that young girls with FAS behave risky by contacting mostly older men via Internet platforms or chat rooms. They quickly declare these men to be their great love and meet up with them, unable to recognise the associated risks and disregarding every objection and advice from their parents. They are easily taken advantage of and completely naive about sexually transmitted diseases, unwanted pregnancy, and emotional stress.

Male adolescents have a higher risk than girls to develop severe criminal behaviour during puberty. Foster parents often report that the boys frequently lie and steal.

At first, they only steal small amounts of money from home, but with increasing age, they sometimes steal larger amounts of money or goods from shops. Because of their low self-esteem and good nature, they want to impress so-called friends and are unable to resist peer pressure. Often, they lack any sense of guilt and are unable to handle money responsibly because they do not grasp the meaning of numbers. They try to cover up their inabilities by "talking big".

5.5 Adulthood ("FAS adult")

It has not been very long that we realised that fetal alcohol syndrome and its variations is a prenatally acquired, teratogenic disability that affects people for the rest of their lives. The diagnosis in adulthood is described in detail in Part III, Chapter 13.

5.5.1 Late diagnosis

In Germany, the diagnosis of FAS in adultshas received little attention in psychiatry so far. In 2012, the psychiatric clinic of the University of Erlangen published for the first time a detailed paper describing FAS in adulthood [7].

FAS is not only a paediatric disease but also a lifelong, persistent physical and neuropsychiatric disorder, which – diagnosed or not – is still present in adulthood.

Conservative estimates assume that in Germany about 3000–4000 children are born with FAS and pFAS/ARND per year [8]. This means that after a period of 20 years 60,000–80,000 of those affected reach adulthood. Today only a small proportion of them have been diagnosed in childhood, and psychiatrists and neurologists have to learn to diagnose and treat this almost "unknown disorder" among their adult patients.

The diagnostic criteria of the 4-Digit Diagnostic Code are, with certain limitations, still applicable to adults. The craniofacial dysmorphia is measurable. Unfortunately, the normative values from Astley et al. [9] only go up to 16 and 18 years, but after this age usually growth is largely completed.

In our longitudinal study [10] we were able to show a persistent microcephaly among 50 percent of the adult patients examined. Body height also remains shorter in many

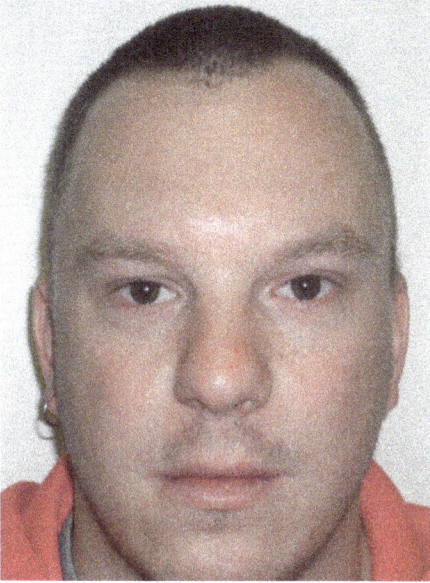

Fig. 5.31: FAS adult, 33 years old.

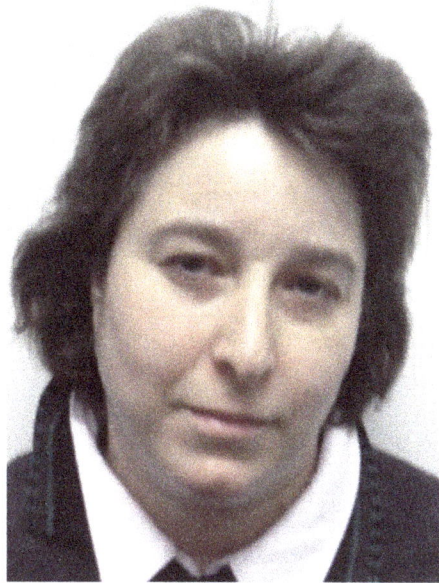

Fig. 5.32: FAS adult, 39 years old.

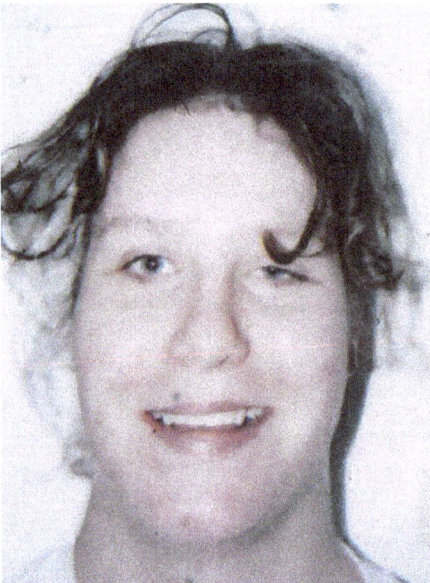

Fig. 5.33: FAS adult, 20 years old.

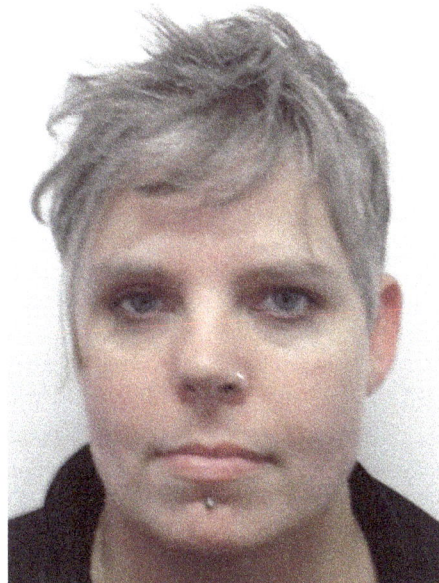

Fig. 5.34: FAS adult, 43 years old.

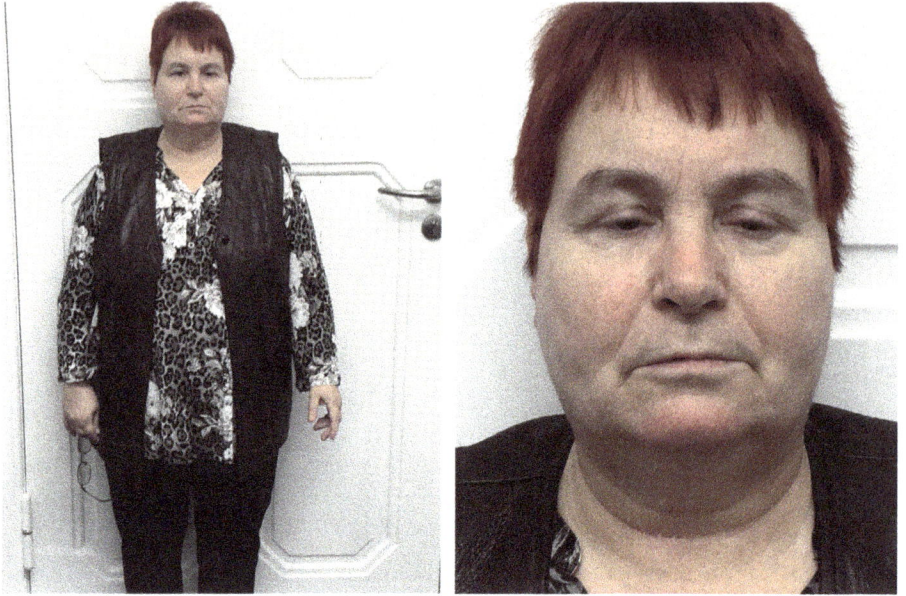

Fig. 5.35: FAS adult, 63-year-old woman.

adult patients; weight is less affected, as previously mentioned and particularly so as women are affected by significant increases in weight in adulthood.

Confirmation of maternal alcohol consumption during pregnancy is often more difficult to obtain in adult patients, but absolutely necessary for the diagnosis (see Section 14.2).

Case report

The foster parents of J. came to our clinic with their adult son, because J. was not able to handle his money and would spend the entire amount within a few days. He asked his former foster parents to give him a quarter of his monthly unemployment benefits every week. The foster parents consented and made an application to the court for legal care. The judge agreed, but asked a psychologist to examine J. shortly before making a decision. After 20 minutes, the psychologist returned and reported that J. is a "completely normal" 20-year-old man, who is perfectly able to handle his money on his own. Therefore, the judge rejected the application.

What happened? After about 2 minutes in the meeting with the psychologist, J. charmingly changed the conversation to his favourite topic about computers and the Internet, and impressed the "unsuspecting psychologist" so much that she rated him as being completely "normal".

Only a later diagnosis of fetal alcohol syndrome finally convinced the judge because then he was able to understand why J. was not able to handle his money although he had "good computer skills", and that he needed the support of his foster parents.

Bibliography

[1]   Little BB, Sell LM, Rosenfeld CR, Gilstrap LC, Grant NF. Failure to recognize fetal alcohol syndrome in newborn infants. American Journal of Diseases of children 1990, 144(10), 1142–46.

[2]   Ipsiroglu OS, McKellin WH, Carey N, Look C. "They silently live in terror". Why sleep problems and night-time related quality-of-life are missed in children with a fetal alcohol spectrum disorder. Social Science & Medicine 2012, doi: 10.1016/socscimed.2012.

[3]   Singer LT, Nelson S, Short E, Min MO, Lewis B, Russ S, Minnes S. Prenatal cocaine exposure: drug and environmental effects at 9 years. J Pediatr 2008, 153(1), 105–111.

[4]   Papousek M. Störungen des Säuglingsalters. In: Esser G (ed). Lehrbuch der Klinischen Psychologie des Kindes- und Jugendalters. Thieme Verlag, Stuttgart, New York 2002, 80–101.

[5]   Jones KL, Smith DW, Ulleland CN, Streissguth AP. Pattern of malformation in offspring of chronic alcoholic mothers. Lancet 1973, 1(815), 1267–71.

[6]   May PA, Gossage JP, Kalberg WO, Robinson LK, Buckley D, Manning M et al. Prevalence and epidemiologic characteristics of FASD from various research methods with an emphasis from recent in-school studies. Dev. Disabil. Res. Rev. 2009, 15, 176–92.

[7]   Walloch JE, Burger PH, Kornhuber J. Was wird aus Kindern mit fetalem Alkoholsyndrom (FAS)/fetalen Alkoholsepektrumstörungen (FASD) im Erwachsenenalter. Fortschr Neurol Psychiat 2012, 80, 320–326.

[8]   Schöneck U, Spohr HL, Willms J, Steinhausen HC. Alkoholkonsum und intrauterine Dystrophie. Auswirkungen und Bedeutung im Säuglingsalter. Monatschr Kinderheilk 1992, 140, 34–41.

[9]   Astley SJ. Diagnostic guide for Fetal Alcohol Spectrum Disorders: The 4-Digit Diagnostic Code. 3rd edn. University of Washington Publication Services, Seattle WA 2004.

[10] Spohr HL, Willms J, Steinhausen HC. Fetal Alcohol Spectrum Disorders in Young Adulthood. J. Pediatr 2007, 150, 175–179.

6 Comorbid disorders and differential diagnosis of FAS

6.1 Sleep disorders

6.1.1 General

Healthy sleep is essential for child development. Sleep disorders cause impairments in physical health, and in cognitive and emotional functions [1]. Newborns and infants are often restless at night and have sleep problems, even without intrauterine alcohol exposure, because regular sleep patterns develop gradually.

A prospective German study, published in 2006, investigated rates of sleep problems in healthy participants older than 4 years of age. It was found that 10% had problems falling asleep and 8% had problems maintaining sleep; taking into account that younger children are affected more frequently [2] (Table 6.1).

Tab. 6.1: Sleep disturbances (in %) in children between the ages of 4 and 10 as reported by their parents with the Child Behaviour Checklist (Lehmkuhl et al.) [3].

Sleep disorders	Boys (n = 496)		Girls (n = 534)	
	sometimes	frequent	sometimes	frequent
General sleep problems	6.5	2.8	6.8	1.7
Insomnia	11.2	2.8	10.5	2.1
Hypersomnia	4.0	0.6	3.9	0.6
Nightmares	13.3	0.8	10.5	1.1
Sleep walking	6.3	1.0	6.7	0.6

A general definition for sleep problems in early childhood is not available at present and, therefore, it is nearly impossible to generalise study findings, particularly regarding prevalence [4]. However, depending on diagnostic criteria, prevalence rates of sleep problems vary from 15 to 30%. Anders et al. (2000), for example, discriminated between problems in falling asleep and maintaining sleep in their studies on general sleep development in the first years of life.

The definition for problems with maintaining sleep in children between the ages of 12 and 24 months in this study was waking up at least twice a night and being awake for more than 20 minutes during the night. Problems falling asleep were assessed as whether infants needed more than 30 minutes to fall asleep even in the presence of their parents or if the parents had to return more than twice during this period of the child being half asleep [5].

https://doi.org/10.1515/9783110436563-006

Fegert et al. (1997) concluded in a prospective multi-centric study that about 40% of children aged 6 to 36 months, woke up at least once a night, and half of the children awakened several times [6].

The more severe sleep disturbances are in the first months of infancy, the more frequently they occur, the more likely they become chronic. Infants, who suffered from severe sleep disorders by the age of 6months, still awakened several times a night at the age of 12 months, and sleep disturbances in 3-year old children persisted into school age [7].

In a large prospective follow-up study ("Maternal Lifestyle Study", 2010) Stone et al. repeatedly investigated children until the age of 12 of 374 women who consumed cocaine, opiates, marijuana, alcohol or nicotine during pregnancy; nicotine was the only consistent predictor for sleep problems during early, middle and late childhood. The effect was dose dependent: sleep problems became more severe with higher nicotine exposure during pregnancy [8].

6.1.2 Sleep disturbances in children with FAS

Many children with FAS suffer from long lasting sleep problems causing more daytime behaviour problems compared to healthy children, and cognitive and emotional impairments. Additionally, the effectiveness of intervention and support for patients with FAS may be significantly reduced if sleep problems are not treated properly.

According to Jan et al. (2007), the severity of the sleep disorders is related more to the severity of the cognitive impairments than to the type of neurological disorder diagnosed [9].

In a study from Stade et al. (2010), sleeping behaviour of 325 Canadian children aged 5 to 8 years by use of questionnares, a 7-day diary and sleep history were analyzed. The reported time to fall asleep averaged 63 minutes and mean sleep duration was 7.2 hours. In the 7-day diary 256 of the 325 caregivers reported sleep problems experienced by their children such as:

- pavor nocturnus/sleep walking ($n = 10$)
- waking more than twice during the night ($n = 169$)
- severe daytime fatigue ($n = 23$) [10]

Chen et al. (2012) reported similar findings. They investigated the sleep behaviour of 33 children with FAS aged 4 to 12 years using the "Caregiver report" and the "Children's sleep habits questionnaire" (CSHQ). Significant sleep problems were found in 85% of the children examined [11].

The occurrence of sleep disturbances in alcohol-damaged children has rarely been examined due to the fact that FAS is difficult to diagnose in newborns [12] and is usually not established until later childhood. Experienced clinicians, foster and adoptive parents agree that in FAS children, sleep disorders are often already present in early infancy. Without intensive treatment, sleep problems tend to persist for a long time, sometimes well into adulthood.

Ipsiroglu et al. (2012) referred to a distinctive feature occurring in sleep disturbances of children with FASD. In an article entitled with the apt description: "They silently live in terror", they were the first to describe the possibility of a "restless leg syndrome" as a cause of severe sleep disorders in children with FASD [13].

The authors examined 27 children with FASD aged 2 to 15 years. The following sleep problems were diagnosed with the "comprehensive clinical sleep assessment" (CCSA):

- insomnia in 27/27 children;
- parasomnia (e.g. sleep walking, nightmares, pavor nocturnus) in 23/27 children;
- Breathing difficulties in 8/27 children; and
- suggestions of Willis–Ekbom disease (restless legs syndrome) in 22/27 children.

Case report of an adoptive mother

"L. came into our family at the age of 11 weeks, in November 2007. In the first couple of days we already noticed that L. slept during daytime and during the night she was awake due to restlessness and jactitation. She was able to quieten down only when lying on the stomach of one of us. These problems continued for several months. She was unable to drink more than 30 to 50 g per meal and, therefore, we had to feed her every 2 hours. When she was 6 months old, she additionally suffered from increased restless legs during the night. At the age of 4, L. complained of pain in her legs and felt the urge to move her legs constantly, not only during daytime but also during the night.

After falling asleep easily, she came to our bedroom every hour and wanted to be held. If we complied, it would take up to 3 hours until all three of us fell asleep; if we denied, she would run to and fro throughout the night without any sleep. During this period, I contacted the Society for Restless Legs Syndrome. I was told that this disorder is very difficult to diagnose in young children and until today there is no medical treatment available for children. Hence, we massaged her legs every night with lavender oil, and at the age of 5 years the symptoms regressed spontaneously."

Circadian rhythm sleep disorders

Difficulties with falling asleep and frequent awakening during the night or in the early morning are classified as circadian rhythm sleep disorders resulting from a misalignment between the timing of the circadian rhythm and the external environment. Circadian rhythms are physiologic and behavioural cycles with a recurring periodicity of approximately 24 hours, generated by the endogenous biological pacemaker, the suprachiasmatic nucleus, which is located in the anterior hypothalamus and responsible for melatonin secretion [9].

Animal models indicate that intrauterine alcohol exposure may disturb sleep wake patterns and particularly affect the suprachiasmatic nucleus, thus disrupting melatonin secretion. Goril et al. (2016) investigated sleep and melatonin secretion abnormalities in children with FASD; they found a high rate of sleep fragmentation and in 79% of the participants an abnormal melatonin profile [47].

The time required for falling asleep may be significantly increased in children with FAS and is possibly due to abnormal melatonin secretion. Because the cerebral cortex also influences the circadian rhythm via the hypothalamus it is possible that excitement, physical stress, anxiety, or an insufficiently darkened bedroom may also change or delay melatonin production [11].

In addition to the severe problems with falling asleep and maintaining sleep seen in patients with FASD, Ipsiroglu et al. described the rarely seen sleep disturbance "hypersomnia" in these children [13].

Case report of a foster mother

From the very beginning, M. suffered from hypersomnia with severe daytime fatigue. At the age of 4 months he was treated with promethazine, but without any improvement. M. was diagnosed with a fetal alcohol syndrome at the age of 18 months and until now, he has difficulties getting up in the morning and he suffers from severe daytime fatigue. Extensive examinations in a sleep laboratory neither confirmed the diagnosis of hypersomnia, nor revealed any evidence for narcolepsy; an adequate treatment was not available. M. literally has to be "pulled out of bed" in the morning by several adults, otherwise he would sleep all day long.

The report continues: "... After 16 hours of sleep he was as tired as after 6 hours.

Once, he did not leave his bed for 4 days because we didn't drag him out of it. He urinated in a bottle and hid his food in his room. He stopped his urgently needed medication and forgot about his personal hygiene. He still has to be pulled out of bed every morning, to make sure he went to his job training, which he really likes. Without our help, he would never reach his goal of completing his training. We need to control and take care of him at every step."

In 2010, Canadian scientists who had been working in the field of FASD for years, combined their clinical experience on sleep disturbances in FAS for the first time and formulated several proposals to optimise sleep hygiene in these children. A shortened summary of these recommendations for sleep hygiene is quoted below [14].

Recommendations for sleep hygiene and healthy sleeping patterns in children with fetal alcohol syndrome

General considerations
- Children with FASD frequently have a melatonin deficiency, which leads to disturbed sleep patterns.
- Sleep disturbances should be treated early and appropriately, as they lead to neurocognitive behavioural and health difficulties.
- Intervention services may be ineffective when sleep deprivation is present.

- The functioning of children with FASD is highly variable; therefore, developmental evaluations help to understand their strengths and weaknesses.
- Sleep hygiene practices designed for typical children are often not useful for children with FASD, as interventions need to be tailored to individual abilities.
- Caregivers and professionals involved should work together in a team.
- Modifying the environment, protection from overstimulation at home, in school. and in social situations are important principles in the general management of children with FASD.
- The rich learning experience that is required for typical children may lead to overloading and disturbed sleep for children with FASD.
- Sleep hygiene interventions are increasingly hard to enforce and are less effective with children with more severe cognitive loss.

Sleep environment
- The children's reactions to the environment should always be carefully observed.
- Their bedroom needs to be quiet, comfortable (temperature, non-irritating clothing and bedding), familiar, secure, consistent and unexciting (minimal furniture without clutter, strong odours, bright lights and colours).
- Their bedroom should not be used for punishment or play.

Preparation for sleep
- Calming behaviour and wind-down rituals promote sleep.
- Beverages containing caffeine or chocolate, excessive mental and physical behaviour, TV, and video games should be avoided in the evening to minimise alertness and delayed sleep onset.
- Bedtime activities require supervision, with emphasis on general hygiene, which is often poor in later life.

Sleep scheduling
- Enforcing rules, structure, routine and consistency are important not just at bedtime but all day.
- Times for bed and getting up need to be consistent, even during weekends and holidays.
- Melatonin replacement therapy for the child combined with sleep health promotion techniques may be useful to establish sleep scheduling.

Sleep hygiene for the caregivers
- Raising a child with FASD is a difficult task, thus the sleep health and emotional needs of the caregivers must always be considered.
- Caregiver sleep patterns are linked to those of the child. Treatment of the child's sleep disturbance with melatonin may lead to better sleep health of the caregivers and reduced burden of care [14].

In Germany, detailed recommendations of the German Sleep Society (DGSM) are used. Similar to the Canadian recommendations for sleep hygiene described above, a structured daily routine, a darkened bedroom, a secure and safe sleep environment and sleeping rituals are recommended. Particularly for small infants, medication like caffeine, theophylline or antiepileptic drugs should be given only if strictly indicated.

If the recommendations are unsuccessful, medical treatment with melatonin should be considered, which is already successfully implemented in the treatment of sleep problems in neurodevelopmental disorders in Canada and the USA [15].

Case report

"At the age of 18 months N. was placed in his new foster mother's home. His foster mother was working at a nursery and was, therefore, able to observe and take care of him in her nursery school. She reported that he suffered from severe sleep problems, that his motor development was delayed and that he became increasingly aggressive. He scratched himself, screamed for hours and masticated or destroyed everything.

Because of his extreme hyperactivity, it was difficult to take care of him. Because of his severe sleep problems, he was medicated with at least 2 mg of melatonin in the evening, and only then did his sleep problems improve significantly."

Quite often birth family contact ordered by the Family Court for children living in foster or adoptive families, especially if placement in these families occurred right after birth, can be very irritating, with subsequent difficulties such as feeding problems, aggressive behaviour, anxiety and increased sleep problems in the afflicted children. Therefore, it should be carefully considered whether these visits are beneficial for the children or have potentially negative influences on their development.

We strongly advise discontinuing these visits if the birth mother is still consuming alcohol, and contact should only be reinitiated after successful alcohol rehabilitation.

Report of a foster mother

"…Birth family visits every 14 days, partly carried out at the hospital where the mother had been admitted in the meantime, interrupted her positive development. After a longer period without visits, her sleeping behaviour improved and her anxiety lessened and finally disappeared completely.

At the age of 14 months L. was able to walk alone. However, during a recent birth family visit the maternal grandfather retained L. against her will and refused to let her go back to her foster mother. After this episode L. stopped walking completely. She became more agitated and restless again for a couple of weeks. Fortunately, the Family Court excluded her grandfather from future visits.

At 18 months of age, L. began to babble cheerfully and to repeat single words, but speech development regressed after several contacts with her grandmother, who was drunk and screamed during the visits. Subsequently, L. meets with her grandmother irregularly and at longer intervals, and in the meantime her speech skills have improved, but nevertheless after each of these arranged visits she becomes 'speechless' again…"

6.2 Congenital malformations

In the decades following the original description of the syndrome in 1973, researchers in many countries reported a wide variety of congenital abnormalities in patients prenatally exposed to alcohol. They were subsumed under the term alcohol related birth defects(ARBD).

Autti-Rämö et al. (2006) investigated 77 children and adolescents participating in a longitudinal study in Finland, who had been prenatally exposed to alcohol. They specified numerous abnormalities and functional disorders, e.g. persistent microcephaly in 45% of the adolescents, strabismus (38%), myopia or hyperopia (40%), tooth displacement (43%), renal/urinary tract infections (22%), heart abnormalities (18%) and hearing disorders (16%) [16].

6.2.1 Alcohol-related birth defects (ARBD)

The National Institute of Alcohol Abuse and Alcoholism (NIAAA) has revised and specified the diagnostic criteria for FAS and ARBD proposed by the Institute of Medicine (IOM) in 1996.

Definition of ARBD
1. Confirmed alcohol exposure during pregnancy: Alcohol exposure during pregnancy is defined as a pattern of excessive alcohol consumption characterised by heavy and frequent alcohol intake or by severe episodic alcohol intake i.e. binge drinking. This pattern can also include evidence of alcohol dependency.
2. One or more congenital abnormalities, including heart defects, malformation of the bones, kidneys, visual and hearing system.

But today, comorbid congenital abnormalities are no longer an important issue for diagnosis of FAS. This fact may be explained by the historical development of the syndrome: In the first years after its discovery only children with classical, "full blown" FAS including the typical craniofacial dysmorphic features were diagnosed, and many patients were born with additional comorbid malformations especially congenital heart abnormalities, which were the most common malformation. Nowadays, we know that these children were only "the tip of the iceberg". Usually, the majority of children (70–80%) are born without craniofacial dysmorphic features, i.e. partial fetal alcohol syndrome (pFAS) or alcohol related neurodevelopmental disorders (ARND); in these cases, heart defects occur significantly less often (Table 6.2).

6.2.2 Congenital heart defects

Apart from pre- and postnatal growth deficiency, CNS impairment and typical craniofacial dysmorphic features, congenital heart defects were one of the most common diagnostic criteria of FASin the past.

Already in 1977, in a paper from the German group of Löser et al. described a total of 16 different congenital heart defects in a sample of 56 children with FAS: 10 patients with atrial septal defects, 2 with ventricular septal defects, 2 with pulmonary stenosis, 1 with an atrial ventricular canal defect and 1 patient with a right pulmonary artery agenesis [17].

Tab. 6.2: Malformations in FAS.

Organ system	Malformation
Heart	Atrial septal defect (ASD)
	Ventricular septal defect (VSD)
	Large vessel malformations
	Tetralogy of Fallot
Skeletal	Radioulnar synostosis (see Fig. 6.6)
	Clinodactyly or camptodactyly (see Fig. 6.5)
	Pectus excavatum
	Hemivertebrae (half-vertebrae)
	Scoliosis
Uro genital system	Aplastic, dysplastic, hypoplastic kidneys
	Horseshoe kidneys
	Duplicated ureter
	Hydronephrosis
	Cryptorchism
	Hypospadia
	Clitoral hypertrophy
Eyes	Strabismus
	Myopia/hyperopia
Ears	Conductive hearing loss
	Sensorineural hearing loss
	Malformations of the external ear
Other	Basically every possible malformation has been described in individual FAS patients.
	The etiological specificity for most of these malformations is however rather uncertain and possibly also a finding by chance.

In 1981, in a study of 76 children with FAS Smith et al. found 32 patients who suffered from heart abnormalities, 20 patients with ventricular septal defect, 4 with Tetralogy of Fallot and 8 patients with an atrial septal defect [18].

In a literature review examining the association between congenital heart defects and FASD, Burd et al. (2007) found a total of 14 retrospective studies with a prevalence rate for atrial and ventricular septal defects of 21%. In this context, Burd described alcohol as a "cardiogenic teratogen agent", emphasising the causal connection between intrauterine alcohol exposure and the occurrence of heart defects [19]. However, how closely they are linked remains unclear, because FAS is typically not diagnosed until later in childhood. The mortality rate as a result of severe congenital heart defects may remain underestimated in patients with FAS, because these children die before being diagnosed with FAS.

Normally heart defects in patients with FAS are not severe. These patients especially suffer from septal defects, which only have to be followed by a paediatric cardiologist and often close spontaneously in the first years of life. Complex heart abnormalities associated with relevant clinical symptoms require surgical repair.

Paediatric cardiologists should keep in mind the fact that FAS may be a cause of congenital heart defects because they will be faced with these more often in possibly undiagnosed patients.

6.2.3 Eyes

In addition to myopia, hyperopia, strabismus and ptosis, children with FAS suffer from further visual impairments. In 1985, the Swedish ophthalmologist A. Strömland described the wide spectrum of malformations of the visual system in human and in animal studies [20].

She reported that retinal fundus abnormalities range from discrete lesions of the optic disc to severe malformations of both the retina and optic nerve.

The most frequent abnormalities are:

1. Optic nerve hypoplasia causing visual impairments with different degrees of severity in affected children.
2. Retinal vessels not straight in their course on the retinal fundus (i.e. displaying slightly curved forms (tortuosity)). This anomaly was found in 49% of children with FAS in the Swedish study and could be possibly used as an additional diagnostic criterion of FAS in uncertain cases [20–23].

6.2.4 Face

Orofacial malformations, midface hypoplasia, epicanthus, low nasal bridge, high-arched palate, cleft palate, low-set and backwardly rotated ears, serious tooth displacement, underdeveloped dental germ of adult teeth and microdontia are often found in patients suffering from FAS.

6.2.5 Ears

Children with FAS often experience recurrent serous otitis media or eustachian tube dysfunction. Sensorineural hearing loss with risk for consequential developmental language disorder occurs quite often. Hearing-loss in FAS is supposed to be associated with embryonal abnormalities of the first and second branchial arches.

According to a literature review by Church and Kaltenbach there are four different forms of hearing loss associated with FAS:
- acoustic problems caused by recurrent serous otitis media
- delay in maturation of the auditory pathway
- sensorineural hearing loss
- central hearing loss.

Ear-related disorders in early childhood may cause sensory deprivation with the risk of irreversible and permanent hearing, speech and mental impairments due to the lack of acoustic sensory input [24].

In a recent study from 2012, Stephen et al. were able to show by using magnetoencephalography (MEG) that patients with FAS suffered from distinct auditory delayed responses compared to healthy children. They recommend this method as an early screening tool for the presence of intrauterine alcohol exposure in children, particularly in cases, where the diagnosis is uncertain due to the lack of typical craniofacial dysmorphic features [25].

6.2.6 Internal organs

In addition to heart defects with a prevalence of about 20%, kidney defects are fairly common (10%), as well as genital and urinary tract defects and hernias.

6.2.7 Skeletal abnormalities

Malformations of the skeleton are generally rare; abnormalities which are more often seen in FAS are pectus excavatum (chicken chest), scoliosis, radioulnar synostosis, clinodactyly or camptodactyly, as well as fovea coccygea.

6.2.8 Skin

Common skin lesions include haemangioma, pathological palmar friction ridge and finger and toenail hypoplasia.

6.2.9 Neurology

In addition to microcephaly, children with FAS occasionally suffer from cerebral movement disorders and epilepsy.

In a Canadian study (2010), a total of 425 subjects aged 2–29 years with a diagnosis of FASD were examined to estimate the prevalence of epilepsy or seizure history. There was a confirmed diagnosis of epilepsy in 25 participants (5.9%) and 50 subjects (11.9%) had at least one documented seizure episode, resulting in an overall prevalence of 17.7% in this sample [26].

Whether brain malformations, such as agenesis of the corpus callosum or neuronal migration disorders, identified by imaging methods as an additional finding in patients with FAS are always caused by intrauterine alcohol exposure, is still uncertain.

6.2.10 Pain sensation

Children with FAS frequently have a significant reduced sensation of pain and even if they experience severe injuries they rarely cry. Furthermore, often they are hardly able to differentiate between heat and cold, and therefore they sometimes put on summer clothes in winter and winter clothes in summer.

Oberlander et al. (2010) examined behavioural responses to an acute pain event in 14 newborns heavily exposed to alcohol during pregnancy and compared them to 14 newborns of abstainers or light drinkers (< 0.5 oz absolute alcohol/day). Acute stress-related markers (cortisol, heart rate, respiratory sinus arrhythmia, heart rate variability, and videotaped facial actions) were collected in a heel lance blood collection at three time points (baseline, lance stick, and recovery). The newborns were additionally examined using an abbreviated Brazelton Neonatal Behavioral Assessment Scale (NBAS).

They found that the heart rate increased with the heel lance stick and decreased during the post-lance period in both groups, but the alcohol-exposed group had lower mean heart rates compared to the control subjects and showed no change in respiratory arrhythmia over time (see Figs. 6.1 and 6.2). Cortisol levels decreased over time in the exposed newborns, but no alteration over time was found in the control subjects. In both groups, facial action analyses revealed no differences in response to the heel lance stich, but the Brazelton Neonatal Scale showed less arousal in the exposed group.

It could be demonstrated for the first time that the reaction to acute pain stimuli is obviously different and reduced in prenatally alcohol-exposed newborns; a pathophysiological explanation for this reduced pain perception is still unknown [27].

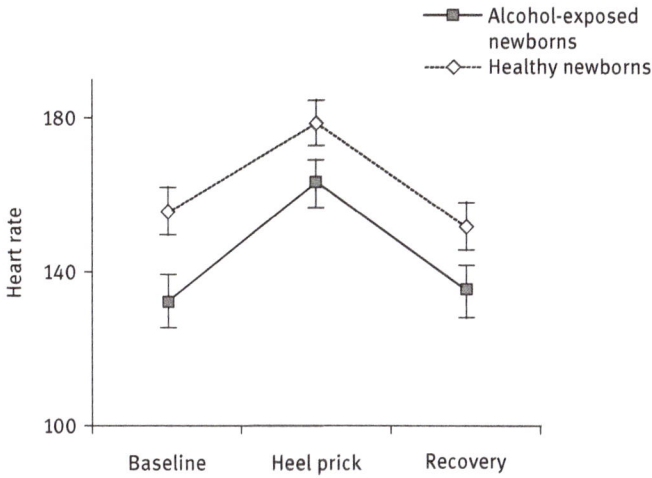

Fig. 6.1: Heart rate [28].

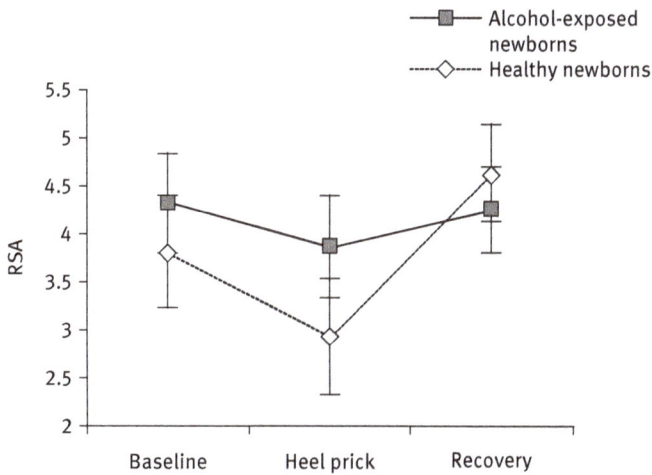

Fig. 6.2: RSA = respiratory sinus rhythm, modified from Oberlander et al. 2010 [27].

6.2.11 Organic malformations

In 2010, as part of a large international study, Jones et al. examined the presence of organic malformations in 245 patients with FASD compared to 342 healthy controls and found many of the minor malformations typically seen in patients with FASD [28], which already had been described years before.

In this study, children with FAS suffered significantly ($p < .001$) more often from:
–   "railroad track" ears (Fig. 6.3)
–   ptosis (Fig. 6.4)

- heart murmurs
- radioulnar synostosis (Fig. 6.6)
- abnormalities in palmar hand lines ("hockey stick crease"), (Fig. 6.7)
- clinodactyly (Fig. 6.5)

In 2010, Australian authors investigated [29] whether the variety of congenital malformations (birth defects) previously described in the classification of ARBD by the Institute of Medicine (IOM) in 1996 is still valid today. This IOM classification comes from a time when malformations were part of the syndrome in high-risk populations.

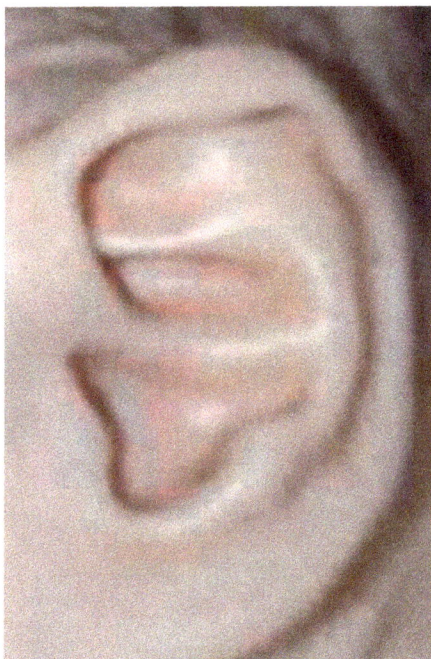

Fig. 6.3: "Railroad track" ears [46]; with approval of the National Human Genome Research Institute.

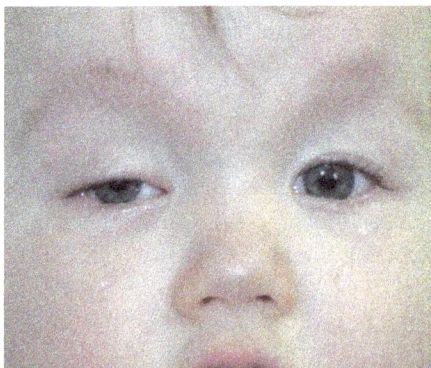

Fig. 6.4: Ptosis.

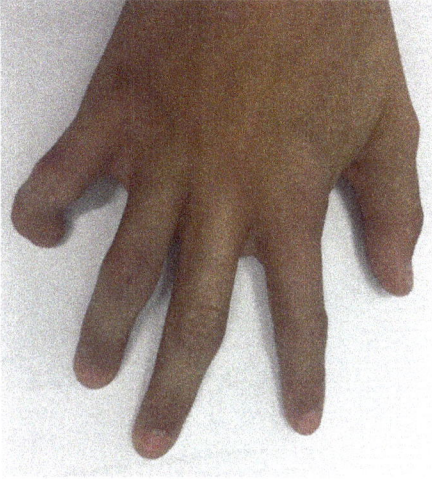
Fig. 6.5: Clinodactyly.

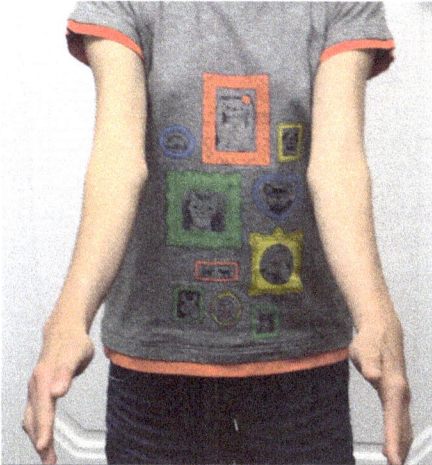
Fig. 6.6: Radio-ulnar synostosis.

Many affected children nowadays do not present with typical facial dysmorphic features, and birth defects potentially associated with FASD cannot be clearly identified, because FAS is usually not diagnosed at birth.

The association between birth defects and prenatal alcohol consumption was examined in an Australian study of children of 4714 women. Despite the fact that many women had reported alcohol consumption during pregnancy, the prevalence for ARBD as defined by IOM was only 2.3%. The authors concluded that ARBD might not occur after prenatal exposure to only moderate amounts of alcohol. Only in the small group of women with high alcohol consumption during pregnancy (i.e. > 140 g alcohol per week), was there a fourfold risk for the presence of birth defects in their offspring compared to abstinent controls. Birth defects in this study were almost lim-

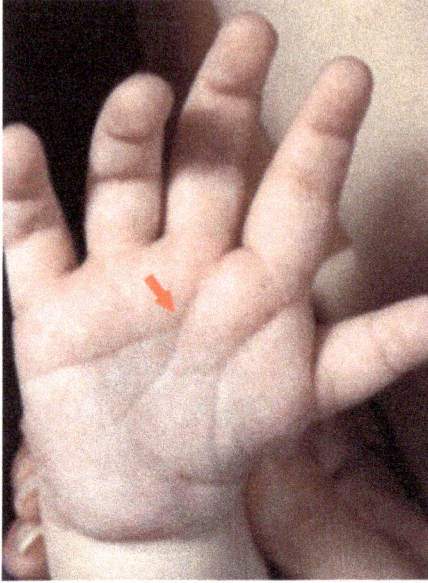

Fig. 6.7: Palm lines and clinodactyly.

ited to congenital heart defects such as ventricular septal defects (VSD) and atrial septal defects (ASD) [29].

In summary: Additional comorbid malformations in FAS have lost significance in the routine diagnostic procedure, particularly in patients without craniofacial dysmorphic features. However, it remains important to check for frequently occurring malformations whilst diagnosing fetal alcohol syndrome, especially for abnormalities of the heart, eyes, ears and teeth, because usually they are not evaluated in the present diagnostic guidelines.

6.3 Differential diagnoses

There are only a few disorders that are actually similar to FAS. Although some are mentioned constantly, they are diagnosed quite rarely.

Nevertheless, every child with an uncertain diagnosis of FAS should be examined by a medical geneticist and undergo extensive genetic testing, including array-CGH (comparative genomic hybridisation) in order to rule out newly detected rare genetic disorders.

For the following selection of potential differential diagnoses for FAS, we decided to show no pictures of the disorders, because there is a high variety and heterogeneity in the expression of the different disorders. Only characteristic symptoms that are different from FAS are listed below.

Aarskog syndrome
- short fingers caused by hypoplasia of the distal phalanges
- males: shawl scrotum, in which the scrotum surrounds the penis

Cornelia de Lange syndrome
- characteristic facial features with long, thick, bushy eyebrows meeting in the middle of the nose (synophrys)
- severe psychomotor developmental delay
- deep, coarse voice
- hypertrichosis

Dubowitz syndrome
- sparse, hypoplastic lateral eyebrows
- epicanthal folds
- thin hair
- external ear dysplasia
- eczema

Fetal hydantoin syndrome
- hypoplasia of distal phalanges
- hypoplastic nails
- hypertelorism

Fetal Valproate syndrome
- high, broad forehead
- medial eyebrow deficiency
- spina bifida (2% of cases)
- increased risk of club foot.

Noonan syndrome
- excess skin on the neck
- often, valvular pulmonary stenosis
- drooping face that appears to lack expression
- freckles, "café au lait" spots

Williams syndrome
- full cheeks, wide mouth
- full, sometimes hanging lips
- dental abnormalities, enamel hypoplasia
- coarse voice
- cardiovascular problems and kidney defects

6.4 Psychiatric disorders

In a follow-up study from early childhood to school age of children with FAS, Steinhausen et al. (1993) described a high rate of persistent psychiatric and cognitive impairments, mainly hyperkinetic disorder, abnormal habits and stereotypic behaviour and affective disorders predominantly in school aged children [30]. Of a sample of 23 children with prenatal alcohol exposure (6 with FAS/pFAS and 17 with ARND), 87% had additional psychiatric disorders as described by O'Conor et al. in 2012; these are listed in Table 6.3 [31].

Tab. 6.3: Psychiatric disorders in patients with FASD.

Psychiatric disorder	Relative frequency in patients
Moderate depressive episode	13%
Adjustment disorder with depressed mood	13%
Bipolar disorder	35%
ADHD	13%
Reactive attachment disorder	9%
Pervasive developmental disorders	4%
Anxiety disorders	none
Psychotic disorders	none

Despite the relatively small sample sizes there were no significant differences between the groups of comorbid psychiatric disorders.

Interestingly, only 26% of patients presented with disorders typically associated with childhood, i.e. reactive attachment disorders, pervasive developmental disorders and ADHD. To the contrary, 61% of patients suffered from affective disorders, particularly bipolar disorder (35%) and depression (26%).

These findings emphasise the unexpectedly high number of psychiatric disorders seen in fetal alcohol spectrum disorders. Only an early diagnosis and immediate specialised care may alleviate later academic failure, problems in vocational training and the inability to live independently. [31].

In contrast to this publication, at our centre we have not seen patients with bipolar disorder in the last couple of years but rather numerous patients with comorbid conduct disorder, often combined with ADHD and emotional disorders, as was already mentioned by Steinhausen et al. in 1993. [30]. Conduct disorder is not mentioned in the study by O'Connor [31].

The authors explained the high incidence of psychiatric disorders in their sample by the fact that these data originated from a specialised FASD clinic – with in and outpatients – which could have potentially increased the chance of psychiatric disorders.

In a literature review from 2009, Paley and O'Connor again referred to a high incidence of psychiatric abnormalities and disorders associated with prenatal alcohol exposure. These psychiatric disorders tend to be long lasting, ongoing from early childhood into adolescence or even into early adulthood [32].

Recently, a systematic review of published literature to estimate prevalence of comorbid mental disorders in FASD and to compare it with general population prevalence estimates, was published by Weyrauch et al. 2017 [48].

The authors compared the prevalence of mental health disorders in the FASD population with rates in the mental health literature. They identified 26 articles reporting more than 5000 cases of FASD. Of 15 comorbid mental disorders, 11 had sufficient data for inclusion in the analysis, which showed significant differences to prevalence estimates of population rates. The most striking result was that ADHD occurred in 50% of persons with FASD, which is 10 times the expected rate. Intellectual disability was the second most frequent comorbid mental disorder, and occurred at 23 times the expected rate.

In five comorbid mental disorders in the FASD population, the rates significantly exceeded the expected rates by 10 to 45%: 1.ADHD, 2. intellectual disability/mental retardation, 3. learning disabilities, 4. oppositional defiant disorder, 5. depression [48].

6.5 FAS and attention deficit and hyperactivity disorder (ADHD)

6.5.1 Introduction

ADHD is the most common behavioural disorder during childhood with significant effects on cognitive, emotional and social development. The disorder persists well into adulthood at a high percentage. Early symptoms are often already present in infancy and become apparent with feeding and sleep problems, as well as excessive crying (so-called "cry-babies") [4]. In nursery school and kindergarten, these children are often outsiders due to their hyperactivity, lack of perseverance, and their inability to play quietly and maintain concentration. The additional impulsivity and difficulties in social interaction raise early problems in daily life.

Concentration deficits and limited impulse control lead to further problems at school age. They subsequently fail in school performance and often are unable to behave appropriately, consequently performing far below their capacity. In adolescence and adulthood hyperactivity mostly decline and difficulties in daily life are focused on inattention and impulsivity. [33].

6.5.2 Prevalence

Nationwide German data collected from May 2003 to May 2006 estimated a prevalence rate for a professionally diagnosed ADHD of 4.8% for children and adolescents. Males were affected significantly more often, 7.9% compared to 1.8% in females. ADHD was diagnosed significantly more often (6.4%) in children from families with a lower social status [33].

According to Peadon and Elliot (2010) the prevalence of ADHD in children in the general population ranges from 5 to 11% [34].

6.5.3 Definition of ADHD

ADHD is defined as a persistent pattern of behaviour, including inattention, hyperactivity and impulsivity. Coexisting symptoms such as unawareness of danger and social rules, defiance of personal limits towards others, low frustration tolerance and emotional problems are often present but not part of the diagnostic criteria (ICD-10, DSM-V).

Clinical symptoms
Inattention. The affected person
(a) does not pay attention to details, makes careless mistakes;
(b) has a short attention span and is easily distracted;
(c) does not like to do things that requires sitting still;
(d) does not appear to be listening;
(e) is unable to carry out instructions;
(f) is unable to stick to tasks that are tedious or time consuming;
(g) often loses things;
(h) is forgetful;
(i) has problems organising daily tasks.

Hyperactivity. The affected person
(a) often squirms, fidgets or bounces when sitting;
(b) is unable to sit still, especially in calm or quiet situations;
(c) is always moving, such as running or climbing;
(d) has trouble playing quietly;
(e) is always "on the go" as if "driven by a motor";
(f) talks excessively.

Impulsivity. The affected person
(a) blurts out answers;
(b) has trouble waiting for his or her turn;
(c) interrupts others.

Studies examining ADHD and FASD

The proportion of children with an ADHD diagnosis who also receive a FAS diagnosis is still unknown and is influenced by underdiagnoses of FAS due to different factors, such as reluctance to ask about alcohol consumption during pregnancy, a lack of knowledge about diagnosing FAS or fear of stigmatisation of the child [34].

Numerous studies have been conducted to examine prevalence and incidence of ADHD, but only a few studies investigated the prevalence or incidence of ADHD as a comorbidity of FAS/FASD [34, 35].

Discriminating between the symptoms of ADHD and FAS is difficult, particularly because many ADHD symptoms (inattention, hyperactivity and impulsivity) are also triggered by prenatal alcohol exposure, and other symptoms, such as mental retardation, executive dysfunction, developmental delay and impairment of social interaction are also present in ADHD. However, children with FAS often present with early onset ADHD, with more severe symptoms and additional striking memory deficits, raising suspicion of intrauterine alcohol exposure as the underlying cause for ADHD.

When diagnosing ADHD, it is always crucial to inquire about possible alcohol consumption in pregnancy

ADHD is the most common psychiatric comorbid disorder in children and adolescents prenatally exposed to alcohol; prevalence reports range from 49% [35] up to 94% [38]. The relationship between ADHD and FAS is still uncertain and overlaps as well as differences are not uniquely defined [34].

In a large explorative study in four states in the USA (Minnesota, North and South-Dakota and Montana), which contain large Native American reservations with high incidences of FASD, Bhatara et al. [35] examined the medical records of 2231 children and adolescents aged 2–14 years (the mean age was 8.7 years) with suspected FASD. The highest number of children included came from South Dakota (73.9%).

With the using of the 4-Digit Diagnostic Code the children were divided into four groups based on the knowledge in their files regarding potential intrauterine alcohol exposure:

- Group 1: no risk
- Group 2: unknown risk
- Group 3: slight risk
- Group 4: high risk

The prevalence of ADHD and other comorbid disorders was also derived from the medical files and divided into four groups.

The ADHD diagnosis was examined following DSM-IV criteria (fourth version of the Diagnostic and Statistical Manual of Mental Disorders by the American Psychiatric Association, 1994 [37]).

In this elaborate study, the authors found ADHD to be present in 41% of the children evaluated, which led to the following distribution:

- Group 1 (no risk for prenatal alcohol exposure): 0.8%
- Group 2 (unknown risk): 15%
- Group 3 (slight risk): 30%
- Group 4 (high risk): 49.5%

This means that half of the children with a high risk of maternal alcohol consumption during pregnancy additionally received a diagnosis of ADHD.

Moreover, other psychiatric problems with a similar distribution were found in each group (Table 6.4).

Tab. 6.4: Psychiatric problems.

	Groups 1–4	Group 4 (high risk)
Learning disabilities	17%	46%
Oppositional behaviour	10%	41%
Sleep disorders (> 3 years of age)	10%	52%
Mental retardation	7.5%	55%

In an Italian field study Kodituwakko et al. described the characteristics of different behavioural disorders seen in school-aged patients with FAS in rural Italy. The authors found attention deficit disorder (ADD) (i.e. attention deficit disorder without hyperactivity) to be the most common behavioural comorbid disorder (55% of children with FAS compared to 2% of healthy children). Attention deficit disorder with hyperactivity was the next most common [38].

There are different theories and hypotheses surrounding the relationship between ADHD and FASD [39–42].

In an extensive literature review examining potential similarities between FAS and ADHD, O'Malley and Nanson [43] proposed five different hypotheses:

1. The prevalence of ADHD in children is high, namely around 3–11% aside from its aetiology, and as such it is a coincidence when both disorders occur in the same person, i.e. there is no relationship between ADHD and FASD.
2. Adults with ADHD tend to consume more alcohol than those without an ADHD diagnosis. Hence, women with ADHD might give birth to children with FASD more often and pass on the genetics for ADHD.
3. There is a common pathogenesis for both disorders in a developing fetus: FASD with ADHD symptomatology and ADHD without FASD. This could be due to a dysregulation of the dopaminergic neurotransmitter system.
4. ADHD is a disorder caused by prenatal alcohol exposure and develops due to the direct teratogenic effects of alcohol on the developing neurotransmitter system.
5. The form of ADHD associated with FASD is a special clinical subtype of ADHD in general.

Unfortunately, there are no plausible arguments given in the discussion of these hypotheses, i.e. they are neither confirmed nor denied.

Mattson and colleagues compared the neuropsychological and behavioural profiles of FASD and ADHD in a literature review in 2011 [44]. For this comparison, the research by Mirski et al. [45] was used to examine both disorders, which developed a four-factor model for attention: focused attention, sustained attention, encoding and shifting attention.

Mattson et al. [44] summarised the similarities and differences between ADHD and FASD graphically (Fig. 6.8).

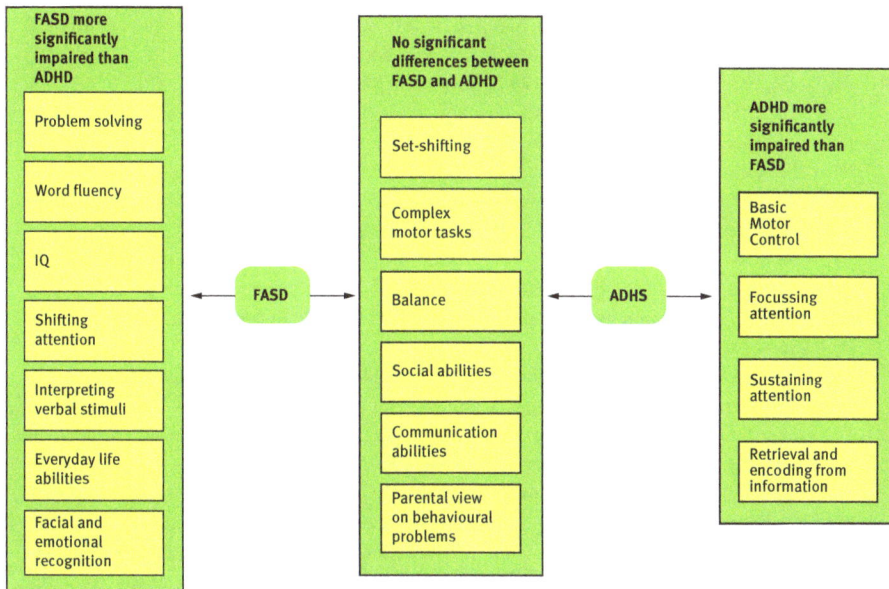

FASD more significantly impaired than ADHD
- Problem solving
- Word fluency
- IQ
- Shifting attention
- Interpreting verbal stimuli
- Everyday life abilities
- Facial and emotional recognition

FASD →

No significant differences between FASD and ADHD
- Set-shifting
- Complex motor tasks
- Balance
- Social abilities
- Communication abilities
- Parental view on behavioural problems

← ADHS →

ADHD more significantly impaired than FASD
- Basic Motor Control
- Focussing attention
- Sustaining attention
- Retrieval and encoding from information

Fig. 6.8: Depiction of the similarities and differences between FASD and ADHD (modified from [44]).

In summary, several studies consistently showed the following two differences in attention problems between ADHD and FASD:
1. Children with ADHD have significantly more problems in focusing and sustaining their attention.
2. Children with FASD, on the other hand, have more significant difficulties to shift attention, to understand information and to solve problems.

Psychopharmacological treatment of FASD is described in Chapter 16.

Bibliography

[1]   Carskadon MM, Acebo C, Jenni OG. Regulation of adolescent sleep: implication for behaviour. Ann N Y Acad Sci 2004, 1021, 276–291.

[2]   Fricke L, Mitschke A, Wiater A, Lemkuhl G. Kölner Behandlungsprogramm für Kinder mit Schlafstörungen. Prax Kinderpsychol Kinderpsychiat 2006, 55, 146–150.

[3]   Lehmkuhl G, Döpfner M, Plück J et al. Häufigkeit psychischer Auffälligkeiten und somatischer Beschwerden bei vier bis zehnjährigen Kindern in Deutschland im Urteil ihrer Eltern – ein Vergleich normorientierter und kriterienorientierter Modelle. Zeitschrift für Kinder – und Jugendpsychiatrie und Psychotherapie 1998, 26, 83–96.

[4]   Papousek M. Störungen des Säuglingsalters. In: Esser G (ed). Lehrbuch der Klinischen Psychologie des Kindes- und Jugendalters. Thieme Verlag, Stuttgart, New York 2002, 80–101.

[5]   Anders T, Goodlin-Jones B, Sadeh H. Sleep disorders. In: Zeanah C (ed). Handbook of Infant Mental Health, 2nd edn. Guilford Press, New York, London 2000, 326–338.

[6]   Fegert JM, Schulz J, Bergmann R, Tacke U, Bergmann KE, Wahn U. Schlaf-Verhalten in den ersten 3 Lebensjahren. Praxis der Kinderpsychologie und Kinderpsychiatrie 1997, 46, 69–91.

[7]   Jenkins S, Owen C, Bax M, Hart H. Continuities of common problems in preschool children. Journal of Child Psychology and Psychiatry 1980, 25, 75–89.

[8]   Stone KC, La Gasse LL, Lester BM, Shankaran S et al. Sleep Problems in Children with Prenatal Substance Exposure. The Maternal Lifestyle Study. Arch Pediatr AdolescMed 2010, 164(5), 452–456.

[9]   Jan JE, Wasdell MB, Reiter J et al. Melatonin therapy of pediatric sleep disorders: recent Advances, why it works, who are the candidates and how to treat. Current Pediatric Reviews 2007, 3(3), 214–224.

[10] Stade BC,Barozzino T, Bennett D, et al. The Nature of Sleep in Canadian Children with Fetal Alcohol Spectrum Disorder. Paediatrics & Child Health 2010, 15, 51A.

[11] Chen ML, Olson HC, Picciano JF, Starr JR, Owens J. Sleep problems in children with fetal alcohol spectrum disorders. J Clin Sleep Med 2012, 8 (4), 421–429.

[12] Little BB, Snell LM, Rosenfeld CR, Gilstrap LC, Grant NF. Failure to recognize fetal alcohol syndrome in newborn infants. American Journal of Diseases of Children 1990, 144(10), 1142–46.

[13] Ipsiroglu OS, McKellin WH, Carey N, Look C. "They silently live in terror". Why sleep problems and night-time related quality-of-life are missed in children with a fetal alcohol spectrum disorder. Social Science & Medicine 2012, doi: 10.1016/socscimed.2012.

[14] Jan JE, Asante KO, Conry JL, Fast DK, Bax MC, Ipsiruglu OS, Bredberg E, Look CA, Wasdell MB. Sleep Health Issues for Children with FASD: Clinical Considerations. Review Article. International Journal of Pediatrics 2010, article ID 639048.

[15] Phillips L, Appleton RE. Systematic review of melatonin treatment in children with neurodevelopmental disabilities and sleep impairment. Dev Med Child Neurol 2004, 46(11), 771–775.

[16] Autti-Rämö I, Fagerlund A, Ervalathi N, Loimu L, Korkman M, Hoyme E. Fetal Alcohol Spectrum Disorder in Finland: Clinical Delineation of 77 Older Children and Adolescents. American Journal of Medical Genetics 2006, 140(2), 137–143.

[17] Löser H, Majewski F. Type and frequency of cardiac defects in embryofetal alcohol syndrome: Report of 16 cases. British Heart Jornal 1977, 39, 1374–79.

[18] Smith DF, Sander GG, Macleod PM, Tredwell S, Wood B, Newman DE. Intrinsic defects in the fetal alcohol syndrome: Studies on 76 cases from British Columbia and the Yukon Territory. Neurobehavioral Toxicology and Teratology 1981, 3, 145–152.

[19] Burd L, Deal E, Rios R et al. Congenital Heart Defects and Alcohol Spectrum Disorders. Congenital Heart Dis. 2007, 2, 250–255.

[20] Strömland K, Miller M, Cook C. Ocular teratology. Survey of Ophthalmology 1991, 35(6), 429–46.

[21] Strömland K. Ocular abnormalities in the featal alcohol Syndrome. Acta Ophthalmol 1985, 63(Suppl), 171–174.

[22] Strömland K, Pinazo-Durán MD. Optic Nerve Hypoplasia: Comparative Effects in Children and Rats Exposed to Alcohol During Pregnancy. Teratology 1994, 50, 100–111.

[23] Strömland K. Contribution of ocular examination to the diagnosis of foetal alcohol syndrome in mentally retarded children. Journal of Mental Deficiency Research 1990, 34, 429–435.

[24] Church MW, Kaltenbach JA. Hearing, speech, language, and vestibular disorders in the fetal alcohol syndrome: a literature review. Alcohol Clin Exp Res 1997, 2(3), 495–512.

[25] Stephen JM, Kodituwakku EL, Romero L, Peters AM et al. Delays in Auditory Processing Identified in Preschool Children. Alcohol Clin Exp Res 2012. doi: 10111/j.1530-0277.2012.01769.x.

[26] Bell HS, Stade B, Reynolds JN, Rasmussen C, Andrew G, Hwang PO, Carlen PL. The remarkably high prevalence of epilepsy and seizure history in fetal alcohol spectrum disorders. Alcohol Clin Exp Res 2010, 34(6), 1084–1089.

[27] Oberlander T, Jacobson S, Weinberg J et al. Prenatal Alcohol Exposure Alters Behavioral Reactivity to Pain in Newborns. Alcoholism:Clinical and Experimental Research 2010, 34(4), 681–692.

[28] Jones KL, Hoyme HE, Robinson LK, del Campo M et al. Fetal Alcohol Spectrum Disorders: Extending the Range of Structural Defects. Am J Med Genet Part A 2010, 152A, 2731–2735.

[29] O'Leary CM, Nassar N, Kurinczuk JJ et al. Prenatal Alcohol Exposure and Risk of Birth Defects. Pediatrics 2010, 126(4), 843–85.

[30] Steinhausen HC, Willms J, Spohr HL. Long-term psychopathological and cognitive outcome of children with fetal alcohol syndrome. Journal of the American Academy of Child and Adolescent Psychiatry 1993, 32(5), 990–994.

[31] O'Connor MJ, Shah B, Whaley S, Cronin P, Gunderson B, Graham J. Psychiatric illness in a clinical sample of children with prenatal Alcohol Exposure. The American Journal of Drug and Alcohol abuse 2002, 28(4), 743–754.

[32] O'Conner MJ, Paley B. Psychiatric Conditions associated with Prenatal Alcohol Exposure. Developmental Disabilities Research Reviews 2009, 15, 225–234.

[33] Schlack R, Hölling H, Kurth BM, Huss M. Die Prävalenz der Aufmerksamkeitsdefizit-/Hyperaktivitätsstörung (ADHS) bei Kindern und Jugendlichen in Deutschland. Bundesgesundheitsblatt Gesundheitsforsch-Gesundheitsschutz 2007, 50, 827–835.

[34] Peadon E, Elliott E. Distinguishing between attention-deficit hyperactivity and fetal alcohol spectrum disorders in children: clinical guidelines. Neuropsychiatric Disease and Treatment 2010, 6, 509–515.

[35] Bhatara V, Loudenberg R, Ellis R. Association of Attention Deficit Hyperactivity Disorder and Gestational Acohol Exposure: An Exploratory Study. Journal of Attention Disorders 2006, 9, 505–522.

[36] Fryer SL, McGee CL, Matt GE, Riley EP, Mattson SN. Evaluation of psychopathological conditions in children with heavy prenatal Alcohol exposure. Pediatrics 2007, 119, e733–e741.

[37] http://dsm.psychiatryonline.org.

[38] Kodituwakku P, Coriale G, Fiorentino D, Aragón AS et al. Neurobehavioral Characteristics of Children with Fetal Alcohol Spectrum Disorders in Communities from Italy: Preliminary Results. Alcohol Clin Exp Res 2006, 30(9), 1551–1561.

[39] Oesterheld RJ, Wilson A. ADHD and FAS (Letter). J Am Acad Child Adolesc Psychiatry 1997, 36, 1163.

[40] Stevenson J. Evidence for a genetic etiology in hyperactivity in children. Behav Genet 1992, 22, 337–343.

[41] Coles CD, Platzman KA, Rashkind-Hood CL, Brown RT, Falek A, Smith IE. A comparison of children affected by prenatal alcohol exposure and attention deficit hyperactivity disorder. Alcohol Clin Exp Res 1997, 1, 150–161.

[42] O'Malley KD, Hagerman RJ. Developing clinical practice guidelines for pharmacological interventions with alcohol-affected children. In: Centers for Disease Control and Prevention, editors. Intervening with children affected by prenatal alcohol exposure: proceedings of a special focus sessions of the interagency coordinating committee on fetal alcohol syndrome. National Institute on Alcohol Abuse and Alcoholism, Bethesda, MD 1998, 145–177.

[43] O'Malley KD, Nanson J. Clinical Implication of a Link between Fetal Alcohol Syndrome and Attention-Deficit Hyperactivity Disorder. Can J Psychiatry 2002, 47(4), 349–354.

[44] Mattson SN, Crocker N, Nguyen TT. Fetal Alcohol Spectrum Disorders: Neuropsychological and Behavioural Features. Neuropsychol Rev 2011, 21, 81–101.

[45] Mirski AF, Anthony BJ, Duncan CC, Ahearn MB, Kellam SG. Analysis of the elements of attention: a neuropsychological approach. Neuropsychology Review 1991, 2(2), 109–145.

[46] http://elementsofmorphology.nih.gov/images/terms/Helix,Crus,Horizontal-large.jpg.

[47] Goril S, Zalai D, Scott L, Shapiro CM. Sleep and melatonin secretion abnormalities in children and adolescents with fetal alcohol spectrum disorders. Sleep Med. 2016, 23, 59–64.

[48] Weyrauch D. Schwartz M, Hart B, Klug G. Burd L. Comorbid mental disorders in fetal alcohol spectrum disorders: A systematic review. J Dev Behav Pediatr 2017, 38, 283–291.

Part II: **Scientific basis of the fetal alcohol syndrome**

7 Epidemiology

7.1 Alcohol consumption in industrialised countries

According to the WHO global status report (2014) [29] the worldwide per capita consumption of alcohol was equal to 6.2l of pure alcohol by persons aged 15 years or older. The highest consumption levels were found in developed countries, in particular in European countries.

Table 7.1 (published by the WHO, 2013) presents data of some comparable WHO countries:

1. The per capita consumption of alcohol from 2003–2008 compared to 2008–2010.
2. Prevalence of heavy episodic drinking (%) in 2010 defined as consumption of at least 60 g or more of pure alcohol on at least one occasion in the past 30 days.
3. Percentage of chronic female alcoholics in 2010 compared to males (in brackets).

Tab. 7.1: WHO – Global status report on alcohol and health 2014.

Country	Alcohol/ capita 2003–2008	Alcohol/ capita 2008–2010	Heavy episodic drinking female % (male %)	Alcohol dependent female % (male %)
Australia	10.1 l	12.2 l	5.1 (6.3)	0.8 (2.2)
Canada	9.8 l	10.2 l	10.9 (25.0)	2.3 (6.0)
England	13.2 l	11.6 l	20.9 (35.5)	3.2 (8.7)
France	13.4 l	12.2 l	17.7 (42.2)	1.3 (4.7)
Germany	12.8 l	11.8 l	5.9 (19.4)	1.1 (4.7)
India	3.6 l	4.3 l	<0.1 (3.2)	0.4 (3.8)
Israel	2.8 l	2.8 l	3.2 (12.7)	1.3 (5.4)
Italy	10.5 l	6.7 l	0.7 (8.0)	0.4 (0.7)
Japan	8.0 l	7.2 l	7.5 (28.1)	0.2 (2.1)
The Netherlands	10.1 l	9.9 l	1.3 (10.5)	0.4 (0.9)
Poland	13.0 l	12.5 l	0.9 (10.1)	1.4 (7.7)
Russia	16.1 l	15.1 l	10.3 (29.8)	3.3 (16.5)
Sweden	10.3 l	9.2 l	15.5 (23.2)	2.8 (6.7)
Switzerland	11.1 l	10.7 l	12.0 (25.8)	1.4 (7.2)
USA	9.5 l	9.2 l	10.9 (23.2)	2.6 (6.9)

Interestingly, the rates of heavy episodic drinking, a well-known risk factor for alcohol consumption during pregnancy, when compared to alcohol dependency are significantly higher, with the highest discrepancy in English females (heavy episodic drinking 20.9% and dependency in females 3.2%) [29].

https://doi.org/10.1515/9783110436563-007

Drinking patterns of women in the last 20 years

The German Nutrition Society defines moderate alcohol consumption for healthy women as a maximum of 10 g pure alcohol per day (20 g for men). At-risk alcohol consumption is defined as more than 10 g/day (21–40 g/day for men) and excessive alcohol consumption is defined as 41–80 g/day; hazardous and harmful alcohol consumption is specified as more than 80 g/day [28].

Drinking behaviour has changed over time. Older women of lower socioeconomic strata and those with unfortunate living conditions have now been partially replaced by younger women who consume high amounts of alcohol within their peer-groups; Saturday night drinking and binge drinking are quite popular today. Presently, female drinking patterns are more similar to male drinking patterns. Some stated causes are better career opportunities and greater financial independence for women. Also, women working outside the home nevertheless more frequently handle a disproportionate share of family issues with greater access to acceptance of drinking alcoholic beverages.

Living in a stable relationship, working in a responsible position and being well integrated in a social environment is likely to protect against alcohol abuse, whereas moderate drinking or at-risk drinking occurs more often in single women or mothers without a supportive social network [2].

Although females are more often lifetime abstainers compared to males, there is an increase of alcohol consumption, including heavy episodic drinking, particularly in young women [1].

A British study examining drinking patterns of English women reported a significant increase in alcohol consumption in young women and girls between the ages of 16 and 24 over a 5-year period from 1998 to 2003 (Fig. 7.1), and studies from the USA and England reported a significant increase of pregnancies and birth rates in teenagers [3] (Fig. 7.2).

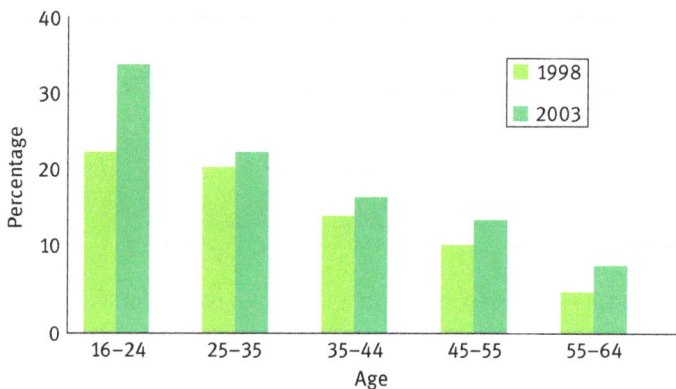

Fig. 7.1: Alcohol consumption (in percentages) of young women in the UK from 1998 to 2003 (with kind permission from R.A. Mukherjee).

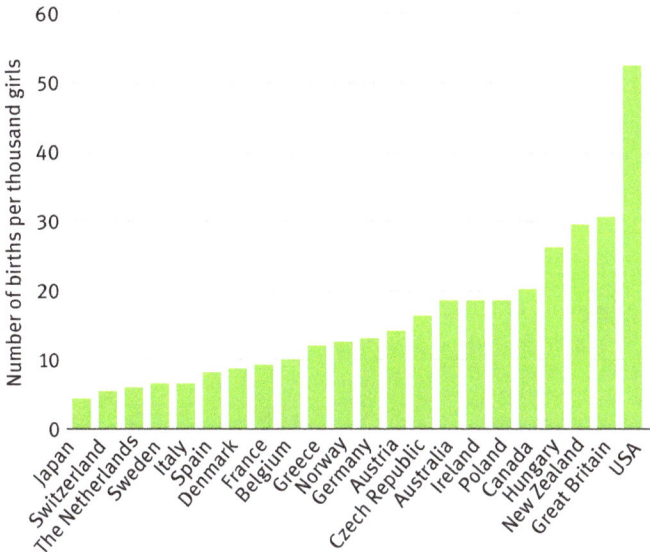

Fig. 7.2: Birth rates of teenage-pregnancies aged 15 to 19 years in 1998 [3].

These facts may predict a higher probability that teenagers addicted to alcohol or teenagers who are heavy episodic drinkers give birth to a child with FAS.

To define the prevalence and predictors of alcohol consumption and drinking behaviour before and during pregnancy, Ethen et al. (2009) collected data by carrying out telephone interviews of 4088 randomly selected women.

About 30% of women reported alcohol consumption at some time during pregnancy, and of these, 8% reported binge drinking. The data showed that 22.5% reported drinking during the first month of pregnancy, 2.7% of women acknowledged alcohol consumption during the entire pregnancy and 7.9% reported drinking only in the last trimester.

Additionally, the authors stated that binge drinking before pregnancy was a particular risk factor for continuous alcohol consumption as well as binge drinking during pregnancy. Other characteristics associated with drinking during pregnancy were smoking and unintended pregnancy [30].

According to a Canadian epidemiological study (2011) of 5882 women, 10% consumed alcohol at some time during pregnancy. Of those, 95% had taken less than one drink a day and only 1.7% of women reported high levels of alcohol consumption during pregnancy with at least one drink per day.

In this study, living with a partner, as well as nicotine consumption, was associated with the probability of alcohol consumption during pregnancy. Furthermore, another significant risk factor was being unhappy or indifferent towards the pregnancy;

these women had a 2.5-fold higher risk for alcohol use during pregnancy. In contrast, immigrants who had moved to Canada clearly drank less [4].

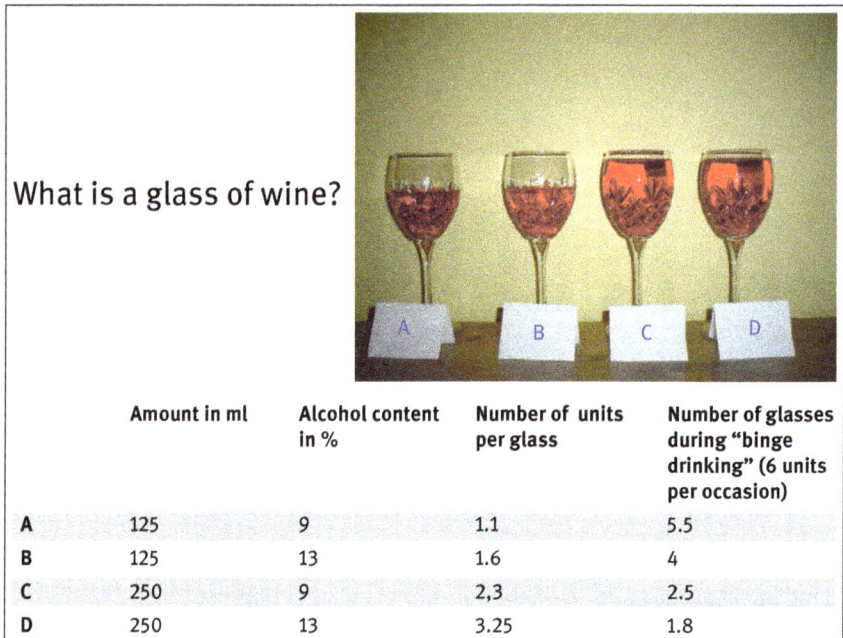

	Amount in ml	Alcohol content in %	Number of units per glass	Number of glasses during "binge drinking" (6 units per occasion)
A	125	9	1.1	5.5
B	125	13	1.6	4
C	250	9	2,3	2.5
D	250	13	3.25	1.8

Fig. 7.3: "What is a glass of wine?" (reprinted with kind permission of R.A. Mukherjee).

To estimate the proportion of women consuming alcohol during pregnancy in Europe, and to analyse whether country variations could be explained by sociodemography and smoking, Marby et al. (2017) conducted an anonymous online questionnaire for pregnant women and new mothers in 11 European countries for 2 months between October 2011 and February 2012 in each country.

The study population consisted of 7905 women, 53.1% pregnant and 46.9% new mothers. On average, 15.8% reported alcohol consumption during pregnancy. The highest proportion of alcohol consumption during pregnancy was found in the UK (28.5%), Russia (26.5%) and Switzerland (20.9%) and the lowest in Norway (4.1%), Sweden (7.2%) and Poland (9.7%).

As the authors stated, almost 16% of women resident in Europe consumed alcohol during pregnancy with large cross-country variations. Education and smoking prior to pregnancy could not fully explain the differences between the European countries. They urged a united European strategy to prevent alcohol consumption during pregnancy, focusing on the countries with the highest consumption [32].

7.2 Light and moderate drinking in pregnancy

One of the most frequently questions asked is: "How much alcohol am I allowed to drink during my pregnancy without potentially damaging my child?"

In the United States, a large population study (Center for Disease Control and Prevention surveillance system) from 2011 to 2013 that examined drinking behaviour in pregnant women aged 18 to 44, reported consumption of any alcohol in 10.2% and binge drinking in 3.1%.

The highest prevalence of alcohol use while pregnant was in women aged 35–44 years (18.6%) followed by black (non-Hispanic) women (13.9%), and women with a college degree (13.0%) and employment (12.0%).

The significant demographic factor for binge drinking during pregnancy in this survey was single marital status. In this group of non-married pregnant women, the prevalence of binge drinking was 4.6 times higher than among married pregnant women [5].

Data from the Avon Longitudinal Study of Parents and Children, a large population-based study reported in 2009, were used to investigate the relationship between binge drinking (consumption of four or more drinks/day) in the second and third trimester of pregnancy and mental health problems in offspring at the ages of 47 and 81 months.

In summary, the results confirmed that any episodes of consuming four or more drinks per day occasionally were independently associated with higher risks for mental health problems (especially hyperactivity/inattention), even in the absence of moderate daily levels of drinking [6].

The same authors re-examined these children at the age of 11 years in 2014 and still found that children who had been exposed to binge drinking as a fetus had a persistently higher risk of hyperactivity and concentration disorders [26].

Animal experiments demonstrated that animals exposed to sudden peaks in blood alcohol levels developed numerous neurotransmitter and neuromodulator impairments, showed clear behavioural problems and deficits in learning, memory and motor coordination [7].

What is moderate drinking?

Over the past 30 years, the opinion about moderate alcohol consumption during pregnancy has changed. Previously it was assumed that only children with intrauterine exposure of constant and high amounts of alcohol during all trimesters of pregnancy would suffer from FAS. Later it was recognised that even occasional alcohol consumption, and particularly moderate alcohol consumption and social drinking, may lead to behavioural abnormalities and developmental disorders in exposed children.

A precise definition of moderate alcohol consumption is difficult. The general recommendation in the USA is that healthy women should not drink more than 10–40 g of pure alcohol per day and one drink per day is considered to be moderate drinking for non-pregnant women [10].

The threshold for teratogenic alcohol effects depends on the total amount of alcohol per day or occasion, on the frequency and timing of alcohol intrauterine exposure, and is highly influenced by the maternal and fetal capacity of alcohol metabolism. In a study evaluating the elimination kinetics of alcohol in pregnant women published in 2004, the authors found that the alcohol elimination rate was higher in women at the beginning of the second trimester compared to non-pregnant women and that the fetal exposure period was extended due to an accumulation of alcohol in the amniotic fluid [8].

Definition of one "drink"

To define a "standard drink" is difficult because the amount of alcohol per drink differs from country to country.

Furtwaengler et al. (2012) [9] investigated the international consensus within guidelines for definition of standard drinks and consumption. Comparing all different guidelines, the authors found a remarkable lack of consensus about what is harmful or excessive alcohol consumption on a daily or weekly basis. Common daily or weekly maximum intake was expressed as a number of "standard drinks" or "units of alcohol". Out of 57 countries whose websites were searched 27 were found to have official low-risk drinking guidelines, but only 10 countries specified alcohol consumption. The recommended maximum intake of alcohol per day was highly variable, i.e. 42 g/d (USA), 12 g/d (Germany) and 10 g/d (Hong Kong and Finland). Out of 27 European Union Member States 8 provide no guidelines for low-risk drinking. Furthermore, the convertibility from units of alcohol into grams of alcohol also differed widely [16], i.e. 1 unit = 14 g (USA), 10 g (Australia), 18 g (United Kingdom) and 12 g (Germany).

'Is moderate drinking during pregnancy harmful to the fetus?'

A systematic literature review reported in 2007 [11] did not identify any consistent evidence for adverse effects of alcohol exposure at low to moderate amounts (i.e. up to 10 drinks/week corresponding to 83 g alcohol/week) during pregnancy. However, many of the studies had methodological weaknesses and, therefore, it cannot be concluded that drinking at these levels during pregnancy is safe.

In the UK Millennium Cohort Study (n = 11,513) Kelly et al. [12, 13] collected data from children examined at ages 3 and 5, whose mothers consumed 1–2 drinks per week or per occasion during pregnancy. These criteria were fulfilled in 29% of pregnant women. Neither clinically relevant behavioural problems nor cognitive deficits were found in this sample compared to unexposed controls.

Of note is a publication from Denmark in 2012 of 1628 women and their children [14] who had been exposed to a moderate amount of alcohol (i.e. 1–8 drinks per week) and who didn't present any reduction in intelligence, attention deficit or impairment of executive functions at the follow-up at age 5. The authors concluded that small quantities of alcohol might not present serious concern to unborn children. This publication was criticised not only from those affected from FAS but also from renowned researchers [15, 16].

Dr. Susan Astley's major point of criticism was the fact that children at 5 years of age were too young to observe the full extent of possible central nervous system damage because the child's brain is not fully developed and mature for complex tasks. According to Astley, 30 years of FAS research has shown that damaging effects of alcohol on the developing brain are most evident when solving complex tasks, and the extent of alcohol damage, particularly due to moderate drinking, only becomes fully apparent in adolescence. More than 2600 children with FASD examined at the Fetal Alcohol and Drug Unit at the University of Washington in recent years by Astley and colleagues still showed almost normal development at age 5, but at age 10 these children had developed severe brain dysfunctions. Attention deficit disorder, for example, were only present in 10% of children at age 5, whereas 60% were affected at the age of 10. Although only 30% of children with FAS had a low IQ, all children examined showed severe impairments in language, memory and motor activity [17].

Parker and Brennan [16] also criticised the early follow-up, because deficits in social behaviour due to low or moderate drinking often are not evident before adolescence.

'Moderate drinking during pregnancy is harmful to the fetus!'

In the recent literature, there are conflicting findings regarding the dangers of moderate drinking during pregnancy. Clinical studies have revealed discrete but lasting psychomotor deficits and behavioural abnormalities after prenatal exposure to low amounts of alcohol. In a longitudinal study with inner city African American children in Michigan, whose mothers drank approximately one alcoholic drink per week during pregnancy, Sood et al. (2001) found, a 3.2-fold risk for aggressive and delinquent behaviour at age 6–7 years compared to unexposed children [19].

In a more recent report from 2012, Bay et al. [20] demonstrated an increased risk of psychomotor deficits as a consequence of low to moderate alcohol consumption during pregnancy.

Besides clinical-epidemiological studies examining the risk for fetal damage by low amounts of alcohol during pregnancy, animal studies with different animal models present a clear picture as well. In several articles, it was shown that after prenatal alcohol exposure to low amounts of alcohol animals had long-lasting behavioural problems, their neurotransmitter systems were damaged and disturbances in neuromodulation and synaptic plasticity were present in several regions of the brain [7, 21, 22].

International recommendations for drinking alcohol during pregnancy

In 2001, the National Health and Medical Research Council (NHMRC) Australian drinking guidelines changed the policy concerning alcohol consumption during pregnancy from abstinence to the recommendation that a woman choosing to drink "over a week, should have less than 7 standard drinks, and, on any day no more than 2 standard drinks". According to this recommendation, drinking in excess of these levels increases the risk for fetal damage. The rationale of the health authorities for modifying the recommendations was based on knowledge that many women in Australia did not comply with the previous, stricter guidelines. However, this new guideline, based on a literature review [31] was not universally accepted across Australian institutes and organisations, and in 2009 the policy was revised, advising that pregnant women should avoid all alcohol consumption.

In 2012, after re-analysing studies of the prior 10 years, 'Leary et al. [23] noted an increased risk of developmental neurological disorders and pre-term birth after alcohol consumption of only 30–40 g per occasion or consumption of not more than 70 g of alcohol once to twice weekly (i.e. two glasses of wine or one large glass of beer). The authors concluded that a lack of evidence of fetal effects due to low amounts of alcohol during pregnancy should not be the deciding factor for recommendations. Furthermore, they raised the question of whether the lack of evidence of fetal effects from low amounts of alcohol should be the deciding factor for recommendations or whether the evidence indicating a relatively low threshold is more important. They concluded that "the safest choice for pregnant women is to abstain from alcohol during pregnancy".

In an editorial in the British Journal of Medicine in 2005, Mukherjee et al. [24] also noted that, in contrast to the recommendation given by the British Ministry of Health stating that 1 to 2 drinks per week during pregnancy was safe, scientific findings demonstrated that there is no safe threshold for alcohol consumption during pregnancy. They concluded that the only safe recommendation for alcohol consumption during pregnancy is complete alcohol abstinence.

In the words of Mukherjee and co-authors [24]:

"Abstinence from alcohol is the only safe message in pregnancy".

The findings of various, more recently published studies support this statement.

The critical threshold for children experiencing damage from alcohol during pregnancy is presently so low that the question arises whether a lack of evidence for damaging effects is more important for a general recommendation than the potential protection of unborn life.

So there is no other option! It is recognised, however, that this definite and unconditional message may engender great fear in women who are unaware of their pregnancy at an early stage. A caveat is that alcohol consumption might not be harmful to the embryo prior to implantation of the fertilised egg into the uterus.

Moreover, even in women who do not recognise their pregnancies until weeks 4 to 8 or later, the following complete abstinence from alcohol during pregnancy might provide protection for the unborn child from further severe damage and prevent development of full-blown FAS [25].

Bibliography

[1] Kraus L, Bloomfield K, Augustin R, Reese A. prevalence of alcohol use and the association between onset of use and alcohol-related problems in a general population sample in Germany, Addiction 2000, 95, 1389–1401.

[2] Berghöfer A, Willich SN. Epidemiologie der Alkoholkrankheit bei Frauen. In: Bergmann R, Spohr HL, Dudenhausen JW (eds). Alkohol in der Schwangerschaft – Häufigkeit und Folgen. Urban & Vogel, München 2006, 9–18.

[3] Tripp J, Viner R. Sexual health, contraception, and teenage pregnancy. BMJ 2005, 330, 500–593.

[4] Walker MJ, Al-Sahab B, Islam F, Tamim H. The epidemiology of alcohol utilization during pregnancy: an analysis of the Canadian Maternity Experience Survey (MES). BMC Pregnancy and Childbirth 2011, 11, 52.

[5] Cheryl H. Tan; Clark H. Denny; Nancy E. Cheal; Joseph E. Sniezek; Dafna Kanny. Alcohol Use and Binge Drinking Among Women of Childbearing Age – United States, 2011–2013. Morbidity and Mortality Weekly Report (MMWR) 2015, 64(37), 1042–1046.

[6] Sayal K, Heron J, Golding J, Alati R, Smith GD, Gray R, Emond A. Binge pattern of alcohol consumption during pregnancy and childhood mental health outcome: longitudinal population based study. Pediatrics 2009, 123(2), e289–e296.

[7] Valenzuela CF, Morton RA, Diaz MR, Topper L. Does moderate drinking harm the fetal brain? Insights from animal models. Trends in Neuroscience 2012, 35(5), 284–292.

[8] Nava-Ocampo AA et al. Elimination kinetics of ethanol in pregnant women. Reprod Toxicol 2004, 18, 613–617.

[9] Furtwaengler NA, De Visser RO. Lack of international consensus in low-risk drinking guidelines. Drug Alcohol Rev 2012, doi: 10.1111/j.1465-3362.

[10] U.S. Department of Human Services and U.S. Department of Agriculture. Dietary Guidelines for Americans, 7th edn. U.S. Government Printing Office, Washington D.C. 2010.

[11] Henderson J, Gray R, Brocklehurst P. Systematic review of effects of low-moderate prenatal alcohol exposure on pregnancy outcome. BJOG 2007, 114, 243–252.

[12] Kelly Y, Sacker A, Gray R, Kelly J, Wolke D, Head J, Quigley MA. Light drinking during pregnancy: still no increased risk for socioemotional difficulties or cognitive deficits at 5 years of age? Int. J. Epidemiol. Community Health 2012, 66(1), 41–48.

[13] Kelly Y, Sacker A, Gray R, Kelly J, Wolke D, Head J, Quigley MA. Light drinking in pregnancy a risk for behavioural problems and cognitive deficits at 3 years of age? Int. J. Epidemiol. 2008, 38(1), 129–140, doi: 10.1093/ije/dyn230.

[14] Kesmodel US, Bertrand J, Stovring H, Denn CH, Mortensen EL. The Lifestyle During Pregnancy Study Group. The effect of different alcohol drinking patterns in early to mid pregnancy on the child's intelligence, attention, and executive function. BJOG 2012, 119, 1180–1190.

[15] Astley S, Grant T. Another perspective on "The effect of different alcohol drinking patterns in early to mid pregnancy on the child's intelligence attention and executive function". BJOG 2012, 119, 1672.

[16] Parker MO, Brennan CH. Low and moderate alcohol consumption during pregnancy: effects on social behaviour and propensity to develop substance abuse in later life. BJOG 2012, 119, 1670–1671.

[17] Astley S, Professor of Epidemiology and Pediatrics, WA State Fetal Alcohol Syndrome Diagnostic & Prevention Network of Clinics, 2012, fasdpn.org.

[18] Alati R, Al Mamun A, Williams GM, O'Callaghan M, Najmann JM, Bor W. In utero alcohol exposure and prediction of alcohol disorders in early adulthood: a birth cohort study. Arch Gen Psychiatry 2006, 63, 1009.

[19] Sood B. Delaney-Black V, Covington C, Nordtrom-Klee B et al. Prenatal alcohol exposure and childhood behaviour at age 6 to 7 years: I. Dose-response effect. Pediatrics 2001, 108, E34.

[20] Bay B, Stoving H, Wimberley T, Denny CH et al. Low to moderate alcohol intake during pregnancy and risk of psychomotor deficits. Alcohol Clin Exp Res. 2012, 36(5), 807–814.

[21] Galindo R, Zamudio PA, Valenzuela CF. Alcohol is a potent stimulant of immature neuronal networks: implication for fetal alcohol spectrum disorder. J. Neurochem 2005, 94, 15001511.

[22] Schneider ML, Moore CF, Kraemer GW. Moderate alcohol during learning and behaviour in adolescent rhesus monkeys. Alcohol Clin. Exp. Res. 2001, 25, 1383–1392.

[23] O'Leary CM, Bower C. Guidelines for pregnancy: What is an acceptable risk and how is the evidence (finally) shaping up. Drug and Alcohol Review 2011, 31, 170–183.

[24] Mukherjee RA, Hollins S, Turk J. Low level alcohol consumption and the fetus.-Abstinence from alcohol is the only safe message in pregnancy. BJM 2005, 330, 375–376.

[25] Larsson G, Bohlin AB, Tunell R. Prospective study of children exposed to variable amounts of alcohol in utero. Arch. Dis. Childh. 1985, 60, 316–321.

[26] Sayal K, Heron J, Draper E et al. Prenatal exposure to binge pattern of alcohol consumption: mental health and learning outcomes at age of 11. Eur Child Adolesc Psychiatry 2014, 23(10), 891–9.

[27] Jahrbuch Sucht 2015, Deutsche Hauptstelle für Suchtfragen (DHS), Pabst Science Publishers, Lengenich 2015.

[28] Deutsche Gesellschaft für Ernährung e. V. Presseinformation: Presse, DGE intern 2/2011 vom 29. November 2011.

[29] WHO global status report 2014.

[30] Ethen MK, Ramadhani TH, Scheuerle AE, Canfield MA, Wyszynski DF, Druschel EM, Romitti PA; National birth defects prevention study. Alcohol consumption by women before and during pregnancy. Matern Child Health J. 2009, 13 (2), 274–285.

[31] Alcohol Guidelines public consultation and submissions (NHMRC) 2001, https://www.nhmrc.gov.au/guidelines-publications/ds9.

[32] Mårdby A-C et al. Consumption of alcohol during pregnancy – A multinational European study, Women Birth 2017, 30(4), e207–e213.

8 Teratogenic effects of alcohol

8.1 Definition of teratology

A teratogen is an intrauterine acting agent that causes permanent damage to an embryo or fetus and has the ability to disturb the healthy and normal intrauterine development. The damage may occur in the form of a malformation, a growth deficit and a functional disorder, and may even result in fetal death [1].

According to the definition of teratology by the World Health Organisation (WHO), it includes all exogenous factors that lead to morphological, biochemical or behavioural abnormalities, which are diagnosed immediately after birth or later [2].

According to Shepard (1982) an agent can be defined as a teratogen when:

1. The teratogen is present during a critical phase of development.
2. The teratogen leads to a congenital impairment in animal studies.
3. There is evidence that the teratogen acts directly on the fetus through the placenta [3].

A teratogenic effect can come from chemicals, drugs, viruses and physical influences or deficiency states. Known teratogens are radiation, infections (e.g. rubella or cytomegaly), maternal illnesses or metabolic disorders (including diabetes or hyperthermia), medicaments (e.g. testosterone, cyclophosphamide, thalidomide, phenytoin and cumarin), environmental chemicals (e.g. 2-chlorophenylthiourea) and, especially, alcohol.

The teratogenic effect on fetal development can happen in a direct or indirect manner. Direct pathways are trans-placental transfers or radiation. Indirect pathways are changes to maternal metabolism or to a maternal coagulation cascade or through reduction of utero placental perfusion. The teratogenic damage of alcohol can take both the direct pathway, i.e. trans placental transfer, and the indirect pathway, i.e. reduced utero-placental perfusion resulting in placental insufficiency [2].

Despite the identification of more than 600 potential teratogens through animal studies, only about 25 teratogens have been proven to have a teratogenic effect in humans. The reason for this large discrepancy is, amongst others, that the animals were given very high doses of a potential teratogen that exceeds the dosage to which a human would normally be exposed.

An important aspect of studying a teratogen is to identify the pathomechanism of the damage. Animal studies can help to explain and demonstrate how a teratogen acts on a developing fetusand to predict the damage that is probably caused by the respective teratogen [3].

The teratogen passes from maternal blood through the placenta and the umbilical cord into the circulation of the fetus (see Fig. 8.1). One of the characteristics of the placenta is the *placental barrier*. It keeps the circulatory system of the mother and fetus

https://doi.org/10.1515/9783110436563-008

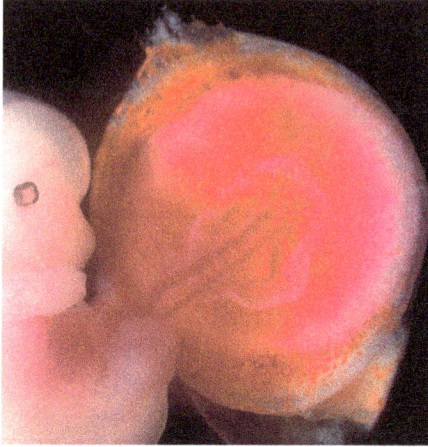

Fig. 8.1: Fetus with placenta.

largely separated and can prevent or permit active transport (diapedesis, pinocytosis) and passive transport (diffusion) of agents. The process of diffusion allows oxygen to transfer easily into the fetal circulatory system. In addition, other agents such as water or vitamins can also pass easily. However, diffusion also allows illegal drugs, nicotine, medication and, in particular, alcohol to pass freely into the fetal circulation.

In a recent publication Burd et al. (2012) demonstrated that 1 to 2 hours after maternal alcohol consumption, the alcohol level of the mother and fetus reaches an equivalent concentration [4]. In contrast to the maternal alcohol elimination capacity, fetal alcohol metabolism is reduced and delayed. This is due to the fact that the fetus is still developing and has lower metabolic capabilities. Another reason is the prolonged exposure period for the fetus due to an accumulation of alcohol concentration in the amniotic fluid (see Fig. 8.2).

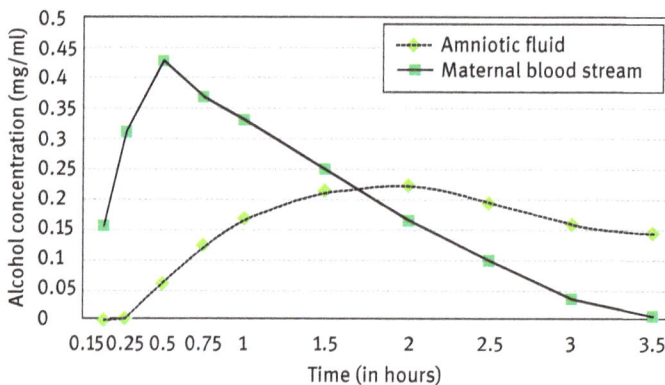

Fig. 8.2: Average alcohol concentration in blood and amniotic fluid of six pregnant women [4].

90–95% of maternal alcohol is metabolised in the maternal liver. The enzyme alcohol dehydrogenase (ADH) degrades alcohol to acetaldehyde. Due to its very limited capacity, fetal alcohol metabolism is crucially dependent on maternal metabolic capacity. This capacity varies strongly and lies between 0.0025 and 0.02 dl/h [4]. The discrepancy in metabolic rates between different mothers could be due to polymorphisms of the ADH enzyme. Moreover, the ADH2*2 allele seems to be a protective factor against the harmful effects of alcohol in both mother and child [5]. This may explain why the expression and variability of FAS in children exposed to the same amounts of intrauterine alcohol can be so different [4].

8.2 Behavioural teratology: evidence from animal studies

Extensive research studies on animals clearly confirmed alcohol as a teratogen during pregnancy. There was a surprising high parallelism between animal studies and epidemiological and clinical findings in affected children [6]. Animal studies have shown that not only severe chronic alcohol exposure, but also moderate amounts of alcohol or episodic drinking may be responsible for teratogenic damage; this can happen in early and in late pregnancy. Similar results were found in humans. Not only children from chronic alcohol dependent mothers were affected by prenatal alcohol exposure; occasional alcohol consumption, i.e. binge drinking ("Saturday night drinking") may also be responsible for severe alcohol-induced damage to a fetus.

Moreover, animal studies demonstrated that alcohol has direct toxic effects on the developing neurons of the brain and that alcohol is responsible, amongst other teratogenic effects, for an increased cell death (apoptosis) [7]. Particularly affected is the cerebrum, but also the hippocampus, cerebellum and corpus callosum. Furthermore, alcohol and its metabolites affect hormonal and chemical regulation processes and influence maturation and migration of neurons [8].

Many of the behavioural problems seen in children with FAS, such as hyperactivity, attention deficit, developmental delays, impaired gross and fine motor skills, gait abnormalities and feeding problems, were also detected in animal experiments [9].

The relationship between brain damage and behavioural problems has been clearly demonstrated in animal experiments. A disrupted brain development is responsible for a pathological behaviour in alcohol-exposed animals. In humans, behavioural disorders are easier to recognise than the underlying brain damage, which so far has only been proven experimentally in animal studies [7].

Animal experiments have also shown individual differences of the teratogenic effects between mothers and their offspring. Goodlett et al. confirmed this "genetic modulation" of the teratogenic damage of alcohol in 1989 [10].

Finally, animal studies have confirmed that prenatal alcohol induced behavioural disorders can persist into adulthood [8].

8.3 Effects of the timing of prenatal alcohol exposure

Each teratogen has a specific individual period of high sensitivity; therefore, possible birth defects depend on the time of exposure during pregnancy. The critical development phases of a pregnancy are depicted in Fig. 8.3.

Over the course of pregnancy, organs and organ systems develop at different time windows. Specific malformations can vary, depending on the time of exposure.

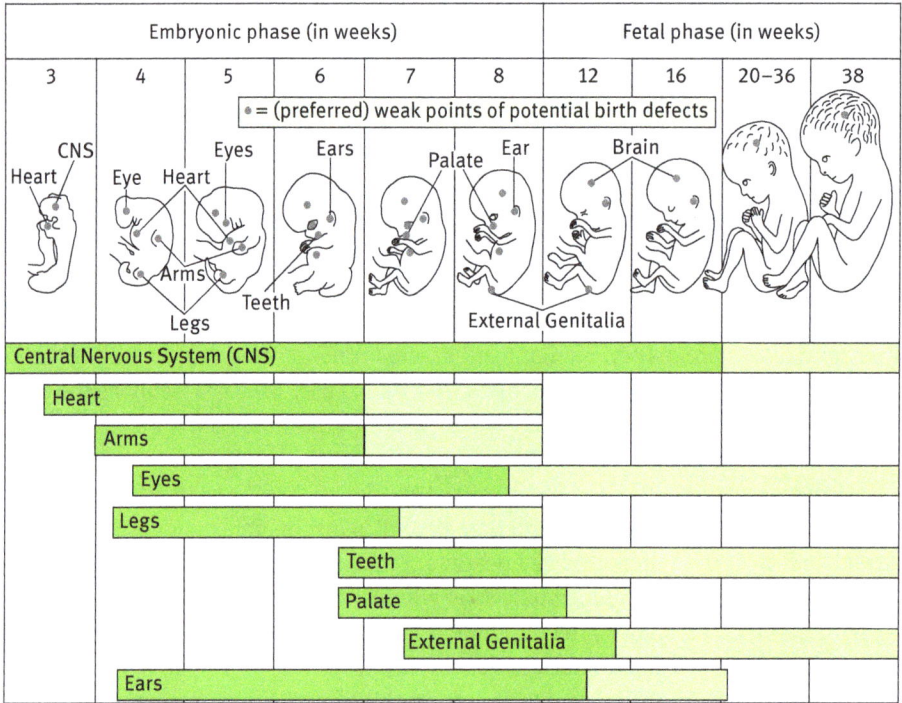

Fig. 8.3: Representation of the fetal organ development. The dark green bars indicate the developmental period with the highest sensitivity to teratogenic agents [11]; i.e. the development of arms and legs takes place between weeks 4 and 7. The highest sensitivity of CNS last from the first week of pregnancy until birth.

Of particular importance with respect to potential damage are days 7 to 10 between fertilisation and implantation of the egg in the uterus (nidation), because women are still unaware of their pregnancy. During this early phase, the fertilised egg cell is supplied by the maternal blood-flow and therefore, alcohol and acetaldehyde easily reach the fertilised egg per diffusion. However, obviously the teratogen will not always cause permanent damage at this early stage. According to the "all-or-nothing principle" the pluripotent cells of the newly formed trophoblast are either still capable of replacing damaged cells or, if the toxic impairment is sufficiently severe, it induces an abortion.

When alcohol exposure happens during the first trimester, organogenesis of the embryo is affected most, leading to possibly serious, especially physical, damage, i.e. congenital heart defects, cleft palate or minor anomalies. Commonly, longitudinal growth occurs primarily during the first trimester, whereas fetal weight gain occurs mainly in the last trimester [11].

During the entire intrauterine development, the brain is the main target of alcohol exposure. The brain grows and develops more rapidly than all other fetal organs and in the middle of pregnancy the head is almost 50% of the total body size; at birth it will be 25% and it is only 12% of the total height in adults. In conclusion, no matter which time of pregnancy the fetal brain is exposed to alcohol, it is the main target of persistent damage. Consequently, brain development can be disturbed in growth and development throughout the entire pregnancy (Fig. 8.3).

Results of studies examining the relationship between the timing of alcohol exposure and the resulting developmental damage have been discussed and debated quite extensively. Day et al. [12] found that children whose mothers drank alcohol only in the first 2 months of pregnancy, have an increased risk of a birth weight, body length and head circumference below the 3rd percentile, depending on the amount of alcohol intake. In contrast, in the "Atlanta-study" Smith and Coles found neonatal growth deficits only in children, whose mothers had drunk alcohol continuously throughout the pregnancy [13].

In their publication "Maternal Health Practices and Child Development Study" (MHPCD), Day et al. [14] suggested a dosage-dependent relationship between maternal alcohol consumption in the second and third trimesters and a reduced postnatal growth between the ages of 8 and 18 months. This growth deficiency persisted significantly compared to age-matched peers 3 and 10 years later [15].

Bibliography

[1]   Wilson JG. New area of concern in teratology. Teratology 1977, 17, 227–228.
[2]   Paulus WE, Lauritzen C. Medikamente und Schadstoffe in der Schwangerschaft; Reproduktionstoxikologie. Spitta Verlag, Balingen 2005.
[3]   Shephard TH. Detection of human teratogenic agents. The Journal of Pediatrics 1982, 5, 810–815.
[4]   Burd L, Blair J, Dropps K. Prenatal alcohol exposure, blood alcohol concentrations and alcohol elimination rates for mother, fetus and newborn. J. Perinatol 2012, 32, 652–659.
[5]   Gemma S, Vichi S, Testai E. Metabolic and genetic factors contributing to alcohol induced effects and fetal alcohol syndrome. Neurosci Biobehav Rev 2007, 31(2), 221–229.
[6]   Driscoll CD, Streissguth AP, Riley EP. Prenatal alcohol exposure: Comparability of effects in human and animal models. Neurobehavioral Toxicology and Teratology 1990, 12, 231–237.
[7]   Kotch LE, Sulik KK. Experimental fetal alcohol syndrome: proposed pathogenic basis for a variety of associated facial and brain anomalies. Am J Med Genet 1992, 44, 168–176.

[8]   Livy DJ, Miller EK, Maier SE, West JR. Fetal alcohol exposure and temporal vulnerability: effects of binge-like alcohol exposure on the developing rat hippocampus. Neurotoxicol Teratol 2003, 25, 447–458.

[9]   Riley EP. The long-term behavioral effects of prenatal alcohol exposure in rats. Alcoholism: Clinical and Experimental Research 1990, 14(5), 670–3.

[10] Goodlett CR, Gilliam DM, Nichols JM, West JR. Genetic influences on brain growth restriction induced by developmental exposure to alcohol. Neurotoxicology 1989, 10, 321–334.

[11] Moore KL, Persaud TVN. Embryologie: Entwicklungsstadien – Frühentwicklung-Organogenese – Klinik. 5. Auflage. Urban & Fischer Verlag/Elsevier GmbH, München 2007.

[12] Day NL, Jasperse D, Richardson G et al. Prenatal exposure to alcohol: Effect on Infant growth and morphologic characteristics. Pediatrics 1998, 84(3), 536–541.

[13] Coles CD, Brown RT, Smith IE, Platzman KA, Silverstein J, Erickson S, Falek A. Effects of prenatal alcohol exposure at school age. I. Physical and cognitive development. Neurotoxicol and Teratol 1991, 13(4), 357–367.

[14] Day NL, Goldschmidt L, Robles N et al. Prenatal alcohol exposure and offspring growth at 18 months of age: The predictive validity of two measures of drinking. Alcohol Clin Exp Res 1991, 15(6), 914–918.

[15] Day NL, Zuo Y, Richardson GA, Goldschmidt L, Larkby CA, Cornelius MD. Prenatal alcohol use and offspring size at ten years of age. Alcohol Clin Exp Res 1999, 23, 863–86.

9 Effects of prenatal exposure to nicotine or illegal substances

9.1 Nicotine use during pregnancy

The most frequently used substance in pregnancy is tobacco, followed by alcohol, cannabis and other illegal substances. Polysubstance abuse in pregnancy is common and almost all alcohol-dependent women are additionally addicted to nicotine, which leads to additional teratogenic effects.

According to information presented by the German Centre for Addiction Issues (DHS) in Hamm, about 36% of men and 22% of women are smoking cigarettesregularly. This amounts to the extremely high number of 22–24 million female smokers, making nicotine the most dangerous teratogenic substance for humans.

According to a current survey conducted by the Center for Disease Control and Prevention, in 2014 16.8% of US adults were cigarette smokers (18.8% male and 14.8% female), with the highest rates in the ages of 25–44, and with 10.7% stated to smoke during pregnancy [1].

In an earlier study from Berlin published in 2006, 23.5% of 293 women reported smoking cigarettes in pregnancy. Of these women, 14.5% consumed nicotine on a daily basis despite a decline in smoking in general and extensive education about negative effects of smoking [2, 3].

Teratogenic effects of nicotine

Teratogenic effects of nicotine and its metabolite cotinine or one of its other teratogenic metabolites are:

1. Vasoconstriction of the umbilical cord blood vessels and the fetal cerebral blood vessels resulting in fetal hypoxia and a reduced supply of nutrients through the blood and consequently to a reduction in birth weight of about 150–250 g [3, 4].
2. Increase of carboxyhaemoglobin in fetal circulation from carbon monoxide rapidly crossing the placenta up to 15% higher compared to maternal concentration, which leads to a further decrease in the oxygen supply for fetal tissues.
3. Rapid diffusion of the water- and fat-soluble elements of nicotine and other components of cigarette smoke into the fetal brain, with nicotine concentration in globus pallidus, N. putamen and thalamus due to the density of nicotine sensitive acetylcholine receptors in the brain stem.
4. Interactions and changes of different brain areas caused by nicotine, such as timing of cell differentiation, synaptogenesis and synaptic activity of multiple neurotransmitter systems in fetal neural circuits [5].

https://doi.org/10.1515/9783110436563-009

In clinical and animal studies it has been shown that nicotine concentration in the placenta, amniotic fluid and fetal blood was up to 15% higher than in maternal serum [5].

Besides the aforementioned effects from nicotine, birth weight is also impacted by nicotine concentration from cigarettes [8], in addition to other factors such as socioeconomic status [6] and age of the mother (> 40 years) [7]. Further, women who smoke during pregnancy are twice as likely to experience a miscarriage, and there is a higher risk for the child dying from sudden infant death syndrome [9].

Moreover, high levels of nicotine exposure may result in psychiatric and cognitive abnormalities. In children whose mothers smoked more than 10 cigarettes per day during pregnancy, a small decline in IQ was seen. After an exposure of 20 or more cigarettes per day a 2.6-fold increase in the likelihood of aggressive and delinquent behaviour was found in comparison to children who were not exposed to nicotine prenatally [10, 11].

The risk of psychiatric disorders after prenatal nicotine exposure in adolescence was examined in a large Finnish population study in which all children born between 1987 and 1989 in Finland were included ($n = 175{,}869$).

In this study, the prevalence for nicotine consumption during pregnancy was 15.3%. The risk of suffering from a psychiatric diagnosis in adolescence was 21% in offspring from mothers who smoked less than 10 cigarettes a day, whereas the risk for the offspring of mothers who smoked more than 10 cigarettes a day during pregnancy was 24.7% (control group 13.7%). This increased risk to suffer from a psychiatric disorder in adolescence was still present after controlling for potential confounding factors such as inpatient psychiatric treatment of the biological mother [8, 12].

High cigarette consumption (> 10/day) additionally can increase mortality rates in childhood and adolescence [12].

In a study published in 2012, women were asked in standardised questionnaires about the behaviour of their children aged 5–18 (e.g. executive function disorders and symptoms of ADHD). Clear abnormalities in different areas of executive functioning were found when maternal nicotine consumption was at 10 cigarettes per day or more during pregnancy. The outcome for executive functioning was significantly worse compared to children without prenatal exposure to nicotine.

The rate of ADHD was 36% if children were exposed to more than 10 cigarettes per day during pregnancy and 25% after exposure of 1–9 cigarettes a day. Compared to children of non-smoking mothers, the rate of ADHD was 17.8%.

Furthermore, this study revealed that mothers who consumed more than 10 cigarettes also had the highest additional consumption of alcohol (12%), marijuana (15%) and cocaine (3%) [13].

In summary, following these recent studies, simultaneous consumption of alcohol and nicotine during pregnancy results in significant cumulative teratogenic effects and, consequently, in behavioural disorders, executive dysfunction, psychiatric diseases and, in particular, in ADHD.

However, compared to nicotine, alcohol remains by far the most significant and dangerous teratogenic substance due to its severe lifelong damage.

9.2 Illegal drugs during pregnancy

Illegal substances, particularly cocaine, heroin and with increasing significance also marijuana or cannabis (psychoactive cannabinoid: tetrahydrocannabinol = THC) and methamphetamine ("crystal meth"), are statistically less common than the two legal substances alcohol and nicotine.

According to the German Centre for Addiction Issues (DHS) the prevalence for cocaine use in Germany (2012) was 0.4% between the ages of 15 and 64 [14].

In contrast to Germany, cocaine consumption in the United States is particularly high. Toxicological screenings of the meconium of newborns whose mothers used cocaine during pregnancy revealed positive rates of cocaine of up to 31% [15]. Urine samples were examined in Boston and revealed the presence of cocaine in 17% and marijuana in 28% [16].

In an English study with 807 pregnant women consecutively examined, a lower number for cocaine usage was found. Only 3 out of the 807 women screened positively for cocaine, whereas the use of marijuana during pregnancy was significantly higher at 14.5%, indicating marijuana as one of the most popular illegal psychoactive substances [17].

For Germany, there are no data available for cocaine use in pregnancy. A comparison of national studies on cocaine use in the period of the last 12 months, showed that Germany was in the average range compared to other European countries (0.8%) [18, 19].

9.3 "Crack baby"

In a study, it was found that women who consume illegal drugs during pregnancy are often older, use drugs for the first time as a teenager, and up to 50% earn their living from prostitution. In addition, up to 75% of these women were infected by hepatitis C and 5% were HIV positive [19]. These women suffered from traumatic childhood experiences, often grew up in families with addiction problems and divorced parents, attained low education levels and experienced mental and physical abuse. Besides nicotine, drug-dependent women used additional psychotropic substances, particularly marijuana and alcohol, but also sedatives and pain relievers [20].

In the early 1980s and 1990s of the last century, taking cocaine in the form of water-soluble cocaine hydrochloride salt or by smoking "crack" was very popular, and cocaine as a possible new teratogenic agent came to be described as leading to the risk of a "coke baby" or "crack baby".

Persistent teratogenic effects of cocaine exposure on specific cognitive functions at the age of 9 years were described, but school achievement was not affected [21]. Children with high prenatal cocaine exposure were likely to manifest behavioural problems at 7 years of age [31].

In an extensive prospective longitudinal study with 200 children up to the age of 7 years, Bandstra et al. 2004 were able to show that severe cocaine exposure during pregnancy could not be the sole risk factor for the behavioural and developmental disorders seen in the children examined [22].

In a critical review of the literature between 1994 and 2000, Frank et al. (2001) identified 37 prospective studies in children up to the age of 6 years. They found no convincing indication that prenatal cocaine exposure was associated with a general developmental disruption or with specific behavioural problems. Many of the symptoms that were originally attributed to the teratogenic effects of cocaine significantly correlated with other factors, such as additional prenatal exposure to nicotine, marijuana and alcohol or with reduced quality of living conditions for these children [23].

In a recent study, Grewen et al. (2014) reported that prenatal cocaine exposure was related to subtle deficits in cognitive and behavioural function in infancy, childhood and adolescence, but concluded that longitudinal studies are necessary to determine whether these early differences persist and contribute to deficits in cognitive function at school age [32].

Prenatal cocaine exposure can lead to a lower gestational age, but is not associated with reduced birth weight, shorter body length and smaller head circumference. The regulation disorders often seen in these infants during the newborn period were no longer present after 1 year [24].

In summary, despite significant perinatal problems in exposed children, the teratogenic effects of cocaine have not been confirmed unequivocally in longitudinal studies.

According to current knowledge, cocaine exposure *in utero* does, indeed, creates a high-risk pregnancy, but cocaine itself seems to create no permanent damage of mental, motor and speech development or behaviour.

9.4 Prenatal cannabis or marijuana exposure

In Germany, cannabis is the most commonly used illegal drug. THC (tetrahydrocannabinol) is the essential psychoactive substance and affects, amongst other systems, the central nervous system through its relaxing and sedating effects. Regular abuse and, particularly, a physical addiction increase the risk of the development of a psychosis.

Signs of cannabis abuse
– overall deterioration of performance in school;
– dramatic mood changes;
– social withdrawal (from friends, parents);
– changes in social behaviour (aggressiveness, impulsivity);
– loss of interest in activities;
– contact with peers with a substance use disorder;
– possession of tobacco products and drugs (plant elements, cigarette paper, etc.).

Cannabis use often is considered to be harmless and its risks are underestimated. In a recent publication from Oregon (USA) it was shown prospectively that continuous cannabis use from early adolescence to the age of 38 leads to a decline in cognitive abilities [25].

Cannabis is the most commonly used illegal substance in young women in Germany today, and the number of hospitalisations for cannabis abuse has tripled amongst adolescents in the last decade.

In a study published in 2012 conducted in a women's clinic in Brisbane, Australia, over a period of 6 years, it was found that out of approximately 25000 pregnant women, 637 (2.6%) were using cannabis during pregnancy. Cannabis consumption during pregnancy resulted in statistically lower birth weight, premature labour and an increased rate of neonatal intensive care treatment [26].

In an American longitudinal study from Pittsburgh that examined the association between school performance and intrauterine exposure to marijuana, 524 children participated in a follow-up examination at the age 14 years. The children were part of a longitudinal cohort, whose mothers had smoked marijuana more than twice a month during the first trimester. The children were examined regularly from birth until adolescence. The authors found that these children scored significantly poorer on a school performance test (WIAT: Wechsler Individual Achievement Test) compared to a control group [27].

In an animal study, Hansen et al. (2008) examined possible toxic effects on the developing brain due to THC alone or in combination with alcohol. The authors found that cannabis application of THC alone did not increase neuronal apoptosis. Given a small dosage of alcohol (3 mg/kg) caused a significant but moderate apoptosis. Neuronal degeneration, however, became disseminated and severe, when cannabis was combined with alcohol. However, when the animals received a combination of cannabis (1–10 mg/kg THC) and alcohol at a low dose (3 mg/kg), there was a significantly higher rate of brain cell apoptosis. This drug combination resembled the massive apoptotic death observed when administering ethanol alone at much higher doses (Fig. 9.1)

The use of cannabis alone during pregnancy might be less harmful, but polydrug use – at least in animal experiments – may have unpredictable consequences [28].

Polydrug use has unpredictable consequences

Cannabis alone does not cause cell death in immature rat brains.

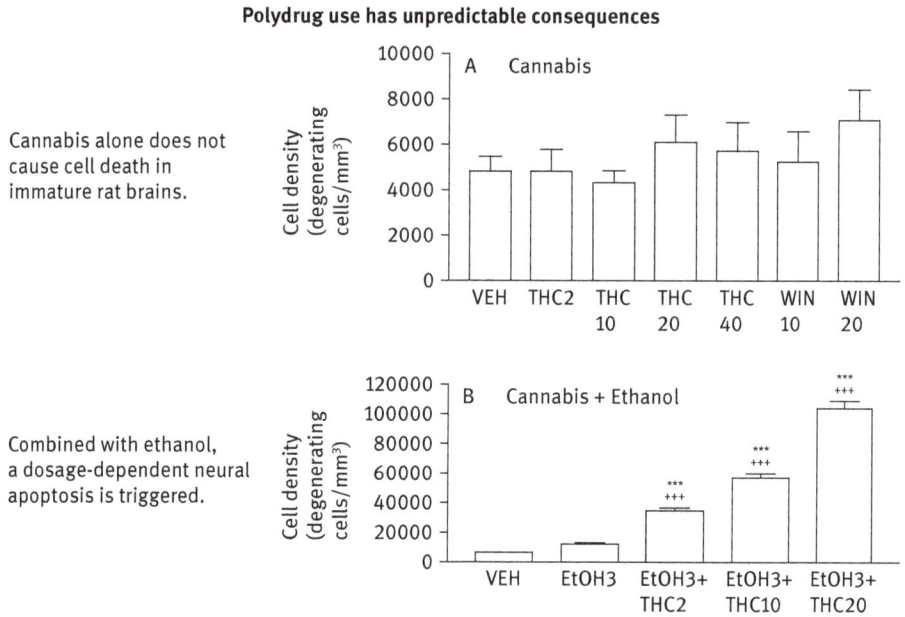

Combined with ethanol, a dosage-dependent neural apoptosis is triggered.

Fig. 9.1: Cannabis in combination with alcohol increases sensitivity to the neurotoxic effects of alcohol on developing rat brains (modified from Hansen et al.) [28].

There are few reliable data on long-term consequences for children exposed prenatally to cannabis only, but the recommendation to be abstinent from cannabis during pregnancy remains.

9.5 Methamphetamine exposure ("crystal meth")

The synthetic drug methamphetamine "crystal meth" is a cheap, fast-working and very harmful drug. It is highly addictive and when used regularly, results in physical decline even at an early stage.

Combined with alcohol intake it leads to:
1. a reduced perception of the effects of alcohol;
2. a significantly impaired reaction time;
3. a significant increase in aggressive behaviour;
4. a pronounced sense of self-confidence.

Sparse literature is available on the effects of methamphetamine during pregnancy. Wright et al. (2015) conducted the first retrospective study in women who used methamphetamine during pregnancy. Of 144 children examined at birth, 29 had been continuously exposed throughout the pregnancy. The authors found that these children had lower gestational ages and birth weights compared to non-exposed children. If use of methamphetamine was discontinued during pregnancy, birth outcomes improved [30].

9.6 Effects of *polydrug* use in pregnancy

The most common combination in polydrug-addicted women is alcohol and nicotine. All alcohol-dependent women are also addicted to nicotine [6].

Several teratogenic effects of nicotine are non-specific and similar to abnormalities seen in fetal alcohol syndrome (e.g. concentration difficulties, motor restlessness, impulsivity); therefore, it is difficult to attribute the effects to a single substance.

Singer et al. (2008) published a study with 180 cocaine-dependent women; 86% of the pregnant women reported that they additionally drank alcohol and 87% that they smoked. Out of the non-cocaine dependent women, 67% reported that they consumed alcohol and 37% that they used nicotine [21].

In an examination of the consequences of prenatal amphetamine exposure (2011), only a small impairment in the development of fine motor skills was detected at age 1 year, but was not detectable at age 3 years [29].

In summary, usage of alcohol and nicotine in polydrug-dependent women leads to permanent damage to offspring. Similar permanent consequences were not found with exposure to heroin, cocaine or amphetamines. Unfortunately, in clinical practice, clinicians are mainly focused on illegal drugs during pregnancy, and additional consumption of alcohol often remains unnoticed.

Bibliography

[1]   Chiriboga CA. Fetal Alcohol and Drug Effects. The Neurologist 2003, 9, 267–279.
[2]   Bergmann RL, Bergmann KE, Schumann S, Richter R, Dudenhausen JW. Rauchen in der Schwangerschaft: Verbreitung, Trend, Risikofaktoren (Smoking in pregnancy, rates, trends, risc factors). Z Geburtsh Neonatol 2008, 212, 80–86.
[3]   Luck W, Nau H. Nicotine and Cotinine concentrations in the milk of smoking mothers: Influence of cigarette consumption and diurnal variation. Eur J Pediatr 1987, 146(1), 21–26.
[4]   Lethovirta P, Forss M. The acute effects on intervillous bloodflow of the placenta. Br J Obstet Gynecol 1978, 85, 729–731.
[5]   Lambers DS, Clark KE. The maternal and fetal physiologic effects of nicotine. Semin Perinatol 1996, 20(2), 115–126.
[6]   Meyer S, Raisig A, Gortner L, Ong MF, BüchelerM, Tutdibi E. In utero tobacco exposure: The rate of SGA/IUGR is modified by socio-economic risk factors. Eur J Ob Gyn Rep Biol 2009, 146, 37–40.
[7]   Fox SH, Koepsell TD, Daling JR. Birth weight and smoking during pregnancy effect modification by maternal age. Am J Epidemiol 1994, 139, 1008–1015.

[8] Fried PA, Watson B. 12-and 24-month neurobehavioral follow-up of children prenatally exposed to marihuana, cigarettes and alcohol. Neurobehav Teratol 1988, 10, 305–313.

[9] Health Canada: Fetal Alcohol Spectrum Disorder. Public Health Agency of Canada, Ottawa 2006.

[10] Olds DL, Henderson CR, Tatelbaum R. Intellectual impairment in children of women who smoke cigarettes during pregnancy. Pediatrics 1994, 93, 221–227.

[11] Freitag, CM. Hyperaktives und aggressives Verhalten bei Kindern nach Rauchexposition in der Schwangerschaft. In: Dudenhausen J (ed). Rauchen in der Schwangerschaft; Häufigkeit, Folgen und Prävention. Urban & Vogel, München 2009, 49–53.

[12] Ekblad M, Gissler M, Lehtonen L, Korkeila J. Prenatal smoking Exposure and the Risk of Psychiatric Morbidity into Young Adulthood. Arch Gen Psychiatry 2010, 67(8), 841–949.

[13] Piper BJ, Corbett SM. Executive Function Profile in the Offspring of Women that smoked during Pregnancy. Nicotine & Tobacco Research 2012, 14(2), 191–199.

[14] Orth B, Kraus L, Piontek D. Illegale Drogen – Zahlen und Fakten zum Konsum. In: Deutsche Hauptstelle für Suchtfragen (ed). Jahrbuch Sucht, Pabst Science Publishing, Lengerich 2012.

[15] Ostrea EM, Brandy M, Gause S, Raymudo AL, Stevens M. Drug screening of newborns by meconium analysis: a large scale, prospective, epidemiologic study. Pediatrics 1992, 89, 107–113.

[16] Frank DA, Zuckermann BS, Amaro H et al. Cocaine use during pregnancy: prevalence and correlates. Pediatrics 1988, 82, 888–895.

[17] Sherwood RA, Keating J, Kavvadia V, Greenough A, Peters TJ. Substance misuse in early pregnancy and relationship to fetal outcome. Eur J Pediatr 1999, 158, 488–492.

[18] Kraus L, Augustyn R. Repräsentativerhebung zum Gebrauch psychoaktiver Substanzen bei Erwachsenen in Deutschland 2000. Sucht 2001, 47, S3–S86.

[19] Klein M (ed). Kinder und Suchtgefahren: Risiken-Prävention-Hilfen. Schattauer, Stuttgart 2008.

[20] Nagel M, Siedentopf JP. Schwangerschaft – Sucht – Hilfe: Ein Leitfaden zum Casemanagement. Charité Campus Virchow-Klinikum, Berlin 2004.

[21] Singer LT, Nelson S, Short E, Min MO, Lewis B, Russ S, Minnes S. Prenatal cocaine exposure: drug and enviromental effects at 9 years. J Pediatr 2008, 153(1), 105–111.

[22] Bandstra ES, Vogel AL, Morrow CE, Xue L, Anthony JC, Severity of prenatal cocain exposure and child language functioning through age seven years: a longitudinal latent growth curve analysis. Subst Use Misuse 2004, 39, 25–59.

[23] Frank DA, AugustynM, Knight WG, Pell T, Zuckerman B. Growth, development, and behaviour in early childhood following prenatal cocaine exposure: a systematic review. JAMA 2001, 285(12), 1613–1625.

[24] Jacobson SW, Jacobson JC, Sokol RJ, Martier SS. New evidence for neurobehavioral effects of in utero cocaine exposure. J Pediatr 1996, 129, 58–59.

[25] Meier MH, Caspi A, Ambler A et al. Persistent cannabis users show neuropsycholological decline from childhood to midlife. PNAS, Proceedings of the Academy of Sciences of the United States of America 2012, 109(40), E2657–E2664, doi:10.1073/pnas.1206820109.

[26] Hayabakhsh MR, Flenady V, Gibbons KS et al. Birth outcomes associated with cannabis use before and during pregnancy. Pediatric Research 2012, 71(2), 215–219.

[27] Goldschmidt L, Richardson GA, Willford JA, Severtson SG Day NL. School achievement in 14-year-old youth prenatally exposed to marijuana. Neurrotoxicology and Teratology 2012, 34, 161–167.

[28] Hansen HH, Krutz B, Sifringer M et al. Cannabinoids Enhance Susceptibility of Immature Brain to Ethanol Neurotoxicity. Ann Neurol 2008, 64, 42–52.

[29] Smith LM, LaGasse LL, Derauf C et al. Motor and cognitive outcome through three years of age in children exposed to prenatal methamphetamine. Neurotoxicol Teratol 2011, 33(1), 176–184.

[30] Wright TE, Schütter R, Tellei J, Sauvage L. Methamphetamines and pregnancy outcomes. J Addict Med 2015, 9(2), 111–117.

[31] Bada HS, Bann CM, Bauer CR, Shankaran S, Lester B, LaGasse L, Hammond J, Whitaker T, Das A, Tan S, Higgins R. Preadolescent behavior problems after prenatal cocaine exposure: Relationship between teacher and caretaker ratings (Maternal Lifestyle Study). Neurotoxicol Teratol. 2011, 33(1), 78–87.

[32] Grewen K, Burchinal M, Vachet C, Gouttard S, Gilmore JH, Lin W, Johns J, Elam M, Gerig G. Prenatal cocaine effects on brain structure in early infancy. Neuroimage 2014, 101, 114–23.

10 Biomarker for the detection of maternal alcohol use during pregnancy

The patient history of maternal alcohol consumption during pregnancy often provides inaccurate and untruthful information about the quantities of alcohol consumed. This may be due to the fact the women do not recall exactly, underestimate the actual amounts of alcohol or deny alcohol consumption because of social pressure. For these reasons, currently used self-report questionnaires give only limited evidence of the real alcohol consumption during pregnancy. Therefore, there is an urgent need for objective biomarkers that can detect and determine the amounts of alcohol consumed during pregnancy.

10.1 Direct and indirect biomarkers

Traditionally used biomarkers are divided into direct or indirect markers. Indirect markers measure alterations that alcohol can cause in humans. Direct makers are metabolites of non-oxidative alcohol degradation.

Indirect biomarkers that can be determined in the maternal serum are the following:

– liver enzymes, i.e. gamma-glutamyl transferase (GGT), aspartate amino transferase (AST)
– mean corpuscular volume (MCV) and carbohydrate-deficient transferrin (CDT).

These indirect markers have a relatively weak sensitivity and specificity, a short time window for measurement, are often only positive in chronic alcohol consumption and can be influenced by other factors that are not caused by alcohol, such as age or illnesses.

Nowadays, indirect biomarkers only play an unimportant role in detecting alcohol consumption compared to direct biomarkers.

The most important direct biomarkers currently used are:
1. Fatty Acid Ethyl Esters (FAEE)
2. Ethyl Glucuronide (EtG)
3. Ethyl Sulfate (EtS) [1]

These biomarkers are products of the non-oxidative metabolism.

In the presence of alcohol, fatty acid ethyl esters (FAEE) result from the metabolism of free fatty acids, lipoproteins and phospholipids under the influence of the enzyme fatty acid ethyl synthase. Due to its delayed half-life elimination in blood and urine, FAEE can be detected up to 24 hours after alcohol intake. FAEE have a high sensitivity

https://doi.org/10.1515/9783110436563-010

and specificity of alcohol consumption during the third trimester in pregnancy in the meconium of newborns.

Ethyl glucuronide (EtG) results from conjugation with UDP-glucoronic acid in the endoplasmic reticulum of the liver cell. It can be detected in urine up to 13–20 hours after consumption of small amounts of alcohol (0.1 grams per kilogram bodyweight) and even up to 80 hours after an intake of large amounts of alcohol (starting at 0.5 grams per kilogram bodyweight). Nowadays, EtG is used as a standard method for detecting alcohol in urine and hair samples.

Ethyl sulphate (EtS) is a direct alcohol metabolite and results after conjugation with sulphuric acid in liver cells. The detection time window is similar to that of EtG, but there is a difference in pathway and degradation. EtS probably has the advantage of no bacterial degradation in stored urine samples even without adding bacterial stabilisers [1]. Nevertheless, in forensic urine analysis, EtS has not become the standard method [2].

Nowadays, FAEE and EtG are used routinely in meconium to prove alcohol consumption during the last trimester of pregnancy. Less commonly, and especially in experimental studies, FAEE or EtG are used in neonatal hair, placenta or the umbilical cord.

In a recent study in 2012, Hastedt et al. demonstrated that FAEE can be routinely used as a valid, non-invasive method to detect alcohol exposure, and that only small amounts of meconium (50 mg) are needed.

They analysed 122 meconium samples of newborns whose mothers were under suspicion of drug abuse during pregnancy. The meconium was analysed in regard to illegal drugs and additionally to alcohol. Unexpectedly, alcohol ranked third after methadone and heroine in this population.

For the first time, detecting FAEE or EtG in the meconium of newborns offers a low-cost screening method to detect alcohol exposure during the last trimester [2].

It should be noted, however, that for ethical reasons, in Germany meconium cannot be examined without the definite agreement of the mother concerned. Therefore, implementation of this procedure cannot be established routinely to date.

Bibliography

[1] Wurst FM, Thon N, Weinmann W. Direkte Ethanolmetabolite in Blut und Urin: Relevanz in Diagnose und Therapie alkoholbezogener Störungen. Journal für Neurologie, Neurochirurgie und Psychiatrie 2009, 10(3), 82–85.
[2] Hastedt M, Krumbiegel F, Gabert R, Tsokos M, Hartwig S. Fatty acid ethyl esters (FAEEs) as markers for alcohol in meconium: method validation and implementation of a screening program for prenatal drug exposure. Forensic Sci Med Pathol 2013, 9(3), 287–295.

11 Neuropathological aspects and pathogenesis of FASD

11.1 Introduction

Prenatal alcohol exposure damages brain structures and leads to impaired brain function in patients affected by FASD, often with persistent lifelong disturbances.

Brain damage and brain dysfunction may be evaluated and confirmed by the following methods:
1. Autopsy of children with intrauterine alcohol exposure;
2. Clinical trials and follow-up studies of patients compared to healthy controls;
3. Imaging methods
   a) structural and functional magnetic resonance imaging (MRI; fMRI)
   b) magnetic resonance spectroscopy (MRS)
   c) positron emission tomography (PET)
   d) animal experiments.

Animal experiments enable us to follow up and document the precise amount of alcohol, the timing of the exposure and the duration of the alcohol intake. Moreover, it is possible to eliminate additional stress factors such as nicotine intake, illegal drugs or medication, psychosocial stress, and nutritional disorders seen in clinical trials.

In general, the following brain regions are particularly affected by prenatal alcohol exposure:
1. *Frontal lobe*: This area of the brain concerns impulse control, is responsible for assessment of the environment, and planning and execution. The most sensitive region is probably the *prefrontal cortex*, which is an important area controlling executive functions.
2. *Corpus callosum*: Exchange of information between the left hemisphere of the brain, responsible for logical thinking, and the right hemisphere, the more emotional side, takes place here.
3. *Hippocampus*: This region of the brain plays a fundamental role in memory processes, learning ability and emotions.
4. *Hypothalamus*: The centre of the autonomic nervous system, the hypothalamus regulates appetite, pain, homeostasis (blood pressure, osmolarity, body temperature), and circadian rhythm, and influences sexual behaviour.
5. *Cerebellum*: It controls motor activity, coordination and movement, but also behaviour and memory.

https://doi.org/10.1515/9783110436563-011

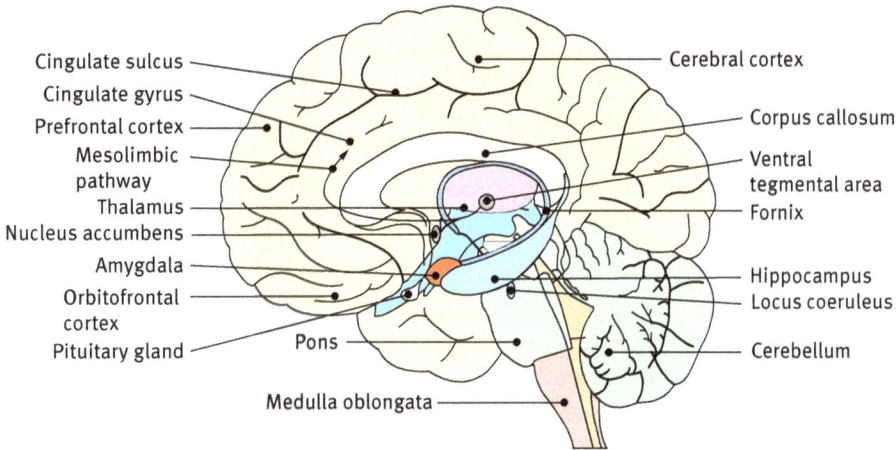

Fig. 11.1: Brain anatomy (modified from Anderhuber F, Pera F, Streicher J (eds). *Waldeyer – Anatomie des Menschen*. 19th edn. Verlag De Gruyter, Boston 2012, 957).

11.2 First descriptions of neuropathological effects

Soon after the discovery of FASD, the first reports on brain malformations and neuropathological findings were published. In 1979, Peiffer et al. reported neuropathological findings in three children and three fetuses with FAS [1]. Wisniewski et al. (1983) published autopsy results of five patients with FAS [25]. These case reports all concerned severely affected children, who died in early infancy due to severe malformations mainly caused by intrauterine alcohol exposure. A large variation of cerebral defects were described, most commonly microcephaly, cerebral dysgenesis and white matter heterotopia.

In his review "Recognition of fetal alcohol syndrome", Clarren (1981) reported on a 4 year-old girl with FAS, who died in a car accident. Her neuropathological findings were remarkably less severe. Besides microcephaly, a reduction in white matter and occasional occurrence of neuronal heterotopia were found [2].

In the vast majority of children with FASD, neuropathological changes are substantially less severe compared to the more serious disorders in the cases described by Pfeiffer and Wisniewski.

In 1984, the Ciba Foundation in London organised a symposium entitled *Mechanisms of alcohol damage in utero* [3]. Clinicians and researchers discussed this topic for several days. One of the results of this symposium was the insight that the damaging effect of alcohol as a teratogen is based on widely different mechanisms and that the timing of alcohol intake is crucial for different neuropathological changes.

At this symposium, Pratt et al. [4] discussed four potential mechanisms of damaging effects of alcohol and its metabolite acetaldehyde on the human central nervous system in the first trimester (Table 11.1).

Tab. 11.1: Time of damage during pregnancy (modified from [4]).

Time of damage	Probable mechanism	Consequences
Shortly after conception	Cell death or chromosomal damage	Early spontaneous abortion or restitutio ad integrum
After week 4 to 10	Cell loss due to cytotoxic processes, abnormal cell migration	Agenesis, heterotopia, brain malformations, microcephaly, characteristic FAS with mental deficits
After week 8 to 10	Delay of neuronal cell migration, resulting in abnormal formations of synapses	Behavioural disorders
Later	Damage of the hypothalamus, resulting in suppression of growth hormone	Overall growth reduction

11.3 Pathogenesis of FASD: evidence from animal studies

Today clinical research and, in particular, animal studies examining intrauterine alcohol exposure and its neurotoxic consequences are accepted worldwide and comprise various neuroanatomical, biochemical, genetic and epigenetic research fields. More than 30 years ago, James R. West (1981), an experienced researcher in neuroanatomy, reported, for the first time, changes of the cytoarchitecture of the hippocampus in animal studies after prenatal alcohol exposure [5].

In 1996, Band and J.R. West published a detailed review of neuropathology of FAS in animal models. They characterised time frames of particular vulnerability concerning development of neuronal populations in the cerebral cortex, hippocampus and cerebellum [6]. Nonetheless, the authors noted: "It is still unknown how the elevated blood alcohol during pregnancy causes permanent CNS damage in offspring".

Many different mechanisms of alcohol-neurotoxicity have been discussed, including hypoxia, glutamate or free radicals. It is still unknown, whether a single neurotoxic mechanism causes damage during different stages of brain development or whether several mechanisms, acting separately or together, are responsible for the brain impairment [6].

In a recent literature review, Berman et al. (2000) pointed out that the damage of the hippocampal structures explains several aspects of neurodevelopmental disturbances seen in FAS, particularly behavioural and attention problems, learning disabilities and disturbance of memory [7].

These neurodevelopmental malfunctions can be reproduced in animal studies. Impairment of the hippocampus, for example, has been documented in a reduced number of neurons, less morphological plasticity and a lower density of dendritic spines on the pyramidal cells.

The evidence of these pathological changes in the development and functioning of the hippocampus, as a central brain structure for memory, learning and emotions, leads to a better understanding of the problems persisting in fetal alcohol syndrome [8].

11.4 Neuroanatomical changes of dendritic spines

The surface of neurons contains small membranous protrusions, predominantly on the dendrites of different neurons, called spines (Figs. 11.2 and 11.3), which are an important connection between dendrites and axons. Dendritic spines are the anatomical correlate for synaptic transmission and enable transmission of electric signals from one neuron to another; they are crucially involved in brain functions like memory and cognition.

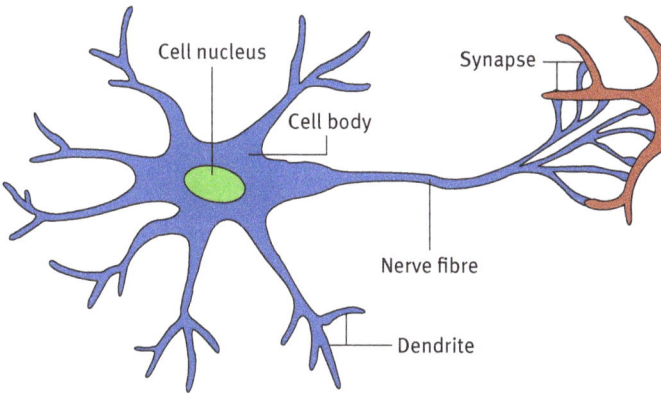

Fig. 11.2: Dendritic spine. A dendritic spine is a bulbous protrusion on the dendrites of a neuron. Spines are typically 0.2–2 µm long. In most cases, a synapse is present at the end of the spine, which transmits signals from one neuron to another. Many neurons have thousands of dendritic spines.

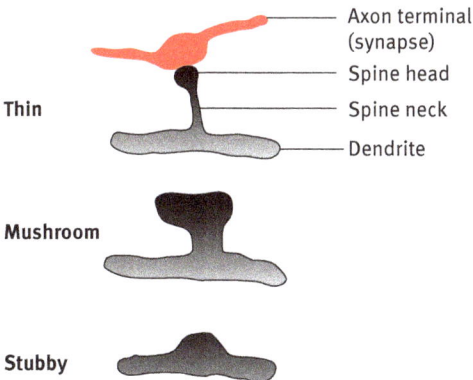

Fig. 11.3: Typical form and length of dendritic spines [9].

11.4.1 Spine dysgenesis

In 1974, Purpura [11] was the first to detect dendritic spines in the cortex of children with mental retardation and to show an irregular development of distortion and entanglement. This abnormal development led to a distinct functional reduction of synaptic connections with reduced neuronal signal transmissions. Purpura called this abnormal development "spine dysgenesis" and suspected that this abnormal dendritic development is responsible for the motor and cognitive deficits seen in acute and chronic neurological disorders. Spine dysgenesis seems to be a pathological microstructural finding common in children with severe mental retardation of unknown etiology (Fig. 11.4).

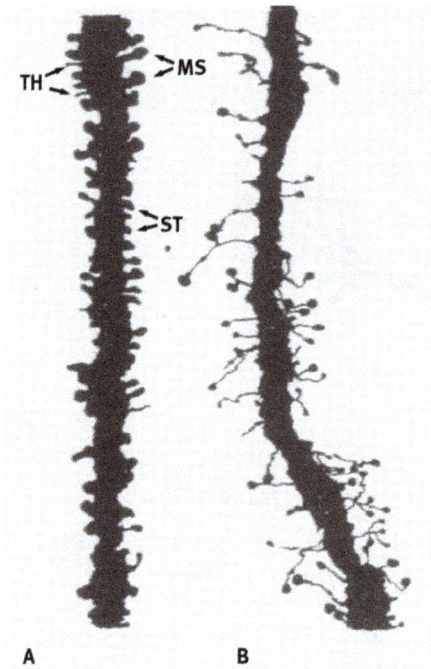

Fig. 11.4: Spine dysgenesis. A) Neurologically healthy 6 months old infant; B) 10 month old infant with severe mental retardation (Golgi stain of an apical dendrite in the motor cortex; camera lucida drawing) [11].

In animal studies, Stoltenburg-Didinger and Spohr (1983) investigated this potential mechanism as a possible explanation for mental retardation seen in FAS [10]. Pregnant Wistar rats received liquid nutrition with 35% of calories replaced by alcohol, and the dendritic spine distribution was examined on proximal apical dendrites of pyramid cells in the parietal cortex of their offspring. Using the Golgi method (Fig. 11.5), microscopic examination revealed a significant abnormal development of the dendritic spines in the brains exposed to intrauterine alcohol compared to healthy controls on days 12 and 40 after birth (Figs. 11.6 and 11.7). The spines were found to be abnormally thin, long, twisted and entangled at both timepoints. These anatomical changes of

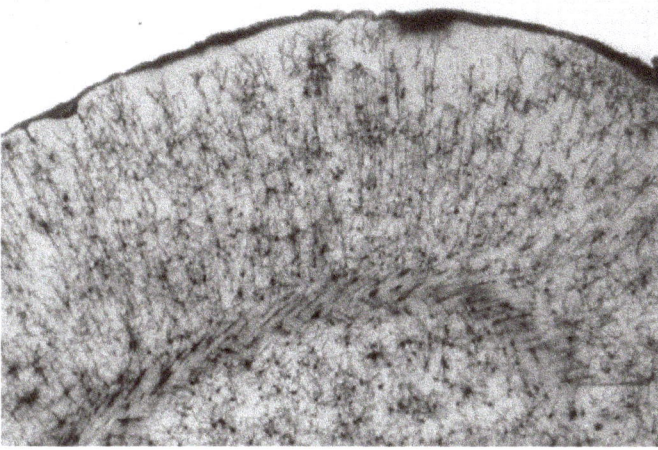

Fig. 11.5: Golgi staining of the motor cortex in an intrauterine alcohol exposed Wistar rat [10].

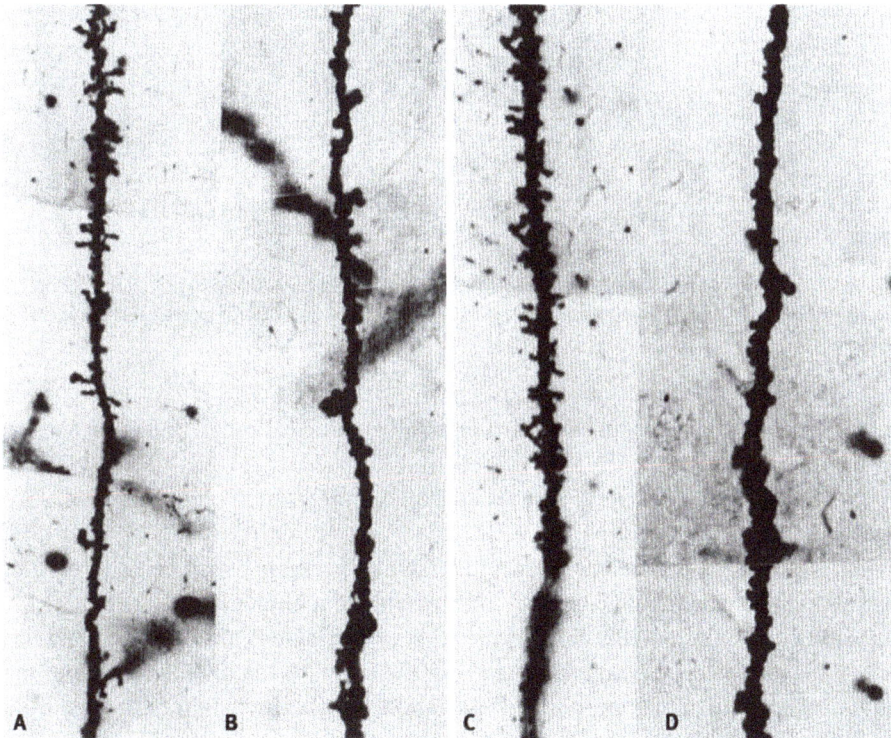

Fig. 11.6: Distribution and shape of dendritic spines in 12 day old rats: A) and C) prenatal alcohol exposed animal, B) and D) healthy animal [10].

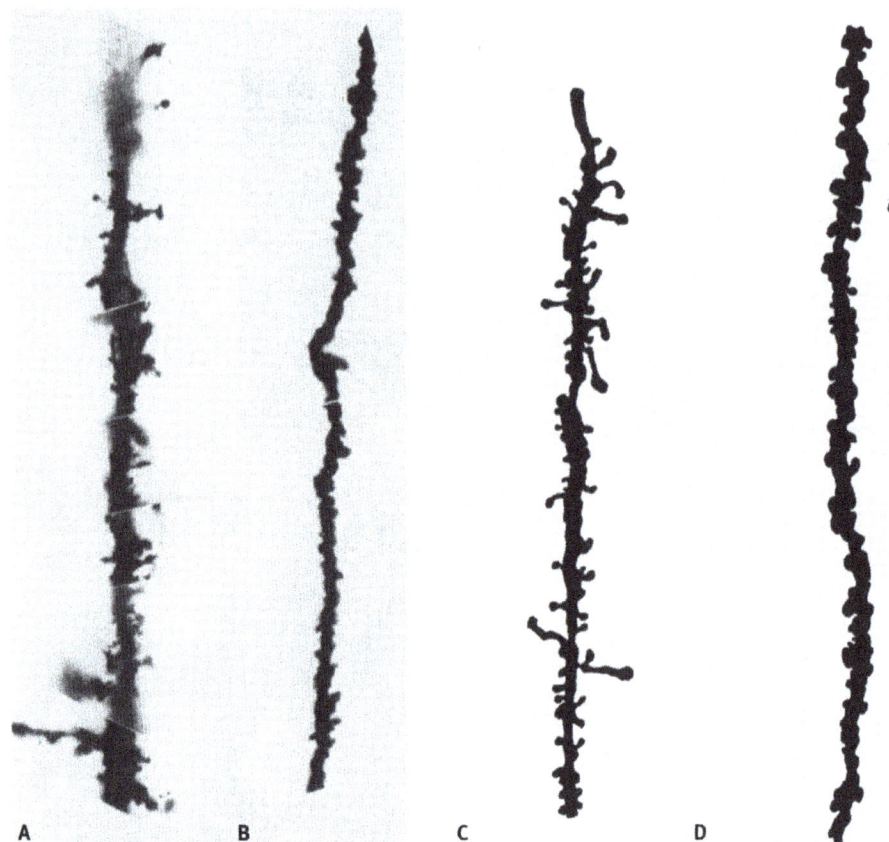

Fig. 11.7: Distribution and shape of dendritic spines in 40 day old rats: A) and C) prenatal alcohol exposed animal, B) and D) healthy animal; right side C) and D) drawn in with camera lucida for clarification [10]

intrauterine alcohol exposure in rats are a clearly in line with the "spine dysgenesis" theory of Purpura [11].

Already in 1981, West et al. described similar findings in the hippocampus of rat brains [5].

In summary, it can be stated that this "spine dysgenesis" may be an important pathomechanism of prenatal alcohol-induced brain impairment.

Ferrer and Galofré (1987) corroborated this hypothesis describing a 5 year old boy with FAS, who died in a traffic accident. For the first time, using Golgi staining, the authors were able to find morphological changes in humans similar to the dendritic spines as described in rats by Purpura (Fig. 11.8) [12].

In a recent study, Halpain et al. (2005) emphasised the importance of dendritic spines being microscopically highly specialised regions of neuronal membranes with a key position for information processing in the brain [13].

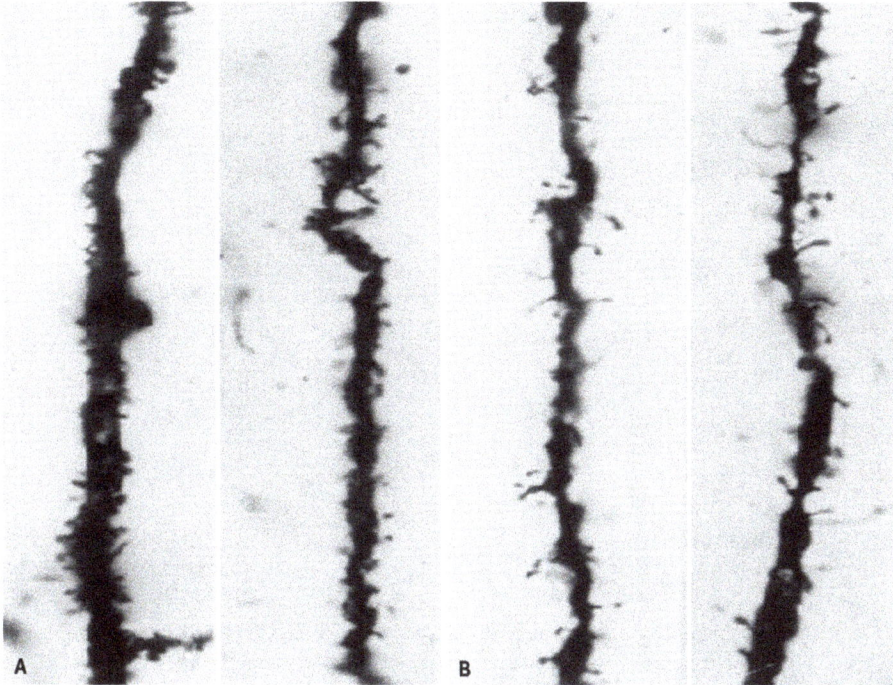

Fig. 11.8: Dendritic spine anomalies depicted with the Golgi method in the brain of A) 3 month old control patient and B) 4 month old child with FAS [12]

11.5 Alcohol-induced apoptosis

Despite intensive research on the pathogenesis of FAS, the underlying causes for the teratogenic effect of alcohol, which results in severe, probably lifelong impairments, are still largely unknown to date.

Ikonomidou et al. (2000) pursued a new research approach towards possible pathogenetic mechanisms explaining the teratogenic impairment. Using alcohol-exposed rats, they found that alcohol acting with a dual mechanism (blockade of N-methyl-D-aspartate glutamate receptors (NMDA) and activation of gamma-aminobutric acid (GABA)) triggers widespread apoptotic neurodegeneration in the developing rat brain [14].

In general, apoptosis is induced by genetically encoded intracellular signals and triggered by a biochemical pathway leading to a programmed "cell suicide".

Neuronal apoptosis is a highly regulated and controlled process in normal brain development and keeps a balance between cell multiplication (proliferation) and destruction (elimination). If this balance is disturbed, for example, due to intrauterine alcohol exposure, apoptotic changes may occur and, subsequently, lead to brain dysfunction [14].

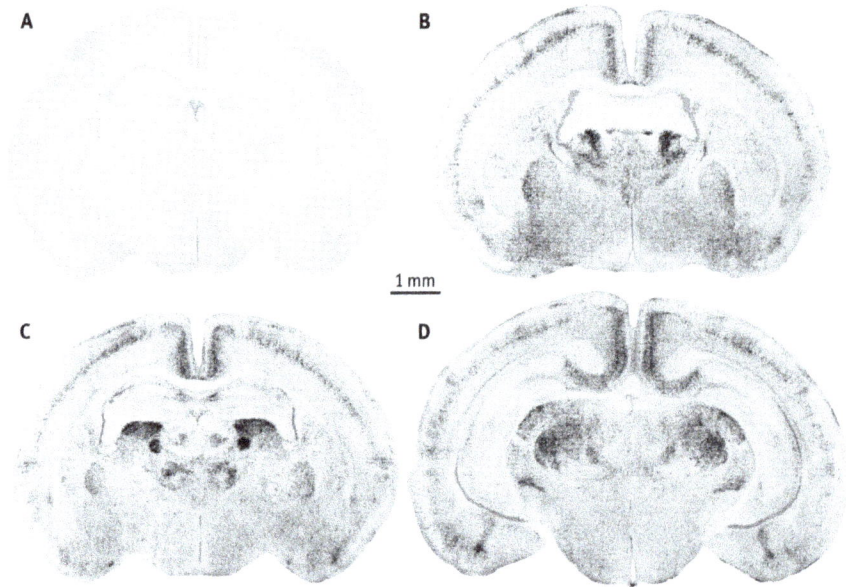

Fig. 11.9: Neurodegenerative pattern of alcohol-induced apoptosis in different slices of the frontal cortex of an 8-day-old mouse, 24 hours after an injection of (A) physiologic saline solution or (B–D) a saline solution with 20% alcohol (with the Olmos' cupric-silver method, which stains dying neurons, black after silver impregnation) [15].

Olney et al. found a clear bilateral staining of dying cells in alcohol-exposed animals compared to non-alcohol-exposed animals (Fig. 11.9), which is a sign of increased alcohol-induced apoptosis in the developing brain of mice [15].

During the spurt in brain growth, a highly sensitive developmental phase (in humans from the 25–26th week of pregnancy until the beginning of the third year of life, and in rats the 6–10th day of life), extensive cell death takes place. During this period of rapid growth, neurons of early synaptogenesis and glial cells responsible for myelination of axons are highly sensitive and susceptible to damage from external factors, e.g. alcohol, nicotine or certain pharmaceutical drugs. In neuronal cells the connection to synapses are apparently programmed genetically following a given time schedule. Deviations in this process trigger intrinsic signals inducing excessive cell death ("suicide").

Apoptosisis an intensive physiological process in the growing brain, and millions of normal neurons perish – in certain brain regions up to 30% of cells.

The authors hypothesised that alcohol-induced extreme neuroapoptosis may be responsible for microcephaly and neuropsychiatric and neurocognitive disorders often seen in FAS. They further assumed that not the total amount of alcohol, but the duration of toxic blood alcohol levels are responsible for the cell damage [14, 15].

Farber et al. (2010), working on alcohol-induced neuroapoptosis in primates (macaque monkeys) found that after 8 hours of fetal alcohol exposure the same severe neuroapoptosis occurred in the primate brain as previously seen in experiments with mice. The apoptosis in the alcohol-exposed animals increased by up to 60-fold compared to control animals. The authors suggest, similar to hypothesis of Iconomidou et al., that this mechanism is the explanation for many neuroanatomical changes and neuropsychiatric disorders associated with FAS [16].

11.6 Brain imaging techniques

With the introduction of magnetic resonance tomography, a new imaging method (MRI) was available to study and diagnose structural changes in the human brain.

In 1996, Johnson et al. were the first to document various CNS-malformations in 10 children with FAS. They demonstrated hypoplasia and agenesis of the corpus callosum and the cavum septum pellucidum, enlargement of the ventricles and brain stem hypoplasia. All children suffered from microcephaly, definite cognitive deficits and problems in motor coordination [17].

From the very beginning of the use of MRI examinations, the abnormal shape of the corpus callosum was noted in patients with FASD. Often it was inconsistently reduced in volume or even absent in some cases, but distinct and consistent changes of the corpus callosum were not observed.

Agenesisor an anomalous shape of the corpus callosum may be associated with mental retardation but also occurs occasionally in healthy individuals of normal intelligence and was also seen in patients suffering from ADHD [18]. The corpus callosum seems to be an area of the brain especially vulnerable to prenatal alcohol exposure [25]; nevertheless, MRI examination of this area is uninformative and not helpful in a definite diagnosis of FASD.

In their review "A decade of brain imaging" Riley et al. (2004) described structural abnormalities in various regions of the brain, including the cerebellum, corpus callosum and the basal ganglia, with different degrees of severity after intrauterine alcohol exposition [19]. The most consistent finding in this review was a reduction in the size of the brain, which was more severe in children with FAS compared to children with pFAS. In addition, the cerebellum showed a greater reduction (15%) in children with FAS than in children with pFAS, and compared to healthy controls the cerebellum was still significantly smaller in children with pFAS.

Furthermore, MRI examinations revealed brain damage caused by prenatal alcohol exposure that fortell the risk of lifelong disturbances in brain development. Particularly affected are the frontal and parietal lobes corresponding to areas associated with neurocognitive deficits and functional disorders. Using novel brain imaging techniques, the authors found "displacements in the corpus callosum, increased gray matter densities in both hemispheres, in the perisylvian regions, and altered gray matter asymmetry in portions of the temporal lobes in the brains of alcohol-exposed subjects". Additionally, they observed a reduction in brain growth in portions of the frontal lobe [19].

In a large multicentre study from 2012, initiated by the Collaborative Initiative on Fetal Alcohol Spectrum Disorders (CIFASD) and supported by the National Institute on Alcohol and Alcohol Abuse (NIAAA), data of 56 adolescent patients with severe prenatal exposure to alcohol and of 43 healthy controls were collected. Participants came from three different areas, i.e. Los Angeles and San Diego (California, USA) and Cape Town (South Africa). Using brain imaging methods (MRI), the authors analysed and examined the relationship between damaged brain regions, neurocognitive dysfunction, facial dysmorphology and the amount of maternal alcohol consumed during the first trimester [20]. They found a highly significant reduction in the FASD group for all regions of the brain evaluated.

In particular, shorter palpebral fissureswere significantly associated with a reduced volume of the ventral diencephalon. Greater dysmorphology of the philtrum predicted smaller volumes in the basal ganglia and diencephalon. Furthermore, lower IQ was associated with smaller basal ganglia volumes and more severe facial dysmorphology.

In patients from Cape Town, detailed data of maternal drinking behaviour were gathered, and the authors found a direct negative correlation between intracranial volume and the total amount of drinks per week.

These striking findings confirm the close relationship between facial dysmorphology and intracerebral changes in the diencephalon and basal ganglia, which seem to be responsible for many of the neurocognitive disorders described in FAS [20].

11.7 Disturbances in brain metabolism

An additional contribution towards neuropathological changes was made by investigation of possible disturbances in brain metabolism. Fagerlund et al. (2006) were the first to use magnetic resonance spectroscopy (MRS) imaging, which determines metabolite concentrations *in vivo* in different tissues. With this method they investigated brain regions particularly sensible to the teratogenic effects of alcohol in a sample of ten adolescents and adults. Metabolite ratios for N-acetylaspartate and choline (NAA/CO) and N-acetylaspartate and creatine(NAA/CR) were determined. They were able to verify disturbances in brain metabolism in alcohol exposed patients compared to healthy controls, i.e. low ratios for NAA/CO and NAA/CR in the parietal lobe, frontal lobe, frontal lobe white matter, corpus callosum, thalamus and the cerebellum – persistent changes in brain metabolism due to prenatal alcohol exposure, which were still measurable in adulthood [22].

Another method for studying brain metabolism is functional magnetic resonance imaging (fMRI). This method uses the different magnetic sensitivities of oxygenated and deoxygenated blood (BOLD-contrast, *blood-oxygen-level-dependent*). Localised neuronal activation in the brain leads to increased hemoglobin concentration and as such to a higher oxygen blood concentration changing the MR-signal (Fig. 11.10).

Using this imaging technique, Spandoni et al. (2009) examined the functional brain activity of 10 patients with prenatal alcohol exposure compared to a sample of healthy controls while processing the same cognitive task (*spatial working memory task*) [23]. Comparing the FAS group to healthy controls, the fMRI examination revealed a much more intensive and widespread brain activity in multiple brain regions in the FAS group (Fig. 11.10). The authors concluded that these current findings could

A Healthy control group

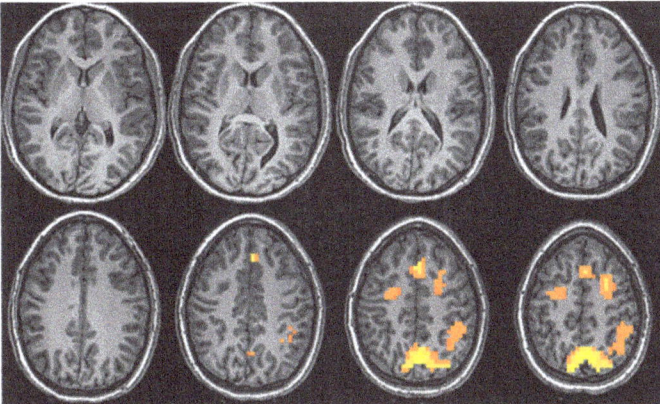

B Intrauterine alcohol-exposed group

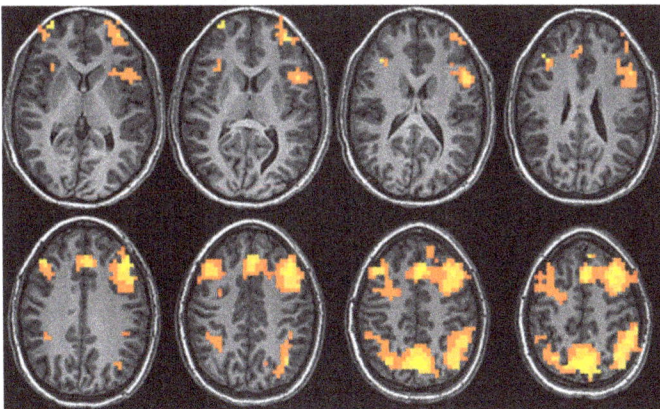

Fig. 11.10: A total of 22 adolescents (prenatal alcohol exposure $n = 10$; healthy controls $n = 12$) between the ages of 10 and 18 processing a spatial working memory task in the MRI scanner (fMRT). Results: The alcohol-exposed group showed an increased activation of the brain, in frontal, temporal, occipital and subcortical regions compared to the healthy control group [23].

either indicate a decreased efficiency of the relevant brain network or function as a compensation mechanism for neuronal and/or cognitive insufficiency. With regard to the existing fMRI evidence of higher prefrontal activation in response to verbal working memory and inhibition demand, the present result may suggest that frontal structures are strained considerably more during cognitive demand in prenatal alcohol exposed individuals.

In a recent study examining children with FAS, Norman et al. (2013) used fMRI and also proved higher activation in the frontal lobe while processing a spatial working memory task. Based on their findings, they concluded that the left middle and superior frontal region seems to be especially affected in intrauterine alcohol-exposed children [24].

Astley et al. (2009) examined 81 prenatal alcohol exposed adolescent and adult patients, selected from a large sample of children, as well as healthy controls. Subjects were categorised in the following three diagnostic groups and one control group:
1. FAS / pFAS n = 16
2. static encephalopathy (SE) n = 22
3. neurobehavioural disorder n = 20
4. healthy control group n = 13.

The participants underwent an extensive neuropsychological, psychiatric examination during fMRI. An extensive neuropsychological/psychiatric battery combined with MRI assessments was implemented. The FAS/pFAS group had smaller frontal lobes compared to other groups. Significant correlations were found between size of the total brain, frontal lobe, caudate, putamen, hippocampus, cerebellar vermis and corpus callosum and the level of clinical CNS deformation. The authors concluded that in patients presenting with more severe symptoms, the MRI results were increasingly pathological. However, fMRI examinations cannot be used as an individual diagnostic tool, as long as normal brain development is undefined [21].

Considering these results, the diverse changes in brain morphology, responsible for the CNS dysfunction, seem to be generally a more local than a global brain impairment [19].

Bibliography

[1] Peiffer J, Majewski F, Fischbach H, Bierich JR, Volk B. Alcohol embryo and fetopathy: Neuropathology of 3 children and 3 fetuses. J Neurol Sci 1979, 41, 125–137.
[2] Clarren SK. Recognition of fetal alcohol syndrome. JAMA 1981, 245(23), 2436–2439.
[3] Ciba Foundation. Mechanism of alcohol damage in utero. Pitman, London 1984.
[4] Pratt OE. Introduction: what do we know of the mechanism of alcohol damage in utero? In: Ciba Foundation Symposion 105. Mechanism of alcohol damage in utero. Pitman, London 1984, 1–7.

[5]   West JR, Hodges CA, Black AC Jr. Prenatal exposure to ethanol alters the organization of hippo-
      campal mossy fibers in rats. Science 1981, 211, 957–959.
[6]   Band LC, West JR. Neuropathology in experimental fetal alcohol syndrome. In: Spohr HL, Stein-
      hausen HC (eds). Alcohol, Pregnancy and the Developing Child. Cambridge University Press,
      Cambridge 1996.
[7]   Berman RF, Hannigan JH. Effects of prenatal alcohol exposure on the hippocampus: spatial
      behavior, electropyhsiology, and neuroanatomy. Hippocampus 2000, 10(1), 94–110.
[8]   Gil-Mohapel J, Boehme F, Kainer L, Christie BR. Hippocampal loss and neurogenesis after fetal
      alcohol exposure: insights from different rodent models. Brain Research Reviews 2010, 64,
      283–303.
[9]   Peters A, Kaisermann-Abramof IR. The small pyramidal neuron of the rat cerebral cortex. The
      perikaryon dentrites and spines. Am J Anat 1970, 127(4), 321–355.
[10] Stoltenburg-Didinger G, Spohr HL. Fetal alcohol syndrome: spine distribution of pyramidal
      cells in prenatal alcohol-exposed rat cerebral cortex; a Golgi study. Developmental Brain Re-
      search 1983, 11, 119–123.
[11] Purpura DP. Dendritic spine 'dysgenesis' and mental retardation. Science 1974, 186, 1126–
      1128.
[12] Ferrer I, Galofré E. Dendritic Spine anomalies in Fetal Alcohol syndrome. Neuropediatrics 1987,
      18, 161–163.
[13] Halpain S, Sprencer K, Graber S. Dynamics and pathology of dendritic spines. Progress in
      Brain Research 2005, 147, 29–37.
[14] Ikonomidou C, Bittigau P, Ishimaru MJ, Wozniak DF Koch C et al. Ethanol-induced apoptotic
      neurodegeneration and the fetal alcohol syndrome. Science 2000, 287, 1056–1060.
[15] Olney J, Tenkova T, Tikranian K, Qin Y-Q, Labruyere J, Ikonomidou C. Ethanol-induced apoptotic
      neurodegeration in the developing C57BL/6 mouse brain. Developmental brain Research 2002,
      133(2), 115–126.
[16] Farber NB, Creeley CE, Olney JW. Alcohol-induced neuroapoptosis in the fetal macaque brain.
      Neurobiol Dis 2010, 40(1), 200–206.
[17] Johnson VP, Swayze VW II, Sato Y, Andreasen NC. Fetal Alcohol Syndrome: Craniofacial and
      Central Nervous System Manifestations. American Journal of Medical Genetics 1996, 61, 329–
      339.
[18] Hynd GW, Semrud-Clikeman M, Lorys AR, Novey ES, Eliopulos D, Lyytinen H. Corpus callosum
      morphology in attention deficit-hyperactivity disorder: morphometric analysis of MRI. J Learn
      Disabil 1990, 24, 141–146.
[19] Riley EP, McGee CL, Sowell ER. Teratogenic Effects of Alcohol. A decade of brain Imaging. Amer-
      ican Journal of Medical Genetics Part C Semin Med Genet 2004, 127C, 35–41.
[20] Roussotte FF, Sulik KK, Mattson SN, Riley EP, Jones KL et al. Regional Brain Volume Reductions
      Relate to Facial Dysmorphology and Neurocognitive Function in Fetal Alcohol Spectrum Dis-
      orders. Human Brain Mapping 2012, 33, 920–937.
[21] Astley SJ, Aylward EH, Olson HC etal. Magnetic Resonance Imaging Outcomes From a Com-
      prehensive Magnetic Resonance Study of Children With Fetal Alcohol Sprectrum Disorders.
      Alcoholism: Clinical and Experimental Research 2009, 33(10), 1671–1689.
[22] Fagerlund A, Heikkinen S, Autti-Rämö I et al. Brain Metabolic Alterations in Adolescents and
      Young Adults with Fetal Alcohol Spectrum Disorders. Alcoholism: Clinical and Experimental
      Research 2006, 30(12), 2097–2104.
[23] Spandoni AD, Bazinet AD, Fryer SL et al. BOLD Response During Spatial Working Memory in
      Youth with Heavy prenatal Alcohol Exposure. Alcoholism: Clinical and experimental research
      2009, 33(12), 2067–2076.

[24] Norman AL, O'Brian JW, Spadoni AD, Jones KL, Riley EP, Mattson SN. A functional magnetic resonance imaging study of spatial working memory in children with prenatal alcohol exposure: contribution of familial history of alcohol use disorders. Alcohol Clin Exp Res. 2013, 37 (1), 132–140.

[25] Wisniewski K, Cambska H, Sher JH, Qazi Q. A clinical neuropathological study of the fetal alcohol syndrome. Neuropediatrics 1983, 14, 197–201.

12 Genetic and epigenetic aspects of fetal alcohol syndrome

12.1 Genetics

Diagnosis of FAS quite often raises some doubt as to whether it is more likely a genetic syndrome rather than teratogenic exposure.

The following example illustrates the importance of such a genetic consultation.

Case report

In our clinic, a 5-year-old male was referred with a question from his foster parents about whether he suffered from FAS, in the presence of his birth mother. Due to his conspicuous facial features, other diagnostic institutions had already suspected the diagnosis FAS. The foster parents had pushed the birth mother to "admit" to alcohol abuse. The biological mother, however, denied any abuse of alcohol during the pregnancy and insisted on suffering from similar conspicuous features since childhood.

Dysmorphic facial features of patient A.:

- a large, slightly bulbous tip of the nose
- large protruding ears
- a long flat philtrum, thin upper lip
- short hands and feet, slight deformation and axis deviation of the fingers
- thin blonde hair
- growth retardation

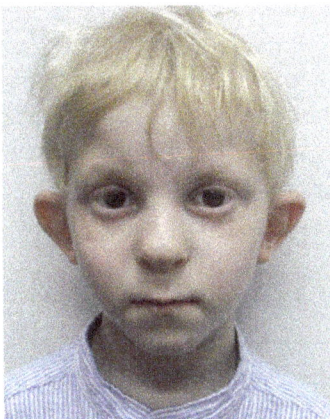

Fig. 12.1: Trichorhinophalangeal syndrome type I.

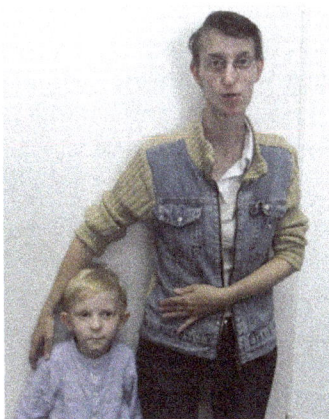

Fig. 12.2: Son and mother suffer from trichorhinophalangeal syndrome type I.

https://doi.org/10.1515/9783110436563-012

Because of the striking similarities between mother and child, a genetic syndrome was suspected, and the child was referred to the Institute of Medical Genetics and Human Genetics, Charité, Berlin. Trichorhinophalangeal syndrome type I (see Fig. 12.1 and 12.2) was diagnosed.

Trichorhinophalangeal syndrome type I

Trichorhinophalangeal syndrome type I is a rare autosomal dominant syndrome with normal life expectancy and with distinct dysmorphic features, including large bulbous tip of the nose, protruding ears, long flat philtrum, thin upper lip, sparse and thin hair; a short stature, short hands and feet, deformed fingers and toes with cone-shaped epiphysis at the phalanges.

In 2013, Douzgou et al. [1] examined 80 children and adolescents with a suspected diagnosis of FAS, who were referred for genetic investigation to the University of Manchester between 2004 and 2010. FAS was confirmed in 20% of the children. Out of 80 patients, 7 (8.75%), however, received diagnoses related to chromosomal disorders, which were all accompanied by additional behavioural and cognitive problems (three patients with 22q11 microdeletion syndrome, one patient with 14q21 syndrome, one patient with 2p16.1-p15 deletion syndrome, one with 15q13.3 microdeletion syndrome and one with 1q21 microduplication syndrome). The authors concluded that chromosome disorders showed phenotypic overlap with FASD and are an important differential diagnosis.

Streissguth and Dehaene [2] investigated a further genetic aspect in their clinical study with twins of chronic alcoholic mothers. The teratogenic effects of alcohol could vary according to fetal genetic sensitivity.

In a sample of 16 twin pairs – 5 monozygotic (identical) twins and 11 dizygotic (fraternal) twins – they found that all monozygotic twins had the same diagnosis, including similar IQ scores, and as such were concordant with each other. The dizygotic twins, on the other hand, were only partly concordant (7 out of 11 twin pairs), the other twin pairs (4 out of 11) were disconcordant with different manifestations of the syndrome (Table 12.1). Despite equivalent alcohol exposure within twin pairs, teratogeni-

Tab. 12.1: Different expression of intrauterine alcohol damage in monozygotic and dizygotic twin pairs (adapted from [2]).

16 Twin pairs		
5 monozygotic twin pairs	11 dizygotic twin pairs	
concordant 5/5	concordant 7/11	disconcordant 4/11
2 FAS/FAS	4 FAS/FAS	2 FAS/FAE
1 pFAS/pFAS	1 pFAS/pFAS	2 pFAS/no visible damage
2 no visible damage	2 no visible damage	

city was more uniform in monozygotic than in dizygotic twins. The authors concluded that modulating effects of genetic background underlie the differential expression of the teratogenic effects of alcohol.

In sum, intrauterine alcohol exposure is etiologic in impaired development, and genetic variation impacts the manifestation in the individual.

12.2 Epigenetics

In the last decade, epigenetics has become a central topic in the field of genetics. Epigenetics investigates cell characteristics that are passed on to daughter cells without alteration in actual DNA sequence. Epigenetic modifications are stable, but potentially reversible and can be triggered by the environment, this connecting external influences with the genome in trait or disease expression. Heritable changes may occur in gene expression resulting from DNA methylation or histone modification.

The recent scientific interest in epigenetics is essentially based on the fact that epigenetics is a crucial link between environmental influences and gene function [3].

This area of study offers new conceptual approaches to understand genetic regulation of developmental processes and disease mechanisms that are potentially reversible and can be influenced by environmental or developmental factors over lifetime. In this way, epigenetics provides new approaches to detect the influence of environmental factors on the genome.

The large variety of symptoms seen in fetal alcohol spectrum disorders suggest that the effects of prenatal alcohol exposure are not only a consequence of the teratogenic effects of alcohol but rather a combined result of teratogenicity, genetics, epigenetics and environmental influences. The complex molecular basis that leads to the development of FASD and the exact mechanisms that induce teratogenic effects are however, still poorly understood.

DNA methylation or modifications of other proteins create epigenetic markers, which are very stable, easy to detect and useful for population-based epigenetic studies.

A wide range of environmental factors, i.e. cigarettes, alcohol, foods, hunger and interpersonal relationships, can influence these epigenetic markers [3].

In a review from 2009, Haycock reported teratogenic consequences of alcohol exposure during specific developmental periods including associated epigenetic reprogramming:

1. genome-wide demethylation during preimplantation
2. genome-wide de novo methylation during gastrulation
3. dynamic epigenetic changes (de novo methylation and demethylation) in the germline.

Haycock indicated that alcohol might induce preconceptual epigenetic changes in the germline and, therefore, the concept of etiology of FASD has to be extended to this period [4].

Results from animal studies

Epigenetic research in the pathogenesis of FASD is largely based on animal studies. These experiments were able to show that maternal alcohol consumption during pregnancy results in an "epigenetic signature" in the genome of the newborn [5]. Although results from animal experiments can only be transferred to humans with caution, epigenetic changes in newborns might be used as a biomarker for the early detection of FAS in humans [6].

In a mouse model for FASD, Zhou et al. (2011) were able to show for the first time that alcohol exposure during early neurulation can induce changes in DNA methylation, resulting in the potentially observed abnormal fetal development [5].

Recent clinical examinations

The possibility to transfer results obtained from experimental animal studies in FAS to humans was the aim of a large Canadian multicentre research project initiated in 2011 [8]. In this study, subjects between the ages of 5 to 18 with confirmed intrauterine alcohol exposure are examined neurologically and compared to healthy controls. In addition, hormonal, geneticand epigenetic analyses are performed. Imaging methods are used to examine the relationship between structural alterations in the brain and functional outcome.

The goal of this comprehensive study is to identify genetic and epigenetic modifications possibly associated with behavioural and neurobiological dysfunction caused by intrauterine alcohol effect. The discovery of genetic and epigenetic markers to predict the severity of behavioural and cognitive deficits would clearly improve identification of children at risk [8].

Finally, Laufer et al. [9] recently reported unique DNA methylation defects in the mucosa of children with FASD, which could be influenced by sex and medication exposure. The authors suggest hopefully, "With future clinical development, assessment of DNA methylation from buccal swabs will provide a novel strategy for the diagnosis of FASD" [9].

Bibliography

[1] Douzgou S, Breen C, Crow YJ et al. Diagnosing foetal alcohol syndrome: new insights from newer genetic technologies. Arch Dis Child 2012, 97, 812–817.
[2] Streissguth AP, Dehaene P. Fetal alcohol syndrome in twins of alcoholic mothers: Concordance of diagnosis and IQ. American Journal of Medical Genetics 1993, 47, 857–861.

[3] Ramsay M. Genetic and epigenetic insights into fetal alcohol spectrum disorders. Genom Medicine 2010, 2, 27–34.

[4] Haycock PC. Fetal Alcohol Spectrum Disorders: The Epigenetic Perspective. Biology of Reproduction 2009, 81, 607–617.

[5] Zhou FC, Balaraman Y, Teng M, Liu Y, Singh RP, Nephew KP. Alcohol alters DNA mythylation patterns and inhibits neural stern cell differentiation. Alcohol Clin Exp Res 2011, 35(4), 735–746.

[6] Kobor MS, Weinberg J. Spectrum Disorders Epigenetics in Fetal Alcohol Spectrum Disorders. Alcohol Res Health 2012, 34(1).

[7] Resendiz M, Chen Y, Oztürk NC, Zhou FC. Epigenetic medicine and fetal alcohol spectrum disorders. Epigenetics 2013, 5(1), 73–86.

[8] Reynolds JN, Weinberg J, Clarren S et al. Fetal Alcohol Spectrum Disorders: Gene-Enviroment Interactions, Predictive Biomarkers, and the Relationship Between Structural Alerations in the Brain and Functional Outcomes. Semin Pediatr Neurol 2011, 1, 49–55.

[9] Laufer BI, Kapalanga J, Castellani CA, Diehl EJ, Yan L, Singh, SM. Associative DNA methylation changes in children with prenatal alcohol exposure. Epigenomics 2015, 7(8), 1259–1274.

Part III: **The fetal alcohol syndrome in adulthood**

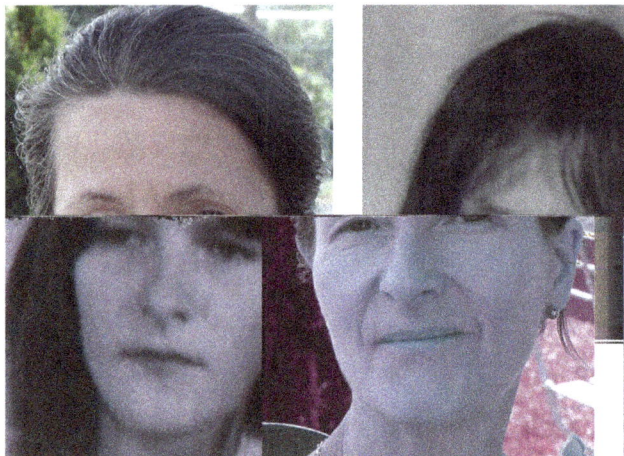

Life story of a 49-year-old women with FAS

Life felt to be always very exhausting to me but I assumed that's quite normal for any-body, and I only need the strength to withstand it. However, with regard to the last years or even the last decades, it seems to me that each damned day has been a struggle to get along with daily demands, and I never felt comfortable, safe or relaxed.

From an early age I was told that I'm too lazy, unmotivated, inattentive and pass-ive without any interest, but I was only unable to deal with the demands of everyday life appropriately – in short: that I could do everything properly if I only would; ac-cording to others, I'm just unwilling. From my point of view, everything was irritating and inscrutable.

I was unable to understand what others expected from me, and I made every effort to meet daily requirements, but nobody noticed it. I was judged on my performance always, and I performed only moderately or even badly. If I sometimes did well, every-one concluded that I was just unwilling to do my best after all.

For years I couldn't understand why I was unable to keep to the point, to man-age time, to comply to appointments and obligations, to plan ahead; why I always loose important things of daily life, why I break appointments, why I neglect a prom-ise or why I'm always getting into dire straits when I have to make a decision. I often wondered, why I'm so slow in understanding, why it is mostly impossible for me to grasp the sense of what is said to me or to follow conversations. I'm wondering, why it is so difficult to learn new things, and to accept responsibility, why I'm easily upset by even little changes in daily routine and why I'm easily fooled into doing something stupid with always the same bad consequences.

Why, why, why – I didn't find any answer. I always tried hard and I always failed miserably, again and again. Finally, I was frustrated, discouraged and depressed.

One day, when I was on the Internet, I found information about disturbances in ex-ecutive functions and I was surprised about the striking similarities with regard to my difficulties. Searching for underlying causes for executive dysfunction, I found pages about alcohol consumption during pregnancy and its far-reaching consequences. I could hardly believe what I read, but for sure all described problems were aligned with my difficulties; this was, indeed, the answer to all my problems.

I remembered that my mother once told me that being pregnant she didn't eat enough but rather had drunken alcohol to console herself for the unwanted pregnancy. My father confirmed that my mother was drinking a lot already before becoming pregnant.

I never attached any importance to these statements. Until now I had been unable to establish a relation between all of my problems and difficulties and the drinking behaviour of my mother especially during pregnancy.

The fact that my mother drank alcohol during pregnancy without considering the developing, unwelcomed child was hard to take and sorrowful.

I now remembered the words of my mother describing me when I was a child: way too little and thin, an always-vomiting child and therefore, feeding me was a torture. Furthermore, she told me that I was delayed in overall development, always hyperactive and restless. She always had to keep sight of me because I ran away from home and behaved riskily. In her words, my head was way too small, with sparse hair, and I was said to have had a baby doll face.

Is it really true that I suffer from symptoms caused by prenatal alcohol exposure?

The overwhelming facts indicated a possible diagnosis of FAS, thus I made an appointment with Prof. Spohr in Berlin.

Finally at the age of 49, I received the diagnosis of fetal alcohol syndrome.

On one hand, it was now a relief to know that I was not responsible for my numerous difficulties since early childhood and, on the other hand, I had to deal with the fact that I had to shoulder the consequences of the misconduct of my mother; I painfully had to accept that my mother who damaged me whilst drinking alcohol during pregnancy, blamed me for being different and for having learning difficulties from the very beginning.

I was hardly able to endure the pain and to deal with the fact that all my difficulties and inabilities are attributable to the underlying brain damage caused by intrauterine alcohol exposure.

But the diagnosis of FAS was also kind of a late acquittal for my inability to behave and act adequately, and I no longer feel guilty about my problems in getting along with the requirements of everyday life anymore.

Tasks necessitating step-by-step procedures are particularly difficult for me. Even when I manage to start a task, I often get stuck at the next step and forget everything again. Hence, a lot of things remain unfinished and I get confused. My apartment is in a permanent state of a complete mess; I'm unable to clean up. I am constantly searching for the things I need, I can't find important documents and I don't know where I leave things. I really want to reduce the chaos and to clean up my apartment but when I'm starting in one corner, the chaos increases in another.

It is very difficult to start on a required task, but once I manage to start an activity it is nearly impossible to interrupt or change task. To manage several tasks one at a time doesn't work at all unless someone instructs me, and I'm always totally exhausted.

I particularly get into difficulties if time management is necessary because it is nearly impossible to prepare myself for an appointment and not forget the time. I'm unable to do things simultaneously. When I am busy, I have no sense of time, which means that I don't realise that time is passing, and I'm unable to estimate the length of time.

If I need to meet a schedule or to keep an appointment, I easily get into trouble and finally I'm unable to notice what is happening in my surroundings.

Years of excessive demands have exhausted me fundamentally. I'm always tired and unable do concentrate. Due to the permanent mental stress and pressure I now also suffer from bulimia and depression and I have to cope with a complex post-traumatic stress disorder.

Every new day is a real effort for me; I'm fully engaged with daily routine and unable to handle any additional tasks.

I'm sure my dream to live a normal live will never come true.

To demand a hurdle race from someone who is physically disabled would be absurd, but this is exactly what happens to me, again and again. This damned disability is invisible to others and, therefore, "non-existent", but nonetheless I'm faced with my disability constantly; day by day from morning till night.

13 Fetal alcohol syndrome in adults ("FAS adult")

13.1 Introduction

About 20 years after the first description of FAS, physicians, caretakers and parents realised that many of the adolescents and young adults diagnosed during childhood still continued to suffer from the syndrome. Despite a reduction of clinical symptomsand especially the craniofacial features, these patients were still struggling with intellectual disability and many behavioural abnormalities. Although many of them had been supported for years, for the most part they were unable to live an age appropriate and independent life.

It became evident that this disorder, previously considered to be a pediatric disease, was in fact a syndrome with long lasting consequences even in adolescence and adulthood. Parents, caretakers and physicians were faced with a great new challenge.

13.2 Longitudinal studies in the United States, France, Finland and Germany

Streissguth et al. (1985) reported the further development of the 11 children who in 1973 were the first to be diagnosed as having FAS. Out of these 11 patients, 8 were re-examined, 2 had died and 1 was lost to follow-up. All eight children were still living with their foster or adoptive parents. The children remained dysmorphic and suffered from growth deficiency. [1].

In 1992, Lemoine et al. re-examined 99 adult patients from their original sample of 1968 [2]. In the meantime, many of these patients lived in psychiatric institutions. Apart from a number of psychiatric disorders, the authors noticed a high rate of suicides. For these adults, intellectual disability and persistent behavioural abnormalities proved to be the most severe problems. Sixteen adults of Lemoine's cohort with behavioural problems and developmental delay in childhood without the characteristic craniofacial dysmorphism, actually suffered from the same distinct behavioural abnormalities and significant concentration difficulties compared to adults with the classic features of FAS. Interestingly, the birth mothers of this sample of patients without clinical dysmorphic features in childhood were proven to be chronic alcoholics. Findings of this re-examination were published in a French scientific journal [2] and went unnoticed, similar to the original description of the disorder. Five years later, it was Ann Streissguth who referred to this excellent and extensive follow-up study [3].

In 2006, Autti-Rämö et al. published a Finnish FASD study examining 77 older children and adolescents aged 8–20 years [14]. In addition to numerous severe or distinct malformations (see Chapter 6.2), the authors described prenatal growth retardationin 70% of the cases and microcephaly in 45%.

https://doi.org/10.1515/9783110436563-013

In a more recent longitudinal study from Sweden (Rangar *et al.*, 2015), the long-term effects of FAS on psychosocial development were examined. Seventy-nine patients with FAS were compared to a control group of unaffected adults [4]. The authors found that adults with FAS more frequently needed special education (25% vs. 2%), were unemployed (51% vs. 15%), received a disability pension (31% vs. 3%), were hospitalised for alcohol dependence (9% vs. 2%) and suffered from additional psychiatric disorders (33% vs. 5%). Interestingly, the frequency of criminal behaviour was not significantly higher in adults with FAS compared to the control population (28% vs. 20%) [4], which stands in contrast to a previously reported follow-up study from Streissguth, 1996 [7].

In 1993, we published a 10-year follow-up study of 60 patients in Berlin who had been diagnosed with FAS or pFAS at initial examination in early childhood. At the time of the 10-year follow-up, craniofacial abnormalities were reduced in this adolescent sample. Microcephaly, short stature and underweight were distinctly visible. Of these patients, 70% suffered from microcephaly, 60% from underweight, and growth deficiency was found in half of the patients. Particularly male patients were affected by growth retardation [5].

In contrast to our expectations, even cognitive abilities were still reduced, although all patients lived with their foster or adoptive parents and had obtained intensive support and assistance.

In fact, re-evaluation of intelligence levels in adolescence suggested a slight reduction compared to that in childhood (Table 13.1). In adolescence, 4 of 16 children with an average intelligence score showed a decline in performance, and also children with subnormal intelligence showed a further decline in intellectual ability [5].The adverse development of intelligence seemed to be caused mainly by disturbance of executive functions, persistent memory deficits, lack of concentration and behavioural problems, including ADHD. Despite the efforts of foster or adoptive parents, a lack of improvement in intelligence was disappointing, but nevertheless in line with results from the USA published by Streissguth et al. in 1991 [6].

Tab. 13.1: Long-term course of intelligence level.

Intelligence quotient (IQ) 10-year follow-up (*n* = 60)							
		Reexamination after 10 years					
Initial presentation		IQ 115–86	IQ 85–71	IQ 70–51	IQ 50–36	IQ 35–21	IQ < 20
IQ 115–86	*n* = 19	14	4	1	–	–	–
IQ 85–71	*n* = 19	1	15	2	1	–	–
IQ 70–51	*n* = 11	–	–	3	6	2	–
IQ 50–36	*n* = 3	–	–	–	2	1	–
IQ 35–21	*n* = 7	–	–	–	1	2	4
IQ < 20	*n* = 1	–	–	–	–	–	1

At initial presentation, 22 of 60 patients had an IQ score under 70. At follow-up examination 10 years later, 26 of 60 patients still showed an IQ score of 70 or below.

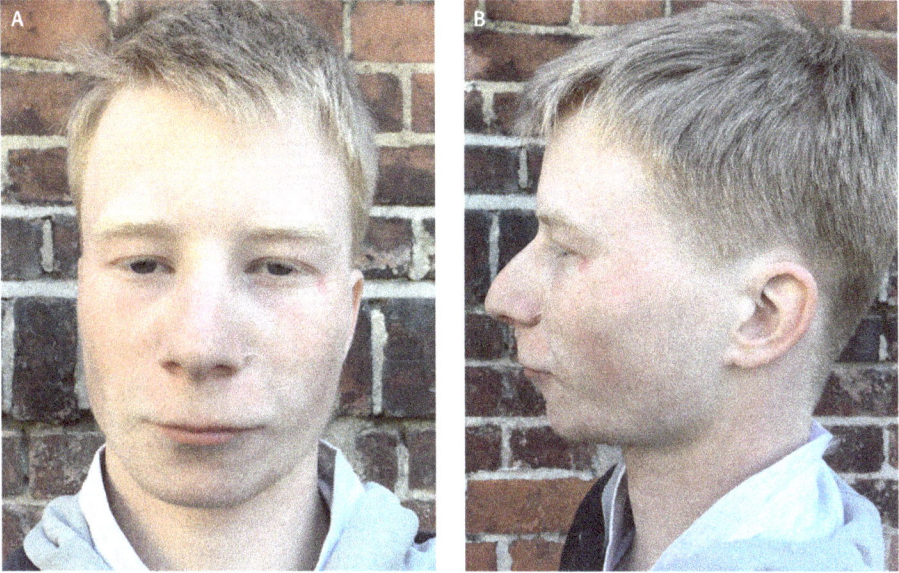

Fig. 13.1: FAS adult, 21-year-old patient (A) full face, (B) profile.

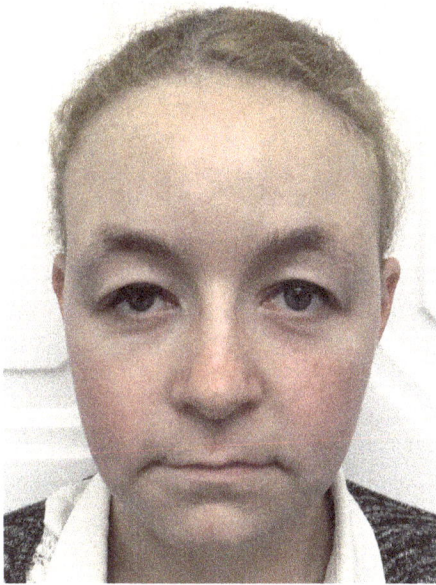

Fig. 13.2: FAS adult, 26-year-old woman.

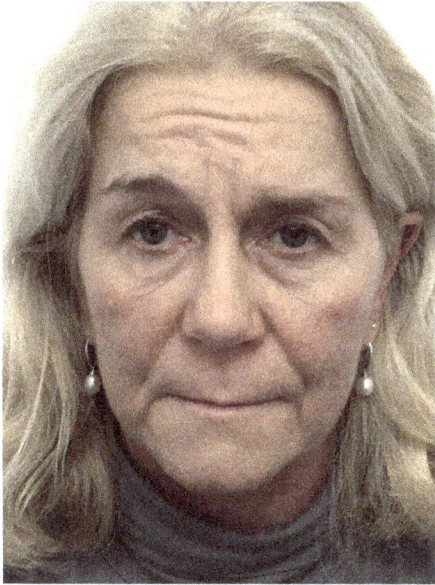

Fig. 13.3: FAS adult, 54-year-old woman.

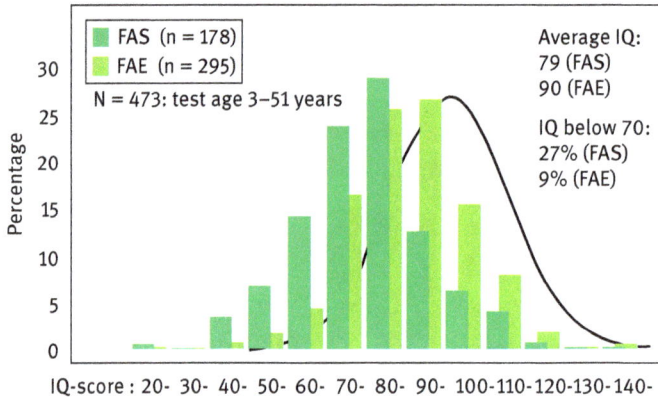

Fig. 13.4: Distribution of IQ between FAS and FAE (fetal alcohol effects) [7].

13.3 Examination into adulthood

To date, there have been only a few reports of follow-up studies examining adult patients with FAS: the French investigation in 1992 [2], a study from Anne Streissguth and colleagues in 1996 called "Secondary disability study" [7] and a follow-up study from Germany in 2007 ("Berlin long-term study") [8].

A. Secondary disability study (1996)

In an extensive cross-sectional study [7] over a 3-year period, Streissguth et al. collected detailed information and data from adult FAS patients who faced difficulties in their everyday lives. Patients (n = 473) aged 3–51 years participated. They were examined using the Fetal Alcohol Behaviour Scale (FABS) [10] and a clinical interview devised particularly for this study by Streissguth et al. [7].

Out of these patients, 178 were diagnosed as having classical FAS and the remaining 295 patients received a diagnosis of FAE (FAE = pFAS). Of the whole sample, 90 patients of the whole sample had already reached adulthood, with a mean age of 25 years. Starting at the age of 6, a wide range of disorders and impairments concerning various aspects of their life were identified (see Fig. 13.4 and 13.5).

The authors called these disorders and impairments *secondary disabilities*. In contrast to primary disabilities (i.e. low IQ, impairments in reading, spelling, mathematical skills or adaptive skills), the secondary disabilities are thought not to be a direct result of intrauterine alcohol exposure. Primary disabilities develop prenatally; whereas secondary disabilities develop later in life, influenced by social environment and the increasing demands of coping with everyday life. The authors classified the multitude of difficulties in patients' everyday lives into eight categories:

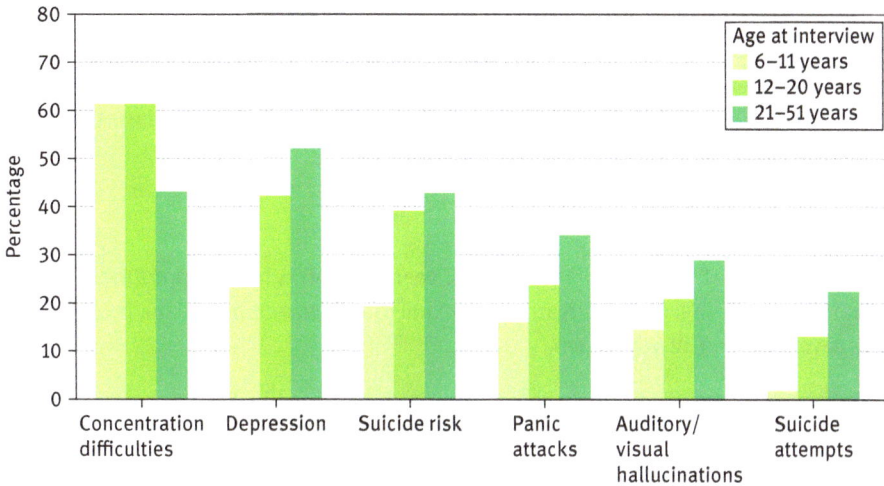

Fig. 13.5: Health problems in different age groups [7].

1. Mental health problems

Psychiatric disorders were found in 90% of patients with FAS/FAE: 61% with ADHD in childhood and 50% with depression in adulthood.

Mental health problems were the most frequent secondary disability occurring in young patients. Of those affected by FAS/FAE, 90% had at least one additional psychiatric diagnosis. In 61% of cases, ADHD was already diagnosed during childhood, and in 40% of cases ADHD was still present in adulthood. In adults with FAS/FAE, the most common additional psychiatric diagnosis was depression (50%). However, 20% had suffered from depression since childhood (see Fig. 13.5) [7].

2. Disrupted school experience

Further, 60% of patients with FAS > 12 years had either been suspended or expelled or had dropped out of school due to learning difficulties and/or behavioural problems. There were hardly any differences between patients with FAS or patients with FAE, but compared to female patients, males had school difficulties more often and particularly in adolescence [7].

3. Trouble with the law

It was found that 60% of patients with FAS/FAE had been accused of or prosecuted for criminal offences: 14% in childhood (> 6 years old) and 58% in adulthood. These patients were either charged with or convicted for a criminal offence. As early as at the ages of 6 and 12, 14% of patients had already experienced a court dispute [7].

4. Confinement

Further, 50% of patients with FAS/FAE (>12 years old) had experienced confinement: 23% mental health inpatient treatment, 15% alcohol/drug inpatient withdrawal treatment and 35% incarceration. Half of the patients with FAS/FAE older than 12 had experienced confinement [7].

5. Inappropriate sexual behaviour

Further, of all patients with FAS/FAE (> 12 years old) 50% had inappropriate sexual behaviour including: sexual advances or sexual touching, exhibitionism, promiscuity, intrusiveness, and/or voyeurism.

6. Alcohol and drug problems

It was found that 50% of patients with FAS/FAE older than 12 suffered from alcohol and/or drug abuse (FAE > FAS). Among these patients, 33% had alcohol problems, 23% had drug problemsand 23% were treated for these problems. There were differences in the degree of dependency. Patients with FAE showed higher rates of alcohol and drug dependency than patients with FAS, and dependency rates increased with age [7].

7. Dependent living

Of patients 21 years and older 80% needed help in daily activities. Females and males with FAS had equivalent rates of problems, whereas males with FAE needed more support in daily activities than females with FAE. Only 20% of individuals with classic FAS were able to live independently.; 80% of those over the age of 21 needed intensive help and supervision in daily life, which was usually provided by family members, friends or care groups. There was no gender difference in patients with classic FAS, but 100% of male patients with FAE, i.e. without dysmorphic features, lived dependently, whereas only one-third of females with FAE lived independently (see Fig. 13.6) [7].

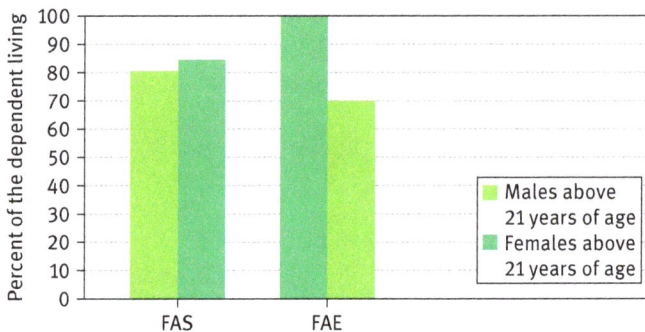

Fig. 13.6: Dependently living males and females with FAS or FAE [7].

8. Problems with employment

The vast majority of adults with FAS/FAE were permanently unemployed or worked temporarily as unskilled workers. As a rule, adults with FAS/FAE were unable to earn sufficient wages to support themselves [7].

Protective factors

The findings of this study, almost 20 years ago, were startling, depressing and in the words of the authors "unacceptable" [7]. It needs to be borne in mind that at the time of examination, these children, adolescents and adults were mainly living under difficult social conditions, often together with their biological families and only a few patients were diagnosed as having FASDin early childhood. At that time, FASD was largely unknown or unrecognised, and treatment or (financial) support was not available. Today, there is an improved knowledge and a greater public awareness regarding this syndrome and its lifelong consequences, largely due to more frequent FASD diagnoses in childhood, with patients receiving earlier treatment and support. Given the demoralising results of their study, the authors tried to identify actions to prevent the development of secondary disabilities:

1. diagnosis before the age of 6 years;
2. a stable and nurturing environment for more than 70% of their lifetime;
3. living in the same place for at least 2.8 years;
4. good quality of home life between the ages of 8 and 12 years;
5. therapeutic interventions and other types of support,
6. more favorable diagnosis of FAS than FAE, because FAS can typically be diagnosed earlier;
7. receiving basic needs at least 13% of their lifetime;
8. no experience of violence in early childhood [7].

B. Berlin longitudinal study (2007)

In contrast to the study of Streissguth at al. [7], which was a cross-sectional study conducted over the course of 3 years, our study in Berlin was a prospective longitudinal study. Adult patients ($n = 37$) were included 20 years after initial examination and diagnostic process [8]. In the period between 1977 and 2003 pediatric, neurological, psychiatric, psychological and sociological data were collected. A total of 37 patients were included; 22 patients presented with classic FAS and 15 had received an FAE diagnosis. There were 22 male patients and 15 female patients. The average age of the patient sample was 21.4 years (age range: 18.1–31.3 years) [8].

Many of the initials symptoms (i.e. growth retardation, microcephaly, developmental delay, hyperactivity, short and upturned nose) declined significantly over the 20-year period. Facial dysmorphic features were even more reduced (see Table 13.2), as

Tab. 13.2: Reversibility of clinical symptomsin 37 adult patients with FAS/FAE [8].

Symptoms	At diagnosis (%)	Follow-up (%)	p
Growth disorder	89	37	<0,001*
Microcephaly	97	49	<0,001*
Developmental delay	89	40	<0,001*
Hyperactivity	73	38	<0,001*
Short nose	62	6	<0,001*
Hypotonia	65	11	<0,001*
Thin upper lip	84	68	NS
midface hypoplasia	62	46	NS

NS = not significant; p = p-value.

described in our 10-year follow up study [5] and by Ann Streissguth et al. in 1991 [9]. This means that many of the symptoms that are helpful in diagnosing FAS in childhood are missing in adulthood, and, therefore, it is more difficult to identify affected adults [8].

However, some features of the FAS facial dysmorphism continued to be present over time, particularly the thin upper lip that remained visible in almost 70% of the adult patients. The midface hypoplasia and the smooth philtrum persisted in about half of the adult patients (46%).

Examination of height, weight and head circumference after 20 years resulted in an overall significant reduction. In our adult patients, short stature, weight deficiency (dystrophy) and microcephaly continued to be detectable. As seen in our previous 10-year follow up study [5], male patients were affected more often than females (See Figs. 13.7–13.9) [8].

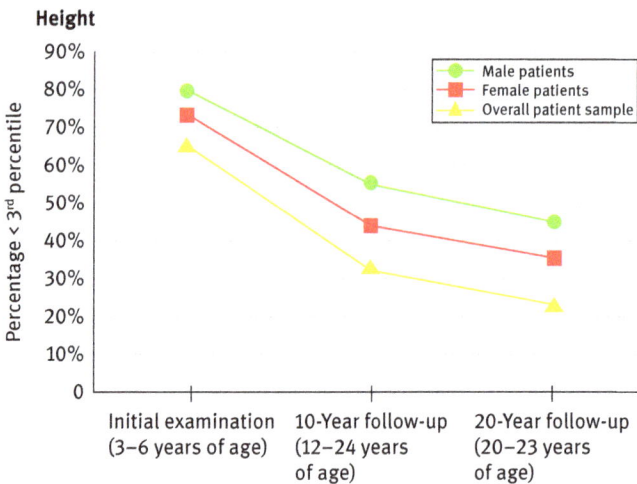

Fig. 13.7: Development of body heightover time in 37 patients with FAS/FAE [8].

Weight

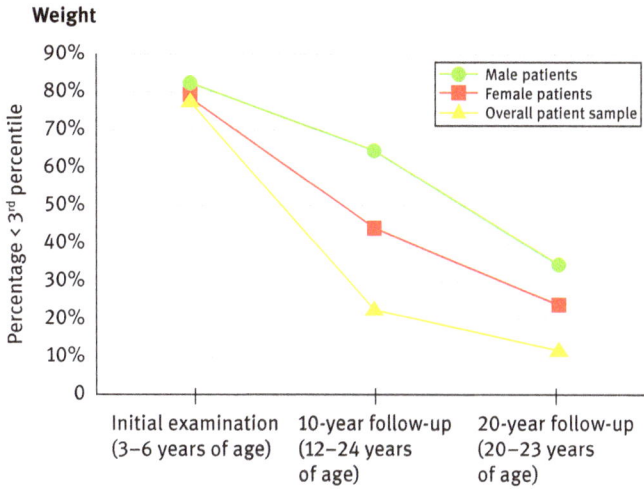

Fig. 13.8: Weight development over time in 37 patients with FAS/FAE [8].

Circumference

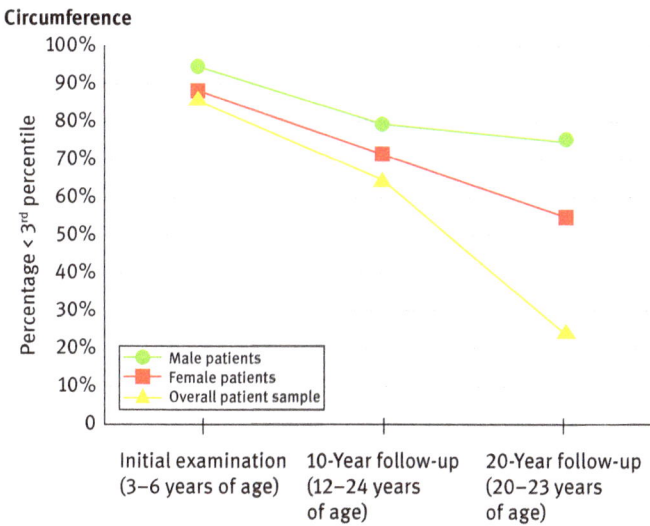

Fig. 13.9: Development of head circumference in 37 patients with FAS/FAE [8].

Microcephaly in adult FASD patients persisted significantly. After 20 years, 75% of male patients and 55% of the female patients investigated still had a head circumference below the 3rd percentile.

In adolescence, the decreased weight seen in childhood often changed to overweight, especially among females, who even became obese. To date, endocrinological studies are unable to explain this phenomenon sufficiently. Dobson et al. described a potential mechanism for the development of obesity in their animal study from 2012 [11]. An animal model was applied to guinea pigs by administering alcohol to pregnant females. As the authors hypothesised, the intrauterine alcohol exposure led to changes in pancreatic tissue and, finally, to obesity in the guinea pigs. The animals were born underweight, but relatively quickly gained weight resulting in obesity at the time of ablactation. Interestingly, although not commented upon by the authors, the weight gain was significantly higher in females compared to male guinea pigs. In addition to the obvious weight gain in this study, there were clear changes in pancreatic functioning, leading to reduced glucose tolerance and increased insulin resistance. This, together with increased visceral fat, leads to a higher risk for the development of metabolic syndrome, type-2 diabetes and cardiovascular disease [11].

Further results

We were able to demonstrate that after 20 years one-third of the adult patients with FAS/FAE had average intelligence and less than half (40%) of the patients suffered from intellectual disability (IQ < 71). If we compare intelligence from the 20-year follow-up sample to that of the 10-year follow-up sample, intelligence seems to remain stable over time in spite of numerical differences (first follow-up in adolescence $n = 60$ vs. $n = 37$). Of the adult patients, 33% had a normal IQ (> 85) compared to 27% after 10 years. Moreover, mental retardation was seen in 30% of patients at the first follow-up and in 40% of patients in adulthood (see Table 13.3). Considering the link between intelligence and head circumference, 80% of our patients (12/15) with mental retardation had microcephaly as to be expected, but 20% of patients with normal intelligence also suffered from a head circumference < 3 percentile [8].

To examine behavioural problems of our adult patients we used the Youth Adult Behaviour Checklist with an observer rating scale of behavioural problems after the age of 18 years. As to be expected, our adult patients had significantly more behavioural problems in domains typically affected by FAS: anxiety, isolation, negative thoughts, attention deficits, intrusion, aggression and delinquency (see Fig. 13.10). It is important to emphasise that there was no significant difference in behavioural problems between patients with FAS and partial FAS (see Fig. 13.11) [8]. Thus, we could prove that patients with partial FAS were suffering from similar severe disabilities as patients with "full blown" FAS.

Tab. 13.3: Intelligence level in the Berlin longitudinal study [8].

Intelligence level (FAS/pFAS)			
	All (n = 37)	FAS (n = 22)	pFAS (n = 15)
IQ > 85	12 (32.9%)	6 (27.3%)	6 (40.0%)
IQ 71–85	10 (26.6%)	5 (22.7%)	5 (33.3%)
IQ < 71	15 (40.5%)	11 (50.0%)	4 (26.7%)

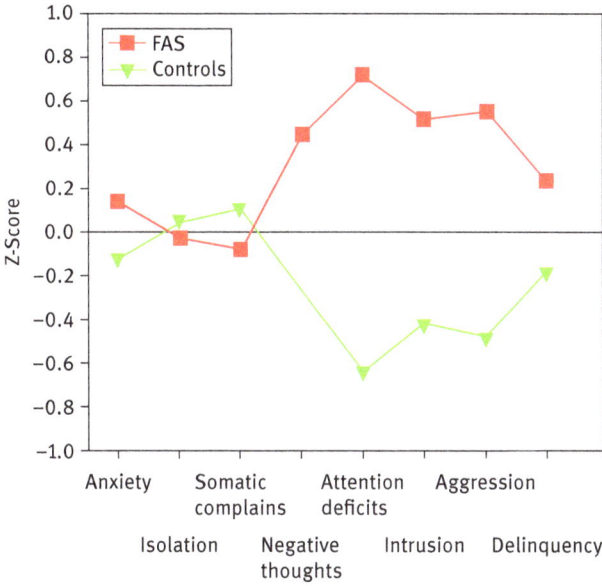

Fig. 13.10: Behavioural problems in adults with FAS measured by the Youth Adult Behaviour Checklist compared to healthy controls [12, 13].

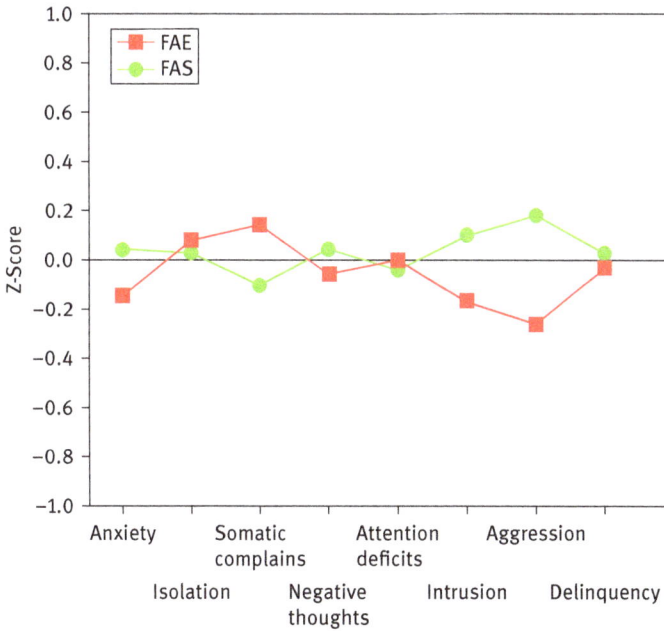

Fig. 13.11: No difference in behavioural problems between adults with FAS (n = 20) compared to adults with FAE (n = 15) measured by the "Youth Adult Behaviour Checklist" [12, 13].

Tab. 13.4: Life perspective(comparison Berlin–Seattle) [8, 7].

	Berlin	Seattle
Life conditions		
Independent living (11/37)	29.5%	
Dependent living (26/37)	70.5%	74%
Profession, employment		
Without profession (5/36)	13.8%	
Without job (31/36)	86.2%	83%

Similar to findings of the "Secondary disability study" from Streissguth et al. [7], 70% of our adults were not able to live independently and needed support; only a very small number of adults (13%) were able to earn their own wages (see Table 13.4).

The convergence of employment status and independent living in both studies are surprising because all protective factors described by Streissguth and colleagues [7] were present in our sample with the only exception being the absence of violence. All children were diagnosed in early childhood before the age of 6; they had been living under stable living conditions with foster or adoptive parents since childhood and had received support and assistance. In our cohort only three cases out of the 37 adult patients had experienced physical violence in early childhood, although this small number may reflect a high rate of unreported cases [8]. Despite more favorable developmental opportunities and the sufficient availability of "protective factors", our 20-year follow-up study clearly indicated similar results compared to the secondary disability study [7]. One explanation could be that the primary disabilities induced by intrauterine alcohol exposure are the underlying cause for the development of secondary disabilities. They additionally may be triggered by increasing burdens and demands in everyday life with only little influence by protective factors.

In 2016, Canadian authors published for the first time a dramatic paper estimating the life expectancy of people with FAS and also specified the causes of death among these patients. The devastating result was that the life expectancy at birth of people with FAS was 34 years (95% confidence interval: 31–37 years), which was about 42% of that of the general population! The main causes of deathfor people with FAS were "external causes" (44%) including suicide (15%); accidents (14%); poisoning by illegal drugs or alcohol (7%); other external causes (7%). Other common causes of death were diseases of the nervous system, the respiratory and the digestive system, congenital malformations and mental and behavioural disorders.

In contrast to our expectations we have to realise that people with FAS may have a considerably lower life expectancy than that of the general population One reason more to diagnose these patients and take care of this vulnerable group of society.

In summary, prenatal alcohol exposure causing FAS or other manifestations of the syndrome will lead to lifelong consequences with persistent impairments concerning

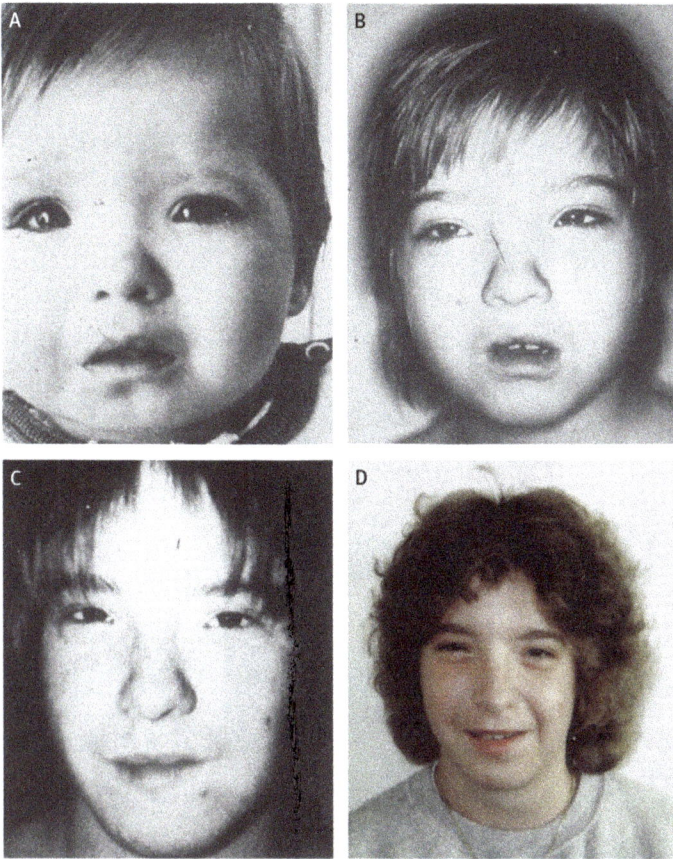

Fig. 13.12: Female patient with pFAS at the age of A) 8 months, B) 3 years, C) 15 years and D) 26 years.

all areas of daily life and risk for additional psychiatric disorders. We still do not know the consequences for elderly patients with FAS, since the syndrome was first described only 40 years ago. It can be assumed however, that the deficits and disabilities, which lead to occupational disabilities, lack of independence and legal incapacity, will continue or even increase with later ages or possibly, at worst, reduce life expectancy. Therefore, it is necessary for physicians and especially psychiatrists to learn to recognise and diagnose this syndrome in adults and become aware of the underlying intrauterine alcohol exposure. As a result of intensive encouragement and support, some of our adult patients in Berlin have, fortunately, been able to create new perspectives for their lives, depending on their individual abilities.

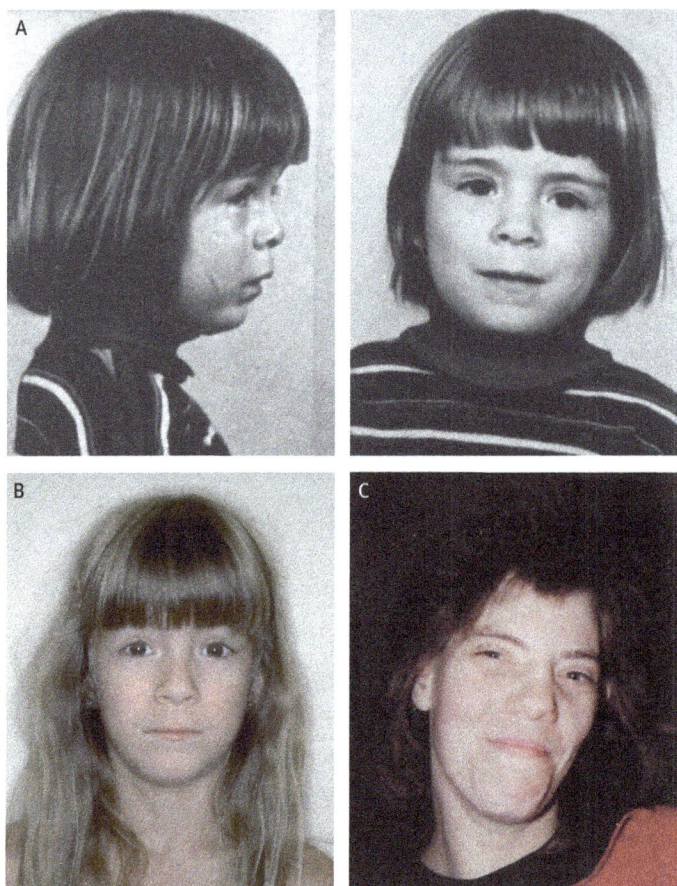

Fig. 13.13: Female patient with pFAS at the age of A) 3 years, B) 10 years, and C) 31 years.

Bibliography

[1] Streissguth AP, Clarren KS, Jones KL. Natural History of the Fetal Alcohol Syndrome: A 10-year-Follow-up of eleven Patients. Lancet 1985, 13(2), 85–91.

[2] Lemoine P, Lemoine Ph. Outcome in the offspring of alcoholic mothers (study of one hundred and fifty adults and consideration with a view to prophylaxis (in French). Ann Pédiatr (Paris) 1992, 39(4), 226–235.

[3] Streissguth A. Fetal Alcohol Syndrome. A Guide for Families and Communities. Paul H. Brookes Publishing Co, Baltimore, Maryland 1997.

[4] Rangar J, Hjern A, Stromland K et al. Psychosocial outcome of fetal alcohol syndrome in adulthood. Pediatrics 2015, 135(1), e52–258.

[5] Spohr HL, Willms J, Steinhausen HC. Prenatal alcohol exposure and long-term developmental consequences. Lancet 1993, 341(8850), 907–10.

[6] Streissguth AP, Randels SP, Smith DF. A test-retest study of intelligence in patients with fetal alcohol syndrome: implications for care. J Am Acad Child Adolesc Psychiatry 1991, 30, 584–587.

[7]   Streissguth AP, Barr HM, Kogan J et al. Understanding the occurrence of secondary disabilities in clients with fetal alcohol syndrome (FAS) and fetal alcohol effects (FAE). Final report to the Centers for Disease Control and Prevention (CDC). University of Washington, Fetal Alcohol and Drug Unit, Seattle 1996, 96–106.

[8]   Spohr HL, Willms J, Steinhausen HC. Fetal Alcohol Spectrum Disorders in Young Adulthood. J. Pediatr 2007, 150, 175–179.

[9]   Streissguth AP, Aase JM, Clarren SK, Randels SP, LaDue RA, Smith DF. Fetal alcohol syndrome in adolescents and adults. JAMA 1991, 265, 1961–1967.

[10]   Streissguth AP, Bookstein FL, Barr HM, Press S, Sampson PD. A Fetal Alcohol Behaviour Scale. Alcoholism: Clinical and Experimental Research 1998, 22(2), 325–333.

[11]   Dobson CC, Mongillo DL, Brien DC. Chronic prenatal ethanol exposure increases offspring adiposity and disrupts pancreatic morphology in adult guinea pig offspring. Nutrition and Diabetes 2012, 2, e57.

[12]   Steinhausen HC, Willms J, Spohr HL. Correlates of psychopathology and intelligence in children with fetal alcohol syndrome. Journal of Child Psychology and Psychiatry and Allied Disciplines 1994, 35(2), 323–331.

[13]   Steinhausen HC. Entwicklungsstörungen im Kindes- und Jugendalter. Kohlhammer Verlag, Stuttgart, Berlin, Köln 2001.

[14]   Autti-Rämö I, Fagerlund A, Ervalathi N, Loimu L, Korkman M, Hoyme E. Fetal Alcohol Spectrum Disorder in Finland: Clinical Delineation of 77 older children and Adolescents. American Journal of Medical Genetics 2006, 140(2), 137–143.

[15]   Thanh NX, Johansson E. Life expectancy of people with Fetal Alcohol Syndrome. J Popul Ther Clin Pharmacol 2016, 23(1), e53–e59.

14 Diagnosing Fetal alcohol syndrome in adulthood

Limited literature is available on the clinical presentation and outcome of fetal alcohol syndrome in adulthood. In addition to previously described articles on long-term consequences of FAS [1–4], Chudley et al. (2007) described the challenges and difficulties of diagnosing FAS in adulthood [5]. In a publication released in 2010, Freunscht and Feldmann published data on live reports of 60 adult patients with FAS, who had been diagnosed during childhood. They also concluded that the affected adults need permanent assistance, support and protection due to their ingenuousness and dependency [6].

In a psychiatric review from 2012, Walloch et al. focused on the question "What happens to children suffering from fetal alcohol syndrome or fetal alcohol spectrum disorder in adulthood?" [7]. This was probably the first publication with detailed and extensive information about FAS in adulthood that emphasised the increasing relevance to psychiatry in Germany.

14.1 Ethical considerations

Today, the large number of adolescents and adults with FAS/pFAS who did not receive a diagnosis in childhood or adolescence is still an unsolved problem. The absence of a diagnosis is often due to the fact that this disorder was largely unknown in the past, and often information about alcohol consumption during pregnancy was not available.

At the second European FASD-Conference in Barcelona (2012), Ilona Autti-Rämö, the renowned Finnish FASD researcher, stated: "diagnosing FAS in adolescence and especially adulthood is an ethical challenge".

It is important to consider risks and benefits when diagnosing FAS in adults, taking into account what the advantages or unpredictable consequences might be to the individual.

For example, should an adult woman, who is leading a relatively content life in line with her somewhat, limited abilities and who is able to hold a job, really receive this diagnosis, be diagnosed with FAS just because her guardians learned that her biological mother was a heavy alcoholic who drank during pregnancy? Should she be informed that she will be disabled for the rest of her life due to the alcoholism of her mother with whom she might have had a positive relationship until now? This question is not easily answered.

Overall, an increasing number of adults with suspected or confirmed alcohol exposure during pregnancy are specifically referred for a FAS diagnosis to the FASD centre in Berlin because they have difficulties dealing with daily routine and job training, and they have few social contacts and suffer from being different. Often they have

https://doi.org/10.1515/9783110436563-014

heard about this "new disorder" through the media and they work out that a wide range of described symptoms and impairments seems to apply to them. They hope this diagnosis will explain the difficulties they are experience in life. In this case, the ethical question is whether a diagnosis is of advantage and perhaps therapeutical (see the case description on page 160).

14.2 Diagnosing adults with the 4-Digit Diagnostic Code

How does one diagnose a 40-year-old person with suspected fetal alcohol spectrum disorder?

We adapted and modified the 4-Digit Diagnostic Code, a diagnostic instrument that has been used until now to diagnosechildren and adolescents and, therefore, normative data and percentiles only related to the ages of 0–18 or 20 [8]. The neuro-psychiatric domains to be examined in the 4-Digit Diagnostic Code are also focused primarily on children and adolescents, but most domains are transferable to adults.

Nevertheless, if maternal alcohol abuse in pregnancy is uncertain, the diagnosis of FAS in adults is possible when facial dysmorphic features are still visible and a growth deficiency, microcephaly or severe brain dysfunction is present. Symptoms are rated corresponding to the criteria of the 4-Digit Diagnostic Code used in children and adolescents. However, if typical dysmorphic features are missing in adulthood and

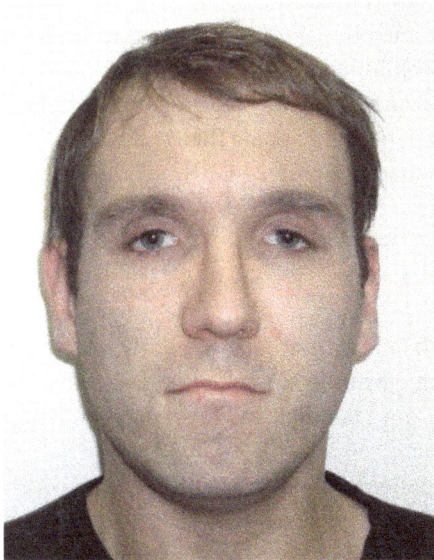

Fig. 14.1: A.M., 30 years old, FAS.

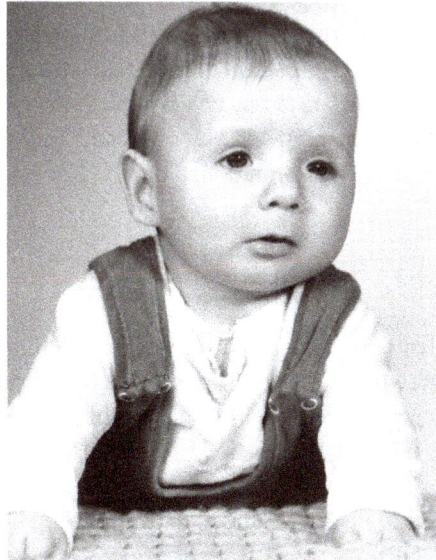

Fig. 14.2: A.M. as a child at the age of 10 months.

Tab. 14.1: Rating criteria for the symptoms in the 4-Digit Diagnostic Code [8].

Growth deficiencies	none 1; mild 2; moderate 3; severe 4
Facial dysmorphia	none 1; mild 2; moderate 3; severe 4
CNS-damage	none 1; mild 2; probable 3; definite 4
Prenatal alcohol consumption	none 1; unknown 2; probable 3; high risk 4

if no photos are available, of both infancy and childhood, a diagnosis of FAS without knowledge of maternal alcohol consumption during pregnancy is very difficult to confirm [5].

14.2.1 Growth deficiency

Adult patients are often not significantly underweight and/or growth restricted. In our longitudinal study [1] only about 20% of patients remained underweight (i.e. below the 3rd percentile), but nevertheless half of the patients were still growth restricted (below the 3rd percentile).

The rank of a maximum of 4 points is transferred if both height and weight are below the 3rd percentile either currently or in the past. More often only one of these symptoms is below the 3rd percentile, and therefore ranked to a total of 3 points in the 4-Digit Diagnostic Code. The rank of 2 points is transferred if one symptom is between the 3rd-10th percentile and the other one is in the normal range.

If height and weight in adulthood are in the normal range, or patients are even obese, it is important to obtain data from their childhood. If no objective data are available, one has to rely on authentic information given by family members or caretakers that the patient was "always small and/or underweight". Using this "unobjective but plausible" information, a rank of 2 or maximum of 3 is assigned.

14.2.2 Facial dysmorphia

Symptoms of facial dysmorphia in adults with FAS are evaluated similarly to those of growth deficiency. The three facial dysmorphic features, i.e. small palpebral fissure lengths, smooth philtrum and thin upper lip, are examined and rated independently from one another.

In a follow-up investigation of 37 adult patients, about 70% still presented with a thin upper lip and smooth philtrum. Midface hypoplasia persisted in 45% of the adults [1].

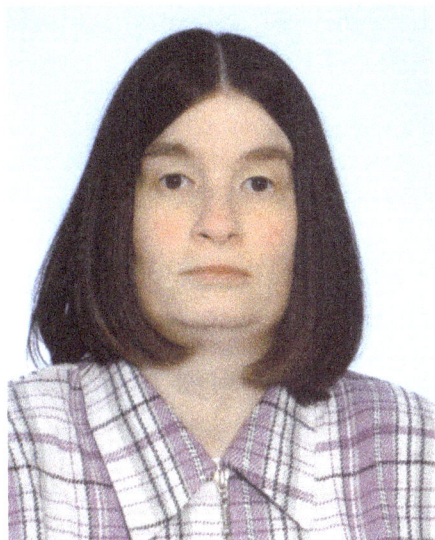

Fig. 14.3: G.W., 38 years old, FAS.

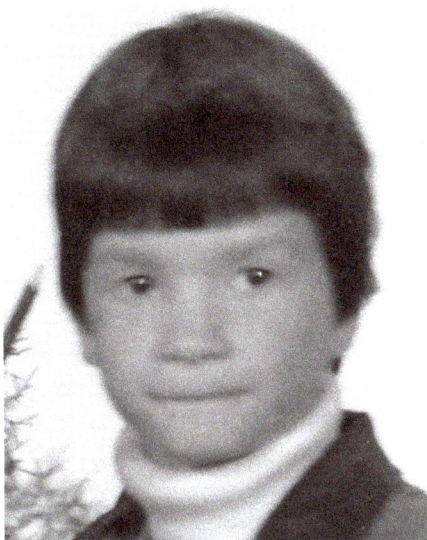

Fig. 14.4: G.W. as a child at the age of 7.

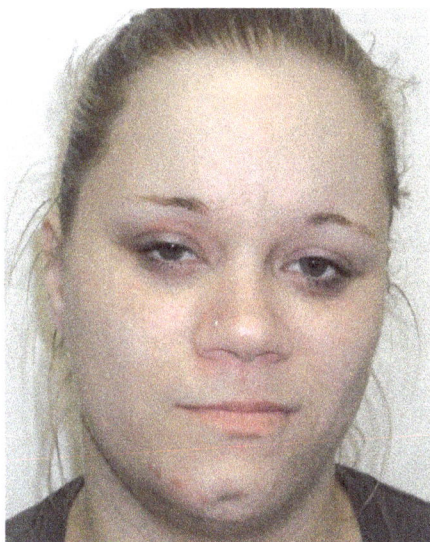

Fig. 14.5: A.G., 28 years old, FAS.

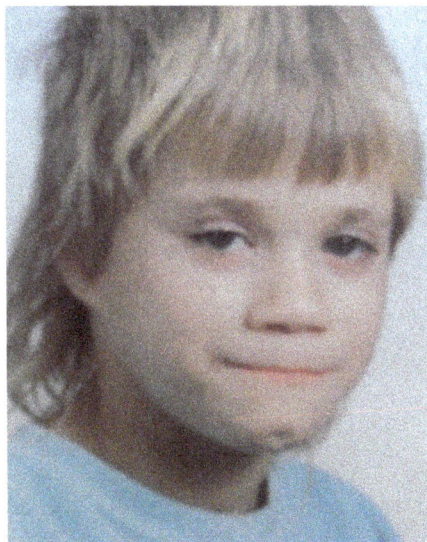

Fig. 14.6: A.G. in primary school.

Palpebral fissure length

According to the 4-Digit Diagnostic Code [8] palpebral fissure length is measured on both sides compared to the normative data from Hall et al. [9]. Although these norms are only standardised up to an age of 16 years, they can still give an indication of the severity of this symptom in older patients, especially because palpebral fissure lengths largely remain the same after the age of 16 years.

This was confirmed in an examination by Cranston, who studied palpebral fissure length in Canadian students and found a mean length of 29.3 ± 1.4 mm [5]. On the standardised percentile curves from Hall et al. [9] the mean for female and male adolescents aged 16 years is 30.2 mm and the 3rd percentile (–2 SD) is 28 mm.

Upper lip/philtrum

We also use the "Lip-Philtrum Guide" (Likert scale) of the 4-Digit Diagnostic Code in adult patients because we experienced that both of these features often persist into adulthood [1]. Similar findings were described by Streissguth et al. [10] and Chudley [5], although as expected, in adult patients the characteristics were less pro-

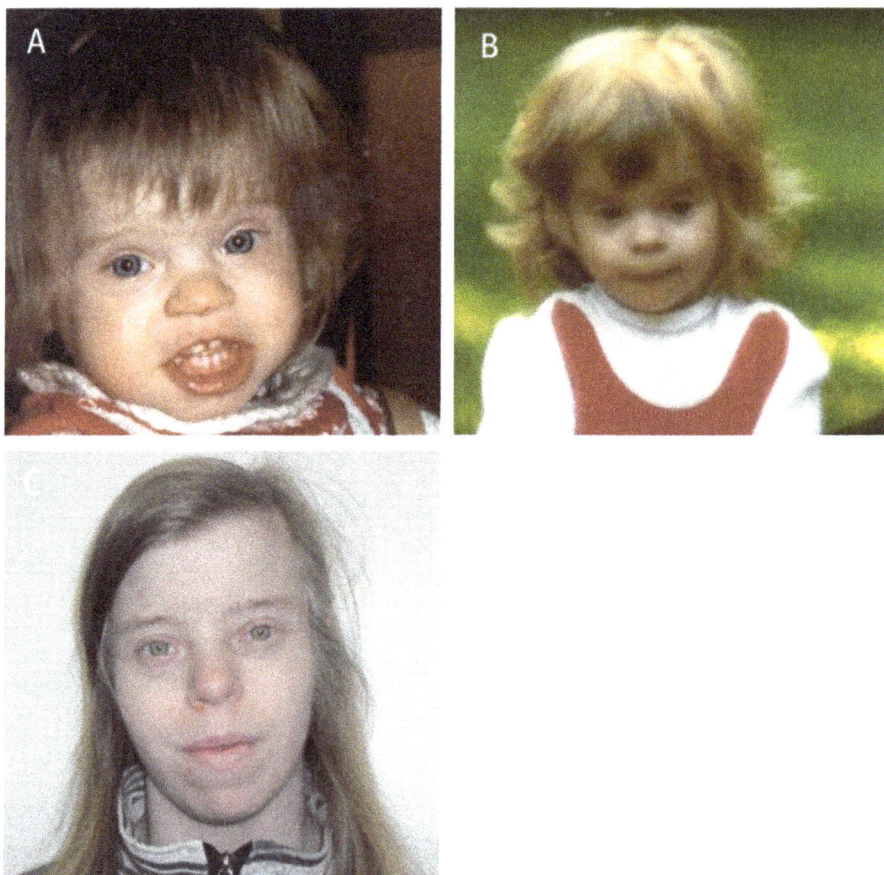

Fig. 14.7: Patient with FAS at A) at the age of 1, B) at the age of 2, C) at the age of 33.

nounced. The older the patients are the more difficult it is to recognise the typical FAS stigmata in a face marked by age, suffering, illness and work.

Therefore, childhood photos should definitely be included whenever possible. This is often accompanied by problems, because many patients do not have photos from their childhood or they are not motivated to locate these earlier photos, since childhood images could potentially remind them of traumatic experiences.

It is important to ask patients well in advance to collect discharge letters, infancy and childhood photos, information about maternal alcohol consumption during pregnancy, evaluation reports and school assessments.

Self-report written by the patient F.

"Facial characteristics are hardly visible anymore. But you can look into my nostrils if you look at my face. My nose is short and the philtrum is long. I have a thick lower lip, but the upper lip is thin. As a young child I had an upturned nose and could not wear glasses without adjustable nose pads. My teeth were crooked, but surgically corrected now. When my girlfriend and I looked at an old photo of me as a child, she asked me where my ears were. My mother used to stick my jug ears to my head with sticky tape. Successfully. One of my classmates tried to find something near my ears once, something that had been discussed right before during biology class apparently, but she couldn't find it. I have no clue what it was, I could not discover anything unusual. My little finger, particularly on my left hand, is bent."

14.2.3 Damage to the central nervous system

Structural damage

Structural CNS damage is the most important finding and is easily detected by measuring the head's circumference. Also in adulthood, particularly in male patients, the head's circumference is often still small [1].

According to the 4-Digit Diagnostic Code [8], a head size on or below the 3rd percentile during childhood is classified as microcephaly; whereas the 10th percentile is defined as microcephaly according to the Canadian guidelines [11] for children and adolescents. Taken together, this suggests that in adults a head size on or below the 10th percentile is categorised as a microcephaly.

In rare cases, it might be valuable to conduct magnetic resonance imaging (MRI), because there are several structural brain abnormalities that occur more frequently after intrauterine alcohol exposure, such as grey matter heterotopia, in particular anomalies of the corpus callosum, cerebellum hypoplasia, basal ganglia and hippocampal hypoplasia. Usually however, findings of MRI in adult patients reveal mostly no abnormalities. It is more crucial to perform an extensive neurological examination, because there are a number of neurological abnormalities that could be present. Besides epilepsy, there could be pronounced difficulties in coordination and balance as well as visual–motor problems.

Functional damage

Although no specific functional CNS-disorder profile in FAS has been confirmed so far, impairments of executive functioning, working memory, information processing, and attention and learning seem very likely to be due to teratogenic damage by alcohol, particularly concerning the prefrontal cortex and hippocampus [13].

In 2011, Temple et al. studied adaptive daily living skills in 15 adult patients with FAS compared to clinical controls with similar IQ scores. They found that patients with FAS showed significantly lower adaptive daily living skills compared to the IQ matched control group [14]. This suggests that IQ is not a good predictor of adaptive daily living skills in adults with FAS.

Affected patients obviously have difficulties in problem solving and planning abilities in their everyday lives; they lack the ability to anticipate and to think in a target-oriented manner, but they are often able to perform a neuropsychological assessment in a calm test situation without any difficulties. They are unable to manage time and money and to control feelings and impulses appropriately [15] (see also life report page 160).

These scientific findings are in line with our clinical observations concerning executive functioning in childhood including that normal intelligence does not seem to be a protective factor against frequent failures in everyday life.

This also applies to adolescents currently in vocational training or professional practices. Trainers and teachers often do not know that adults with FAS fail in performance and behaviour despite a normal intelligence level simply because they have executive function disabilities, and it has little to do with a lack of motivation and oppositional behaviour, although this is often assumed.

This misunderstanding has an even more severe impact on adult patients because they are often unable to make themselves understood properly and to take appropriate steps to receive the support and assistance from social services, employment agencies or public health officers to which they are entitled.

Usually parents or caretakers do not guide them in their everyday life anymore and, therefore, they often do not receive the support and help needed. Even with normal intelligence and acceptable school reports, they are unable to successfully complete vocational training, to deal with stress resulting from work pressure and to deal with daily life demands without understanding their failure. Therefore they "take refuge in sickness" at a young age, especially developing depression, addictive disorders or getting into problems with the law.

According to the 4-Digit Diagnostic Code, significant (two or more standard deviations below the mean) functional brain impairment in three or more domains must be proven by neuropsychological and developmental tests.

The functional domains for children and adolescents are:
1. intelligence
2. school achievements

3. adaptive behaviour/social skills
4. executive functioning
5. motor and sensory integration
6. speech development and social communication
7. mental health
8. behaviour/attention

These functional domains of the central nervous system should also be examined in adults in whom the assessment of speech development, motor and sensory integration and maybe even school achievements presently is not useful or necessary. However, possible existing test results describing developmental language or motor disorders as well as earlier school assessments, revealing academic difficulties, should be included in the evaluation of the eight functional domains, and as such, potentially be rated as a significant problem.

When examining adult patients, it is important to consider that the pathological symptoms revealed during the examination could also have been influenced by other postnatal factors, i.e. the age of a patient, other acquired diseases, poverty, social isolation, broken familial structures, abuse, violence and childhood neglect. Not all pathological symptoms found in the functional domains are necessarily caused by alcohol-induced prenatal brain damage.

Many of the neuropsychological impairments and behavioural problems found in childhood and adolescence do not change for the better with the passing of years [1, 3]. Moreover, many behavioural problems even tend to increase, sometimes with severe consequences such as criminal behaviour, getting into debt, alcohol dependency, suicidal tendencies.

Therefore, behavioural difficulties, social problems and communication impairments are no longer assessed as developmentally delayed problems, but rather as permanent damage [14].

So far, there are only a few psychotherapy studies that show an improvement in social skills and neuropsychological impairments by specialised intervention programs (see Chapter 4). Particularly stable environmental factors such as, employment, a solid partnership and governmental support lead to an improved continuity and increased contentment in individual cases and probably induces a reduction of behavioural problems [14, 16].

Some neuropsychological impairment is less evident in adulthood, but other impairments persist. This particularly applies to the executive function disorder, difficulties in social interaction and to social behaviour. To date we do not know which factors lead to a better prognosis and if certain positive developments are long lasting. It remains an important and central research area, which hopefully will improve the treatment and support of patients with FAS [17].

Information on maternal alcohol consumption during pregnancy is difficult to assess, and sometimes almost impossible in adult patients, as described in the following case reports.

Case report

At the funeral of her mother, a 30-year old woman who had hardly had any contact with her mother before she died, met the sisters of her mother. It was 20 years ago that she had seen her aunts. At the funeral, they told her that her mother had always been a chronic alcoholic and that she had also drunk intensively during her pregnancy. It was only then that she realised that the alcohol abuse of her mother during pregnancy might be responsible for the numerous difficulties and failures in her former life.

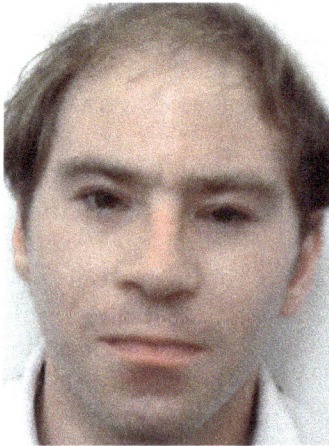

Fig. 14.8: 25-year old patient, FAS adult.

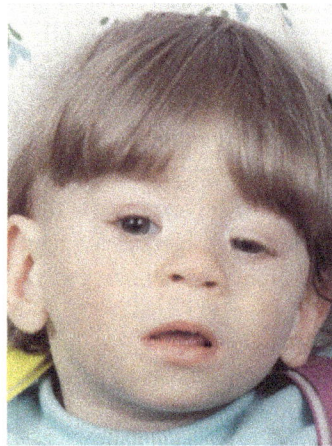

Fig. 14.9: The same patient at the age of 18 months.

Case report

A 41-year old woman had several clinical symptoms pointing to the possibility that she might suffer from FAS. Unfortunately, she did not know anything about her mother and, additionally, she had neither contact with her hometown, nor to relatives or her previous foster parents. The only slight clue to her childhood was a small black-and-white photo depicting her on her first day at school with a large bag of candy; on this photo there was a little girl with a very distinctive and typical FAS-face.

Of interest is the first Japanese case report of an adult FAS-patient published in 2004 [18]:

Case report

A 35-year old woman who was hospitalised for 15 years due to multiple neuropsychiatric abnormalities is described. Besides mental retardation, the woman suffered from schizophrenic symptoms, bipolar disorder, severe ADHD and impulsive behaviour. She had had a low birth weight and showed distinctive facial dysmorphic features. Because her biological mother and the family had always denied alcohol abuse during pregnancy, she had not been diagnosed with FAS. It was only recently that the family of the patient admitted the previous denial of severe alcohol abuse during the pregnancy and, therefore, the diagnosis was finally confirmed in adulthood.

These examples demonstrate that information about potential maternal alcohol consumption during pregnancy must be investigated thoroughly in order to classify the fourth section of the 4-Digit Diagnostic Code as accurately as possible.

14.2.5 Final interpretation of the diagnostic criteria

The diagnostic criteria of the 4-Digit Diagnostic Code can also be used in adulthood and, consequently, adults can receive the diagnoses FAS, pFAS or ARND according to the diagnostic code combinations of the 4-Digit Diagnostic Code. [19].

14.3 Secondary disabilities in adults with FAS

Since Streissguth et al. described the secondary disabilities in patients with FAS in 1996 [3] comorbid disorders are part of the diagnostic process of FAS in adults. They must be assessed, investigated in detail and, when possible, treated.

About 10 years after this first description, Clark et al. (2004) once again investigated the presence of "secondary disabilities" in 62 adult patients in British Columbia, Canada [20].

The incidence of the secondary disabilities corresponded to the findings of A. Streissguth [3]. For example, the rate of *mental health* disorders was very high (92%); in this study, ADHD (61%) and depression (47%) were also frequent comorbid disorders, and 34% of the patients had an IQ-score below 70, while about 70% were unable to live independently. Similar findings were also described in our study from 2007 [1].

In their study, Clark et al. described the high vulnerability to manipulation (92%), which may lead, amongst others, to falsifications of the truth, i.e. a risk of false statements, distortion of facts in court or when agreements or warnings are not understood.

Another interesting finding of this study was that secondary disabilities were not dependent on reduced intelligence, but rather had an impact on the degree of problems in adaptive functioning.

In the Seattle study of A. Streissguth et al. [3], about 90% of patients had mental health problems; ADHD was the most frequent comorbidity in childhood and adolescence, and with increasing age more than half of adult patients suffered from depression with high rates of suicide threats (43%) and suicide attempts (23%). It remains unclear whether numerous postnatal psychosocial problems like physical and emotional abuse, unemployment, poverty, trouble with the law, substance abuse or the brain damage caused by intrauterine alcohol exposition itself are responsible for the increased rate of suicidality.

14.3.1 Children of adult patients with FAS

Raising children is always a challenging task for all parents. Parents need the ability to show patience and provide an unconditional positive influence for their child. When their child misbehaves, parents have to be able to have consequences for inappropriate behaviour but still maintain a positive attitude.

If mothers suffering from FAS have attention and perception problems, cognitive deficits and limited judgement, they are, as expected, soon unable to cope with the care of their newborn. Despite the multitude of difficulties of these twofold-burdened women, they are quite capable of parentingtheir children but need additional intensive help and support, especially in a setting of alcohol or drug problems or other mental health diseases.

Experience shows that women with FAS usually have many children, although they often live under socially difficult conditions. It is not uncommon that foster or adoptive parents of children presented for a diagnosis of FAS report that the biological mother herself comes from a family with alcohol abuse, neglect or violence. Often, these women also grew up in a sheltered home or with foster or adoptive parents and were probably damaged by alcohol exposure during their mother's pregnancy as well. Many of these women start drinking alcohol already in early adolescence, which means that it is not uncommon that woman with undiagnosed FAS will herself deliver a child possibly suffering from fetal alcohol syndrome.

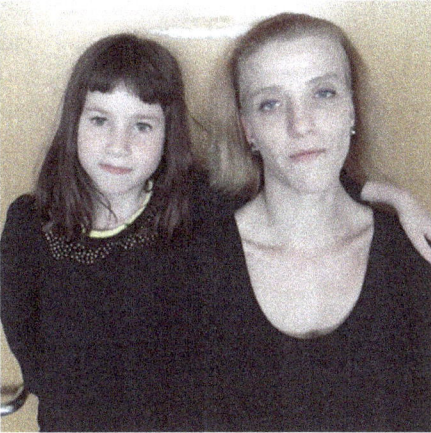

Fig. 14.10: A mother and her child, both suffering from FAS.

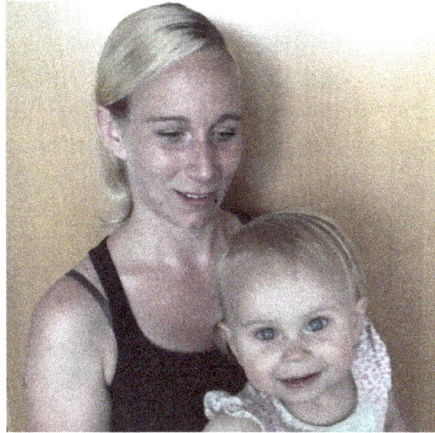

Fig. 14.11: Mother and daughter with FAS.

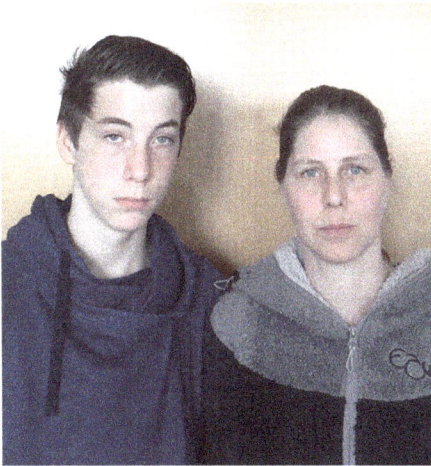

Fig. 14.12: Mother and son with FAS.

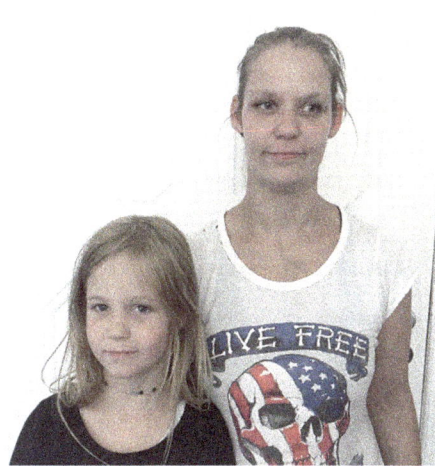

Fig. 14.13: Mother and daughter with FAS.

In the large Streissguth study [3], 17% of the patients were parents with an average age of 18. An impressive percentage of the female patients (40%) had consumed alcohol during their pregnancies, and 17% of their children showed symptoms indicative of FAS at follow-up.

In summary, it can be stated that mothers of alcohol-damaged children are a large and often undiagnosed group with risk of FAS, which has to be taken into account in prevention strategies.

14.4 FASD and the legal system

Adolescents and adults with FAS are more likely than their peers without a prenatal alcohol exposure to have conflicts with the law; as plaintiff, witness or victim and especially as a defendant in a crime. The criminal justice system needs to know the impairments and cognitive deficits of patients with fetal alcohol spectrum disorder when dealing with people suffering from this disease.

Example taken from a lecture held by a judge at the 3rd International FASD Conference in Vancouver in 2004

The judge interrogates a young man who has stolen a bicycle. The defendant admits in a friendly manner that he "took the bike with him". The judge lets him go with a kind and firm warning.

Six weeks later the same young man and the same judge are again in a court hearing for a stolen bicycle. This time, the judge is clearer and instructs the young man that the theft is a big violation of the law. The young man again admits friendlily and openly that he took the bike with him. He states: "It was standing against a tree and didn't belong to anyone". He was sentenced to a couple of hours of community service in a home.

Again 6 weeks later, the young man is arrested again and re-presented to the same judge, because he has stolen a bike for the third time. The judge asks him with harsh words as to why he has again stolen a bicycle despite previous warnings and the sentence. The young man answers, again in a friendly manner, that right at that moment he needed a bicycle and that the bicycle obviously didn't belong to anyone.

According to his own report, the judge lost his temper at this point; he felt disrespected and not taken seriously by the young man. He could not condone this remorseless behaviour and sentenced the young man for this theft in the case of recurrence and imposed a high fine, which the accused young man accepted with a smile and without any contradiction.

Because the young man remained friendly even at a third court appearance and because he always apologised for what he had done and did not defend his behaviour, the judge became suspicious and wanted to make sure that his behaviour was not due to an illness and referred him to a medical specialist.

In this particular case, the result of the examination was the diagnosis of FAS in adulthood, characterised by typical difficulties in social interaction and executive functioning.

It was obvious that the patient had no sense of wrongdoing and was unaware of the consequences of his misconduct. He did not understand the warnings of the judge, neither at the first, nor at the second or third time, and with his friendly behaviour, he probably wanted to oblige the judge.

The report of the judge ended with the insightful recommendation that in the case of doubt that an FAS diagnosis might be present, an assessment in a specialised centre should be conducted before starting a criminal process or issuing a judgement.

Learning and behavioural problems associated with FAS, as well as difficulties in social interaction make those affected more prone to criminal behaviour [21].

This example shows what kind of problems and challenges may arise for the legal system and criminal defence due to impairments of a patient with FAS [22]. A person with FAS can be misunderstood in court, harassed in prison and with the wrong impression be released from prison back into society. Therefore, it is important that those professionals who deal with FAS know the syndrome and its consequences in order to be able to react appropriately.

In a legal paper published in 2013, Mela and Luther used the term "invisible disorder"; a term, that exactly describes the problem: Undiagnosed adult FAS patients seem inconspicuous and normal at first, but they are not [23].

Typical offences committed by people with FAS are usually not violent crimes, but rather offences that are committed repeatedly due to lack of insight and memory deficits, and sentences and penalties usually do not have any long-term effects.

It is unclear to date how many people with a known diagnosis of FAS have been sent to prison. The numbers are most likely small, since most of those affected are without a diagnosis. In a survey in 2004, Burd et al. [24] calculated that there are nearly 100-fold less offenders with a FAS diagnosis in prison compared to the incidence of the syndrome in Canada and the USA (0.087/1000 compared to 1–9/1000).

In a Canadian study by Popova et al. from 2011, it was found that the probability to be in prison during a prespecified period of time was about 19 times higher for adolescents with FAS compared to adolescents not affected by FAS [25].

In their article on secondary disabilities in adult FAS patients Streissguth et al. [3] found an incidence of 35% for incarceration of offenders with FAS. With increasing age, adult FAS patients report more criminal offences, particularly theft, fraud and drug-related crimes.

Characteristic difficulties that predispose people with FAS to criminal offences
- Lack of impulse control;
- inability to predict future consequences of current actions and behaviour;

- difficulties with planning and with understanding cause and effect and in assuming responsibility;
- lack of empathy and low frustration tolerance;
- no power of judgement to evaluate their own behaviour;
- tendency for explosive episodes;
- vulnerability to peer pressure, e.g. conduct a crime to impress friends;
- often simplicity and easy manipulation.

Characteristics that people with FAS display in court
- Limited ability to understand the legal process and a sentence or conviction;
- limited ability to evaluate their own offence, e.g. they admit an offence only to please the judge;
- tendency to repeat offences despite convictions! ("I want. I take").

In a criminal case concerning a person affected by FAS, the court has only three options:
1. conviction
2. acquaintance
3. preventive detention.

It is important not to withhold judgement due to the insignificance of the current crime, but it is desirable to obtain an acquittal because of a confirmed diagnosis of FAS!

This is the only way that the FAS diagnosis will be documented in court files, and in consideration of a potential future offence, the diagnosis of FAS will be known for the next trial.

Recommendations to the court in the situation of criminal offences by FAS-patients:
1. familiarity with patients with a confirmed FAS-diagnosis;
2. initiating full legal support;
3. retention in a specialised 24-hour supervised therapeutic facility;
4. initiating possible necessary psychiatric out-patient treatment;
5. intensive care with 1:1 support if necessary.

In summary, there have been few studies investigating the association between FAS and criminality or studies describing the treatment of delinquent FAS patients by the legal system from the USA and Canada. In our justice system, the term *invisible disorder* still holds true, describing the situation of patients with fetal alcohol spectrum disorder. Adults with FAS are usually undiagnosed; neither judges, nor prosecutors or prison staff know enough about the syndrome. Improved general education and acceptance of this neuropsychiatric disorder in our legal system, particularly the criminal justice system, is highly necessary. If a neurocognitive disorder is suspected, a medical assessment should be initiated before a defendant is potentially convicted.

Bibliography

[1]   Spohr HL, Willms J, Steinhausen HC. Fetal Alcohol Spectrum Disorders in Young Adulthood. J. Pediatr 2007, 150, 175–179.
[2]   Autti-Rämö I, Fagerlund A, Ervalathi N, Loimu L, Korkman M, Hoyme E. Fetal Alcohol Spectrum Disorder in Finland: Clinical Delineation of 77 Older Children and Adolescents. American Journal of Medical Genetics 2006, 140(2), 137–143.
[3]   Streissguth AP, Barr HM, Kogan J et al. Understanding the occurrence of secondary disabilities in clients with fetal alcohol syndrome (FAS) and fetal alcohol effects (FAE). Final report to the Centers for Disease Control and Prevention (CDC). University of Washington, Fetal Alcohol and Drug Unit, Seattle 1996, 96–106.
[4]   Lemoine P, Lemoine Ph. Outcome in the offspring of alcoholic mothers (study of one hundred and fifty adults and consideration with a view to prophylaxis (in French). Ann Pédiatr (Paris) 1992, 39(4), 226–235.
[5]   Chudley AE, Kilgour AR, Cranston M, Edwards M. Challenges of Diagnosis in Fetal Alcohol Spectrum Disorder in the Adult. Am J Med Genet Part C semin Med Genet 2007, 145C, 261–272.
[6]   Freunscht I, Feldmann R. Young Adults with Fetal Alcohol Syndrome (FAS): Social, Emotional and Occupational Development. Klinische Pädiatrie 2011, 223, 33–37.
[7]   Walloch JE, Burger PH, Kornhuber J. Was wird aus Kindern mit fetalem Alkoholsyndrom (FAS)/fetalen Alkoholsepektrumstörungen (FASD) im Erwachsenenalter. Fortschr Neurol Psychiat 2012, 80, 320–326.
[8]   Astley SJ. Diagnostic guide for Fetal Alcohol Spectrum Disorders: The 4-Digit Diagnostic Code. 3rd edn. University of Washington Publication Services, Seattle WA 2004.
[9]   Hall JG, Froster-Iskenius UG, Allanson JE. Handbook of Normal Physical Measurements. Oxford University Press, New York 1989.
[10] Streissguth AP, Aase JM, Clarren SK, Randels SP, LaDue RA, Smith DF. Fetal alcohol syndrome in adolescents and adults. JAMA 1991, 265, 1961–1967.
[11] Chudley AE, Conry J, Cook JL, Cook C, Rosales T, LeBlanc N. Fetal alcohol spectrum disorder: Canadian guidelines for diagnosis. CMAJ 2005, 172(5suppl), S1–S21.
[12] Landgraf M, Heinen F. S3-Leitlinie; Diagnostik des Fetalen Alkoholsyndroms. AWMF-Registernr: 022-025, 2012.
[13] Mattson SN, Schoenfeld AM, Riley EP. Teratogenic effects of alcohol on brain and behaviour. Alcohol Res Health 2001, 25, 185–191.
[14] Temple V, Shewfelt L, Tao L, Casati J, Klevnick L. Comparing Daily Living Skills in Adults with Fetal Alcohol Spectrum Disorder (FASD) To An IQ Matched Clinical Sample. J Popul Ther Clin Pharmacol 2011, 18(2), e397–402.
[15] Mattson SN, Crocker N, Nguyen TT. Fetal alcohol spectrum disorders: neuropsychological and behavioral features. Neuropsychol Rev 2011, 21(2), 81–101.
[16] Streissguth AP, Kanter J (eds). The challenge of fetal alcohol syndrome: Overcoming secondary disabilities. University of Washington Press, Seattle 1997, 2539.
[17] Kerns, KA, Don A, Mateer CA, Streissguth AP. Cognitive deficits in nonretarded adults with fetal alcohol syndrome. Journal of Learning Disabilities 1997, 30(6), 685–693.
[18] Suzuki K. Adult fetal alcohol syndrome (FAS) with various neuropsychiatric symptoms. Nihon Arukoru Yakubutsu Igakkai Zasshi 2004, 39(5), 474–481.

[19] http://depts.washington.edu/fasdpn/htmls/4-digit-code.htm.

[20] Clark E, Lutke J, Minnes P, Quellette-Kuntz H. Secondary disabilities among adults with fetal alcohol spectrum disorder in British Columbia. J FAS Int 2004, 2, e13.

[21] Fast DK, Conry J. Fetal alcohol spectrum Disorders and the Criminal Justice System. Developmental Disabilities Research Reviews 2009, 15, 250–257.

[22] Fast DK, Conry J, Healthy J. The challenge of fetal alcohol syndrome in the criminal legal system. Addiction Biology 2004, 9, 161–166.

[23] Mela M, Luther G. Fetal alcohol spectrum disorder: Can diminished resposibility diminish criminal behaviour?. International Journal of Law and Psychiatry 2013, 36, 46–54.

[24] Burd L, Selfridge RH, Klug MG, Bakko SA. Fetal alcohol syndrome in the United States corrections system. Addiction Biology 2004, 9, 164–176.

[25] Popova S, Lange S, Bekmuradov D, Mihic A, Rehm J. Fetal alcohol spectrum disorder prevalence estimates in correctional systems: a systematic literature review. Can J Public Health 2011, 102(5), 336–340.

Part IV: **Intervention, prevention, and social law issues**

15 Treatment and intervention programs

15.1 General aspects

If parents or caregivers receive a FAS diagnosis for their child, a common response is: "Why do we actually need a diagnosis when there is obviously no treatment available?"

Diagnosing FAS is a critical and sensitive moment for everyone concerned. Caregivers or parents often believe that "something is wrong" with their children, and often it is a long and difficult way to find the final diagnosis. They have consulted many different doctors in a diagnostic odyssey and often received the message that the developmental delay of their child will disappear over time or will be compensated by dedicated care. Parents trust these reassurances and try even harder to educate and support their handicapped child.

With aging of the child, the parental concern did not diminish. It became evident that cognitive deficits and increasing behavioural problems cannot be explained only by developmental delay, difficult neonatal conditions or insufficient education.

Often, information from the socioenvironment, (e.g. Internet or family doctor) raises the suspicion that FAS could be the cause of the problems. Finally, the child is referred to specialised centres to receive a correct diagnosis according to FAS-guidelines [1].

With this diagnosis, the sobering prognosis of FAS needs to be explained to the caregivers: lifelong physical and mental disability, probably with reduced independence and a need for constant supervision and support.

Many foster and adoptive parents are completely unprepared for this diagnosis and think, that "years of effort and support, with the hope of improvement seem to be for nothing". Deep disappointment and the anxious questions of what to do now and what the appropriate treatment is are often the first reactions.

At this initial encounter following the diagnosis of FAS, there is an important need for a detailed consultation:

- *The first message*: There is no longer any doubt; the difficulties and problems of the child are not the result of insufficient education, which often is quickly suggested by neighbours, social environment and educators. The cognitive deficits and behavioural problems can be attributed to be the consequence of maternal alcohol consumption during pregnancy resulting in irreversible damage to the developing brain.
- *The second message*: Presently, there is no convincing treatment available, and it is likely that there will ever be one.
- Interventions that are frequently implemented today, such as physiotherapy, speech therapy or occupational therapy, are generally indicated and are helpful

https://doi.org/10.1515/9783110436563-015

for treatment of developmental delay but cannot cure the damage caused by the intrauterine insult of alcohol.

–   Psychotherapeutic interventions are recommended in single cases, particularly when a child was additionally exposed to traumatic experiences in early childhood. However, in overview there is no evidenced psychotherapeutic intervention tailored specifically to FASD disorders.

–   Foster and adoptive parents shoulder the main burden of living with affected children; 24 hours a day, 7 days a week and for at least 18 years! This burden is particularly hard for the first few years of child's life.

–   Only the protective care of foster parents or other caregivers for these affected and often neglected, potentially physically and sexually abused children, may help them to gain self-confidence and trust.

–   *The third message*: It requires patience to endure the difficulties and problems of these children for an extended time. Due to the diversity of symptoms, a prognosis can only be made on an individual basis and with great caution. Parents often know better than professionals what is convenient for their children and which treatment may be helpful.

–   Last but not least, the parents have to look for "allies" who will support them individually; this may be child services, support groups or professionals experienced with FAS.

15.2 Pharmacotherapy

15.2.1 Treatment of ADHD in FASD patients

The efficacy of pharmaceutical treatment in patients with FAS is for the most part based on the treatment of comorbid ADHD. The literature is limited to only a few publications.

After the study of Peadon [3], there were only two randomised trials, published with very small number of subjects until 2009. Oesterheld et al. (1998) [6] only examined four children aged 4 to 12, and Snyder (1997) [7] explored 12 children, who were treated with different medications over a short time period. Overall, these studies reported a significant improvement in hyperactivity and impulsivity, but not in attention.

In 2008, Doig et al. [8] published a retrospective study of 27 children diagnosed with FASD and ADHD, treated in the FASD clinic in the Alberta Hospital in Calgary. The researchers studied the pharmaceutical effects in ADHD in general and their response to drug treatment considering which type of ADHD (hyperactive/impulsive, inattentive, oppositional defiant behaviour) responded best. In 18/27 patients the hyperactivity/impulsivity improved significantly. Similar results (19/27) were found for ADHD with oppositional behaviour. In contrast, only 9/27 patients showed significant improvement in their attention ability; the medications used were: atomoxetine (6), dextroamphetamine (10) and methylphenidate (18) [8].

Despite the poverty of data, we believe that medication is useful, particularly in FAS patients suffering from hyperactivity and impulsivity, and if symptoms are severe, treatment is indicated already before the age of 6. Contrary to previous findings, we observed significant improvements even in attention.

Pharmaceutical drugs approved for ADHD are listed below:

Stimulants
- **methylphenidate**:
- immediate-release (IR): duration of peak action around 2–4 hours, i.e. Ritalin®, Medikinet®, generics;
- sustained-release (SR): duration of peak action 3–8 hours, i.e. Ritalin LA/SA®, Equasym retard®, Medikinet retard®;
- extended-release (ER): duration of peak action 8–12 hours, i.e. Concerta®
- **amphetamine**:
- Several currently prescribed amphetamine formulations contain both enantiomers: Adderall® and lisdexamphetamin: Elvanse®.

Other substances (nonstimulants)
- **atomoxetine**: Strattera®
- **guanfacine**: Intuniv®

In our clinic, we commonly begin treatment with methylphenidate due to its fast effects on hyperactivity and impulsivity. Indication for the substance is based on individual symptomatology, requirements in everyday life and potential side effects. Treating children as young as 3 to 4 years old, we always start with methylphenidate IR at low dosage (0.25 mg/kg body weight) and with a careful increase in dosage (maximum 1 mg/kg body weight).

Treatment of aggressive behaviour and conduct disorder
In addition to ADHD, children with FAS often suffer from conduct disorder (CD) or oppositional defiant disorder (ODD) also. These patients often need pharmaceutical treatment to participate in school or in daily social activities. Although there are no studies available, FAS patients with a diagnosis of ADHD and CD are currently treated with Risperidone, which is an atypical antipsychotic (Risperdal®).

In 2015, Ozsarfat and Koren published the first study investigating the effectiveness of treating FASD children with Risperidone in combination with stimulants or atomoxetine. Data were collected from a FASD clinic in Tel Aviv.

Ten children with FASD (5–16 years of age; 3 female, 7 male) suffering from ADHD were treated with stimulants (methylphenidate/amphetamine) or atomoxetine. They received Risperidone due to an additional impulse control disorder with aggressive behaviour (DSM-IV: ODD or CD). All patients, except for one 10-year-old boy, responded successfully to the co-medication with Risperidone (dosage of 0.5–1.5 mg/d, see Table 15.1) [10].

Tab. 15.1: Efficacy of Risperidone in children with FASD (modified from Ozsarfati und Koren, 2015) [10].

Patient	Gender	Age	Diagnosis	Daily dosage of Risperdal®	Additional medication (Other drugs)	Response (Reaction) to Risperdal®	Side effects
1	f	16 years	ADHD, ODD, CD	1 mg	Ritalin SR®	yes	none
2	m	6.5 years	ADHD, ODD	1 mg	Concerta®	yes	none
3	m	11 years	ADHD, ODD	1 mg	Concerta®, Aderall®, Ritalin®	yes	none
4	m	10 years	ADHD, ODD	0.5 mg	Concerta®	no	creatinine increase
5	m	16.5 years	ADHD, ODD, CD	1.5 mg	Concerta®	yes	none
6	m	13.4 years	ADHD, ODD	1.5 mg reduced to 1 mg	Stratera®	yes	depression, suicidal ideation (not after the reduction to 1 mg of risperdal)
7	m	5 years	ADHD, ODD	first: 0.2 mg, then: 0.3 mg, reduced to 0.25 mg	Ritalin®	yes	very calm, depressed at 0.3 mg, not anymore at 0.25 mg
8	m	5 years	ADHD, ODD	first: 0.1 mg then: 0.3 mg	Ritalin®	No yes	none
9	f	9.5 years	ADHD, ODD	0.5 mg	Concerta®, Lamictal®, Zyprexin®	yes	none
10	f	7.5 years	ADHD, ODD	0.5 mg, 1.5 mg	Ritalin®, Concerta®	no information provided	increased anger with Ritalin®

In summary, pharmaceutical treatment of cognitive deficits and behavioural disorders is essential for patients with FAS, because non-pharmacological interventions have not been very satisfying to date.

Behavioural problems, serious conflicts with teachers, parents and peers contribute to additional severe emotional distress. Therefore, pharmacological treatment including restricted indication and intensive therapeutic drug monitoring should be started early, despite general justified reservations against pharmaceutical treatment in young children.

15.3 Psychotherapeutic interventions

The majority of children, adolescents and adults with FAS show little response to psychotherapeutic treatment, and some of them seem to be almost resistant to any therapy. The lack of success is due to the fact that patients receive therapeutic interventions, which are not tailored to specific cognitive and emotional deficits of FAS [2]. Intervention models and treatment programs treating FASD are not sufficiently validated.

Apart from improvement of disabilities, it is important for the patients to promote their cognitive, emotional and social recourses, in order to increase self-confidence and improve trust in their own abilities.

Informative dialogues are necessary for general understanding of impairments and deficits associated with FASD before starting therapeutic intervention, and this should be the basis for every psychotherapeutic program [2]. To date, many different intervention models have been studied, but the evidence has been proven only occasionally.

In 2009, Peadon et al. [3] analysed the few available randomised controlled studies, examining the efficacy of a completed intervention.Out of 475 studies, only 12 met the previously determined quality criteria, but only 3 had a sample size (60–100 children) large enough for general conclusions. The interventions were targeted at mathematical abilities, speech and social skills and were implemented for a period of 6 to 12 weeks. These three treatment studies found significant improvements in mathematical abilities, speech and social skills, but the follow-up was very limited in time, sometimes lasting only a few weeks [3].

Kodituwakku and Kodituwakku [4] conducted an extensive literature review in 2011 and found only 12 publications that complied with the criteria of evidence-based intervention studies and showed significant improvements. Interventions examined in these studies were, for example, training programs for social skills, for speech, for neurocognitive abilities, for working memory and parent–child interaction therapy as well as for cognitive behavioural therapy. However, in this literature review there was also a distinct lack of longer follow-up periods.

In a pilot study in 2004, Grant et al. examined the effects of a modified PCAP program (Parent-Child Assistance Program) at the University of Washington; 19 young women with FAS participated in this study for 1 year. The supervisors in this study were non-professional case managers. The researchers were able to show that intensive supervision led to significant improvements in daily life activities. The women drank less alcohol, consumed illegal substances to a lesser extent, used contraceptives more regularly, used health care services more often and became more domestic in general [5].

In summary, presently there are no evidence-based therapeutic strategies, except for a few pilot studies. Hence, there is a continuous great need for research, examining effective long-lasting therapeutic intervention programs in children, adolescents and adults with FAS. This holds particularly true for deficits in executive functions, which create so many difficulties in everyday life and result in a loss of independence.

15.4 Vitamin A supplements

It is recognised that ethanol and its metabolites interact in many ways with the metabolism of folate, choline and vitamin A, and especially with retinoic acids.

In 2011, Ballard et al. [9] introduced supplementation with vitamin A, folate and choline during pregnancy as preventative measures that might reduce the risk of developing FAS.

The authors speculate that ethanol alone is not responsible for the entire spectrum of teratogenic abnormalities; nutritional deficiencies, exacerbated by alcohol may also have an additional contributing effect in developing FAS.

Deficiencies in vitamin A (all-trans-retinal deficiency), folate and choline are found in individuals living under conditions of poverty and are common in alcoholics, particularly in alcohol-dependent women during pregnancy. Alcohol has a direct impact on retinoic acid-metabolism; it lowers the level of retinoic acids, which are necessary for normal neural development in a fetus.

The authors proposed that supplementation of vitamin A, choline and folate during pregnancy in alcohol-dependent women may mitigate the negative consequences of intrauterine alcohol exposure. At present however, this treatment approach seems unrealistic [9].

15.5 Social services

Depending on their individual needs, children and adolescents with FAS and their families have the possibility of receiving single case support or family assistance. If more training and education in self-sufficiency is necessary, single case support seems to be more effective. If main priority is focused on severe family problems due to behavioural difficulties of the child, individual family assistance is the therapy of choice.

If community services are not successful, foster parents sometimes have to accept institutional placement of their child. It must be emphasised that the development of such a situation is normally not the fault of caregivers but rather the result of intrauterine alcohol damage.

Because patients with FAS often have pronounced difficulties in social interactions, living in large groups is problematic for them and this has to be taken into account in choosing an appropriate institution.

Generally, to improve any support, professional caregivers, single case managers and family assistants need to be educated much more about the deficits of FAS. Therapeutic and pedagogic intervention programs should not be costly for patients. Similar to autism spectrum disorder, certain symptoms are not treatable; therapeutic success can only be expected by constant repetitive training opportunities.

15.6 Assisted living communities and assisted living for single adults

FAS in its different manifestations is a lifelong physical and mental disability. The permanent damage needs intensive supervision and support beyond the age of 18, in order to complete job training and to at least find a position in a disability work programme.

When adultpatients are not severely disabled, support by a single caseworker or placement in assisted living housing is a reasonable choice. A model for an assisted living community for adults with FASD is provided by "Sonnenhof e.V" in Berlin, one of the first institutions of this kind in Germany. The intention is to enable patients to live as independently as possible and to work in a job, depending on their individual skills (for detailed description, see Appendix A).

Support in daily life by a case worker includes, for example, individual support whilst learning practical life skills; daily assistance in structuring daily routines; promoting the ability to make new contacts, hold relationships and manage conflicts; resource-oriented support to allow personal development and finally, to help during crisis situations and daily conflicts.

Bibliography

[1] Astley SJ. Diagnostic guide for Fetal Alcohol Spectrum Disorders: The 4-Digit Diagnostic Code. 3rd edn. University of Washington Publication Services, Seattle WA 2004.
[2] Paley B, O'Connor MJ. Intervention for individuals with fetal alcohol spectrum disorders: treatment approaches and case management. Developmental Disabilities Research Reviews 2009, 15(3), 258–267.

[3] Peadon E, Rhys-Jones B, Bower C, Elliott E. Systematic review of interventions for children with Fetal Alcohol Spectrum Disorders. BioMed Central (BMC) Pediatrics 2009, 9, 35.

[4] Kodituwakku PW, Kodituwakku EL. From Research to Practice: An Integrative Framework for the Development of Interventions for Children with Fetal Alcohol Spectrum Disorders. Neuropsychol Rev 2011, 21, 204–223.

[5] Grant T, Huggins J, Connor P et al. A pilot Community Intervention for young Women with Fetal Alcohol Spectrum Disorders. Community Mental Health Journal 2004, 40(6), 499–511.

[6] Oesterheld JR, Kofoed L, Tervo R, Fogas B, Wilson A, Fiechtner H. Effectiveness of methylphenidate in Native American children with fetal alcohol syndrome and attention deficit/hyperactivity disorder: A controlled pilot study. J Child Adolesc Psychopharmacol 1998, 8, 39–48.

[7] Snyder J, Nanson J, Synder R, Block G. A study of stimulant medication in children with FAS. In: Streissguth AP, Kanter J (eds). The challenge of Fetal Alcohol Syndrome: Overcoming Secondary Disabilities. University of Washington Press, Seattle 1997, 64–7.

[8] Doig J, McLennan JD, Gibbard WB. Medication Effects on Symptoms of Attention-Deficit/Hyperactivity Disorder in Children with Fetal Alcohol Spectrum Disorder. J Child Adolesc Psychopharmacol 2008, 18, 365–371.

[9] Ballard MS, Sun M, Ko J. Vitamin A, folate, and choline as a possibe preventive intervention to fetal alcohol syndrome. Medical Hypothesis 2012, 78, 489–493.

[10] Ozsarfati J, Koren G. Medications used in the treatment of diruptive behavior in children with FASD – A Guide. J Popul Ther Cin Pharmacol 2015, 22(1), e59–e67.

16 Prevention of FAS and FASD

Jan-Peter Siedentopf and Manuela Nagel

16.1 Introduction

Fetal alcohol syndrome, i.e. the congenital consequences of maternal alcohol consumption during pregnancy (FASD) are often referred to as "the most common preventable congenital malformations".

Although this assumption holds true for the frequency, it is unclear whether this disorder is preventable when dealing with pregnant addicts whose substance abuse is not regulated by their free will or by rational decisions. The approaches and concepts necessary to prevent the negative consequences of alcohol consumption in this rather small population should also target the prevention of addictions in general, which, however, goes far beyond the topic of the current chapter.

As described previously in the section on epidemiology and FAS (see Chapter 7), there is a large research and knowledge gap regarding the incidence and prevalence of FAS and FASD in many countries, including Germany. The estimated incidence for FAS of about 4000/700 000 live births [1] suggests that a tremendous study population is required in order to prove the efficacy of a preventive measure. Therefore, it is almost impossible to provide a scientific assessment of the effectiveness of preventive measures specifically created to prevent FAS and FASD.

Consequently, most of the concepts for prevention that will be described do not aim to reduce the incidence and prevalence rates of FAS/FASD, but rather try to target populations with a large majority of women of childbearing age. This approach is in line with more recent studies from English-speaking countries, in which the avoidance of *alcohol-exposed pregnancies* (AEP) is the main goal of their prevention campaigns. Since the prevention of alcohol consumption during pregnancy is the only certain method to prevent FAS and FASD completely, we took on the same goal and decided to start using the term alcohol-exposed pregnancies in the context of this chapter – and for our future work – as well.

A total of 208 alcohol prevention projects for children and adolescents in Germany were examined in a Health Technology Assessment (HTA) report from the German Institute of Medical Documentation and Information (DIMDI) in 2012. In summary, the report concluded that the alcohol prevention projects used in Germany are, for the most part, not properly evaluated [2].

https://doi.org/10.1515/9783110436563-016

16.2 General prevention programs

If alcohol consumption would be perceived as a social phenomenon with one of its "side effects" being alcohol consumption during pregnancy, then it should be possible to achieve the prevention of AEP through a general reduction of alcohol consumption.

Following this reasoning, the approach to put warnings on alcoholic beverages or in stores that sell alcohol does not have a large short-term impact, but with consistent labelling of all alcoholic beverages could, however, in the long run, reduce the social acceptance of or reduce the ignorance regarding pregnant women consuming alcohol [3, 4].

Studies with highly controlled conditions in secluded populations were able to significantly reduce AEP by forbidding the sale of alcohol to pregnant women [5]. However, transferring these positive findings from rural Alaska to regions with easier access to alcohol is most likely to fail.

Similarly to the successful reduction of cigarette consumption, a reduction of AEP could be expected through banning the advertisement of and a price increase for alcoholic beverages [6].

In this context, the importance of internet-based advertising in influencing drinking behaviour should not be overlooked. The European "AMPHORA" research project described the influence of online alcohol marketing or alcohol branded sports sponsorship on the drinking behaviour of adolescents (http://www.drogenbeauftragte. de/fileadmin/dateien-dba/DrogenundSucht/Alkohol/Downloads/Abschlussbericht-AMPHORA-Veroeffentlichung_200114.pdf). Internet-supported prevention projects must, often with little financial means and not enough staff, compete against well thought out advertising campaigns on television, the Internet and social media formats. This competition seems almost futile without consistent, well-coordinated and cooperative prevention campaigns, since just one expired link quickly leads to disinterest or a loss of credibility.

16.3 Substance abuse prevention for children

Already in early childhood, the way alcohol is handled within the family, as well as the effects of alcohol consumption, can be observed by children.

Common practices such as raising a glass and toasting with others before a meal is already keenly observed and imitated at the early age of less than 2 years. In best-case scenarios, this can be used to teach the child certain restrictions or taboos ("for adults only", "not for mama", etc.). In order to establish long-term prevention strategies based on these early interfamilial scenarios, which can be highly diverse, the rest of the child's life must be filled with reinforcing and additional strategies. One special caveat should be the consumption of alcohol reduced or alcohol free beer. While the alcohol content poses no risk, young children get accustomed to the very special taste of beer. This may lead to earlier consumption of beer containing alcohol without the "need" to get accustomed to the bitter taste.

Langeland and Hartgers pointed out in a review that women who experienced sexual or physical abuse as a child more frequently displayed problems with alcohol consumption [7]. Up to 70% of women who drink during pregnancy have experienced sexual, physical and/or emotional abuse during childhood. Moreover, experiences of abuse increase the risk of mental and psychiatric disorders, in particular depression. Since these, in turn, increase the risk of uncontrolled use or abuse of addictive substances, the prevention of sexual or emotional abuse, violent experiences and neglect is at the same time an effective prevention of AEP [8, 9].

Intrauterine alcohol exposure leads to increased rates of problematic drinking behaviour and psychiatric disorders in young adults [10]. Hence, the risk of repetition by the next generation is clearly present [11].

16.4 Prevention programs for adolescents and young adults

Despite the fact that prevention campaigns in schools focus on one's individual approach to alcohol, it would be beneficial to point out the dangers of alcohol consumption during pregnancy early on, for example during sex education.

The results on the efficacy of school prevention campaignssummarised in the HTA report by the German Institute of Medical Documentation and Information (DIMDI) from 2012 are, unfortunately, very sobering [2]. According to the authors of the report, of the 208 projects examined, only 11 were examined for efficacy. Of these, partly very large-scale projects, only four were able to achieve a reduction in alcohol consumption/binge drinking or a delay in the start of alcohol consumption. With regard to the current aim here, i.e. the prevention of AEP, a relevant effect can only be expected of the two projects "Tingling in my stomach" ("Kribbeln im Bauch") and "Project crystal clear" ("Aktion Glasklar") – if they are also effective beyond the duration of the prevention campaign (until 16 years of age). The HTA report describes the effects of "Project crystal clear" as "short-term and little".

The use of new media is clearly an important enrichment of the different possibilities for educational and prevention campaigns. Drug and Addiction report from 2012 by the Federal Drug Commissioner described several projects that were funded by the Federal Ministry of Health and made use of social networks [12]. According to the HTA report, however, the largest of these projects, "Alcohol? Know your limit" did not have any prevention effects.

Besides these general prevention strategies developed for school settings and as such, without or with little gender-specific adaptations, there is an increase in questions regarding the association between alcohol consumption and sexuality in the "girls' hour" at gynecologists. In this setting, not only the increased risk of unsafe sexual behaviour under the influence of alcohol should be addressed but also the dangers of alcohol consumption during pregnancy. This approach is implemented in the project "Pregnant? Your child drinks with you! Alcohol? No sip – No risk!" by the "Medial Association for Health Support e.V." (http://www.ÄGGF.de), funded by the Federal Ministry of Health and aimed to provide medical information on alcohol consumption during pregnancy in school classes for adolescents aged 14–18. Previous evaluations of a similar project on sex education suggests positive long-term effects.

One aspect of the project "Responsible from the start!" which was initiated by the working group Alcohol and Responsibility of the "Federal Association of the German Spirits Industry and Importers, is a brochure with the subtitle "What girls should know about alcoholic drinks during pregnancy" [13]. Since the main information is transferred via a brochure, the effectiveness of the prevention is limited by the ways the brochure is made available to the public. When information is given during counselling, there is a higher probability that the brochure will be read afterwards.

16.5 Before conception: women and couples

Women who use contraceptives and who want to get pregnant, only need to go and speak to a gynecologist when they are using permanent contraceptives, particularly in the case of an IUD (intrauterine device). It is much more common for women, however, to stop using their current contraceptive on their own (usually the "pill", oral hormonal contraceptives, less often condoms). Only after her period stops and a pregnancy test turns out positive, do women go and seek the advice of a gynecologist again (see Section 16.6 "Prevention programs targeted to pregnant women"). Therefore, it is usually not possible for physicians to intervene in the period between planning a pregnancy and the early phases of a pregnancy. Hence, in order to avoid AEP, it is urgently advised to address the wish to have children or the topic of alcohol and pregnancy at every regular visit for, for example, a contraceptive renewal or pap smear [14].

In the study "Health in Germany: current situation" upper class women between the ages 30 to 44 years and 45 to 64 years presented the two groups with the highest percentage of dangerous alcohol consumption [15]. In light of the increased risk for AEP and for giving birth to children with FAS/FASD for mothers of higher age, it seems urgent to develop specific prevention strategies targeted at this specific patient group.

Alcohol consumption during the early stages of pregnancy leads to a significantly increased rate of miscarriages compared to complete alcohol abstinence [16, 17]. With this knowledge, it seems completely incomprehensible why the topic "alcohol use during pregnancy" is not given more attention in the context of reproductive medicine [18].

16.6 Prevention programs targeted to pregnant women

On the website of the Federal Commissioner on Drugs the focus on "new policies to prevent drug use during pregnancy and nursing" is emphasised [19]. Seven projects that were funded over the period of 1 year present their final reports on the website. The most important finding seems to be the crucial need for networks and integrated care approaches. Difficulties in the interaction between gynecologists and counselors are pointed out repeatedly. In particular, gynecologists who were offered additional training on the topic alcohol use during pregnancy only seldom participated. A major problem is the detection of pregnant women who consume alcohol (see Section 16.7 "Risk assessment during pregnancy").

The specifically developed Internet-based intervention for alcohol and nicotine-consuming pregnant women called the "IRIS Platform" by the University of Tübingen is worth a special mention (http://www.iris-plattform.de). This highly text-based intervention was evaluated in a research project from April 2014 to April 2015. However, "due to its high demand" it was continued independently from the research project.

The above-mentioned project initiated by the working group Alcohol and Responsibility of the Federal Association of the German Spirits Industry and Importers is based on the brochure "Responsible from the Start!" and as such, largely dependent on passive information transfer. In systematic reviews, these types of approaches are judged to have little effect, although the results might be more positive in individual cases [20].

Overall, it is of crucial importance that all those coming in contact with and advising pregnant women, especially midwives and gynecologists, clearly advise to completely stay abstinent from alcohol during the complete course of the pregnancy.

16.7 Risk assessment during pregnancy

It is common in Germany to make use of medical services specifically designed to pregnant women early on in the pregnancy, i.e. already 1 to 2 weeks after the period stops or directly after a positive pregnancy test. Pregnant women who are subsequently informed early on about FAS/FASD and the possibility of preventing it via complete alcohol abstinence, will, for the most part, halt their alcohol intake.

According to guidelines for mothers, the first examination of the fetus should happen "as soon as possible" after finding out about a pregnancy [21]. One part of this first examination should be patient history (of the mother) and as such, collecting (implicitly) potential risk factors for an AEP.

In Germany, the joint Federal Committee of Physicians and health insurance companies (www.g-ba.de) has expectant mothers document their prenatal and natal care ("Mutterpass"). In this document, it should be recorded if they received a consultation regarding the use of stimulants and, when applicable, there is the option to document

Name   Date

CHARITÉ

CharitéCentrum für Frauen-, Kinder- und Jugendmedizin mit Perinatalzentrum und Humangenetik

Evaluation of Alcohol consumption in pregnancy (Berliner EvAS)

1.) Gestational age today (week or due-date)? _____

2.) When did You realise You are pregnant? _____
(gestational week or date)

3.) Did You drink alcohol during this pregnancy?

- never
- once
- less than once a month
- 1 – 4 times per month
- 2 – 3 times per week
- 4 times per week or more

4.) On the days when you drank alcohol, how many drinks did you have per day?
(one unit (10g) of alcohol equals approximately 0,33 l beer, a small glass of wine or champagne (0,1 l), or a standard serving of liquor

- 1 unit
- 2 units
- 3-4 units
- more than 4 units

5.) Did You change your alcohol consumption after realising you are pregnant?

- No
- Yes, I stopped drinking alcohol
- Yes, I reduced alcohol consumption.
- Yes, I increased alcohol consumption.

Evaluation (Please mark the appropriate box according to the answer to questions 3 and 4)

	never 0	once	less than once a month	1 – 4 times per month	2 – 3 times per week	4 times per week or more
1 unit (A)		1	1	2	3	4
2 units (B)		1	2	3	4	5
3 – 4 units (C)		2	3	4	5	6
More than 4 units (D)		3	4	5	6	6

Fig. 16.1: Recommendations for the therapeutic consequences following the evaluation of the questionnaire.

Berliner EvAS – Risk stratification

Group 0/1
(Positive feedback, counselling)

If the pregnant women did not drink alcohol in pregnancy she should be encouraged to maintain abstinence throughout pregnancy.
Although there is **no proven safe level** of alcohol consumption in pregnancy, less than one unit per month *appears* to be safe.
The women should be counselled towards complete alcohol abstinence for the rest of pregnancy.

Group 2
(Thorough counselling)

Amount and/or interval of alcohol consumption do not indicate a high risk for FAS or FASD. Many patients in this group will have reduced drinking pattern after diagnosis of pregnancy, they should be supported to achieve and maintain abstinence throughout pregnancy.
Patients that did **not** reduce their drinking habits after diagnosis of pregnancy should be counselled towards abstinence.

Group 3
(Intensive counselling, referral to specialist)

In non-regnant women the amount of alcohol consumed in this group is within a widely accepted "normal" range. Male and female peers will consume alcohol in a similar fashion, taking little or no risk to develop alcohol dependency in future.
Within pregnancy the amount of alcohol consumed by this group (per occasion and/or per week) lies just below a margin where alcohol related birth defects are statistically *detectable*. Non-detectable cognitive or behavioural deficits (below "genetic ability") may occur.
Intensive, in some cases repeated counselling is necessary to achieve abstinence. Close monitoring of alcohol consumption throughout pregnancy is essential.
If in doubt, refer to a specialist in addiction medicine.

Group 4 - 6
(Referral to specialist)

Fetuses and children of women in this group are at **high risk** for alcohol related birth defects. Intrauterine growth retardation, especially reduced head circumference, is a warning sign.

The patients have a **high risk** to suffer from or develop alcohol dependency and should be referred to addiction specialists - for their own and the fetuses sake.

Psychosocial situation can include **child-deprivation, violence and poverty**. Siblings should be evaluated for developmental deficits, signs of violence or deprivation and FAS/FASD.

Continuous developmental monitoring and support is essential to reduce the burden of FAS/FASD.

For scientific evaluation use additional groups A-D, giving further detail about the mount of alcohol consumed per occasion.

Fig. 16.1: (continued)

"substance abuse" in the section "Special diagnostic findings during pregnancy". Additional requirements regarding the documentation are not given.

According to our own findings, it seems unlikely that it is possible to reliably detect alcohol consumption during pregnancy without a structured interview or questionnaire [22]. Suitable questionnaires to identify alcohol intake such as the TWEAK, AUDIT-C or T-ACE are available in English, but have not yet been validated for German-speaking populations. In a comprehensive review in the year 2009, Burns *et al.* concluded that these commonly used questionnaires are, indeed, able to detect risk behaviour, alcohol abuse and alcohol dependency, but their ability to detect AEP is questionable [23]. The biggest limitation of these questionnaires is, in our opinion, that only high amounts of alcohol consumption are recorded. The first question on tolerance in the TWEAK-questionnaire is: "How many units can you drink, before you are intoxicated?". The third question in the AUDIT asks about occasions where the interviewee consumed six or more glasses of alcohol [24]. Since these questionnaires were originally developed for people who are not pregnant, it is understandable that these questionnaires focus on alcohol amounts that are dangerous for the consumer herself. However, in light of the complete abstinence that is required during pregnancy to protect the fetus, these amounts are obviously too high.

In the survey that we developed to systematically assess alcohol consumption (see Fig. 16.1, "Berliner EvAS") during pregnancy, we chose to include the assessment of any form or amount of alcohol consumption [25]. In addition to an individual risk assessment, the survey evaluation includes clinical recommendations.

One possibility for early risk assessment during pregnancy could be a FAS diagnosis in older siblings. Hence, guidelines like the German S3-guideline on the diagnosis of FAS/FASD could also be of significance for the prevention of FASand FASD.

16.8 Identification of women at risk of prenatal alcohol exposure

An important and particularly difficult aspect of prevention is the identification of pregnant women with a high risk for an AEP. Mothers of children with FAS/FASD seem to have, amongst others, the following characteristics that could act as risk factors: physical abuse during childhood (see Section 16.3 "Substance abuse prevention for children"); the presence of psychiatric disorders; substance disorders; advanced maternal age; a lack of social support; and five or more previous pregnancies [11]. Women who have already given birth to one child with FAS/FASD have a high risk of repetition [27, 28]. Therefore, any pregnancy of a mother who has already given birth to a child with a FAS or FASD diagnosis should be seen as a high-risk AEP pregnancy and as such, the prenatal care should be very intensive. However, since another risk factor is the relatively late and unreliable usage of prenatal care services, other institutions/ services such as child services or general physicians should be prepared to intervene early on.

Therapeutic interventions for women with known alcohol problems should always include a consultation on safe contraceptive methods. When these patients express a wish to become pregnant, their treatment should, on the one hand, be adapted to a possible pregnancy and, on the other hand, relapse prevention strategies as well as crisis intervention strategies should be established in accordance with the patient. A potential relapse should be approached differently in pregnant patients compared to non-pregnant patients, since the occurrence of binge drinking episodes, typical during a relapse, pose a high risk for the development of FAS/FASD.

The use of medication for relapse prevention, e.g. naltrexone, should be evaluated carefully before being used by pregnant women [29, 30].

Therapeutic interventions that could prevent the development of FAS or FASD after prenatal alcohol consumption or reduce its consequences have not surpassed a stage of purely hypothetical theories [31].

Bibliography

[1]   Pötzsch O. Geburten in Deutschland, 2012. In: Statistisches Bundesamt (ed). Statistisches Bundesamt, Wiesbaden 2012.
[2]   Kaskutas LG, Lee ME, Cote J. Reach and Effects of Health Messages on Drinking During Pregnancy. J. Health Educ. 1998, 29(1), 11–20.
[3]   Hankin JF, Sloan JJ, Ager JW, Sokol RJ, Martier SS. Heeding the Alcoholic Beverage Warning Label During Pregnancy: Multiparae Versus Nulliparae. J. Stud. Alcohol 1996, 57(2), 171–177.
[4]   Korczak D. Föderale Strukturen der Prävention von Alkoholmissbrauch bei Kindern und Jugendlichen. Deutsches Institut für Medizinische Dokumentation und Information (DIMDI), Köln 2012.
[5]   Bowerman RJ. The Effect of a Community-Supported Alcohol Ban on Prenatal Alcohol and Other Substance Abuse. Am. J. Public Health 1997, 87(8), 1378–1379.
[6]   Stanley FD, Daube M. Should industry care for children? Public health advocacy and law in Australia. Public Health 2009, 123, 283–286.
[7]   Langeland WH, Hartgers C. Child Sexual and Physical Abuse and Alvoholism: A Review. J. Stud. Alcohol 1998, 59, 336–348.
[8]   Norman R, Byambaa M, De R, Butchart A, Scott J, Vos T. The Long-Term Health Consequences of Child Physical Abuse, Emotional Abuse, and Neglect: A Systematic Review and Meta-Analysis. PLOS Medicine 2012, 9(11), e1001349. doi: 10.1371/journal.pmed.1001349.
[9]   Bensley LS, Van Eenwyk J, Simmons KW. Self-reported Childhood Sexual and Physical Abuse and Adult HIV-Risk Behaviors and Heavy Drinking. Am J Prev Med 2000, 18(2), 151–158.
[10] Baer JS, Sampson PD, Barr HM, Connor PD, Streissguth AP. A 21-year longitudinal analysis of the effects of prenatal alcohol exposure on young adult drinking. Arch Gen Psychiatry 2003, 60(4), 377–85.
[11] Sayal K. Alcohol consumption in pregnancy as a risk factor for later mental health problems. Evid Based Ment Health 2007, 10(4), 98–100.
[12] Die Drogenbeauftragte der Bundesregierung, Drogen- und Suchtbericht. Bundesministerium für Gesundheit, Berlin 2012, 168.

[13] Feldmann R. Verantwortung von Anfang an! "Arbeitskreis Alkohol und Verantwortung" des BSI e. V., Bonn 2012.

[14] Dudenhausen JW. Prävention fetaler Alkohol-Spektrum-Störungen durch Aufklärung. Geburtsh Frauenheilk 2012, 72, 981–982.

[15] Lange C, Ziese T. Daten und Fakten: Ergebnisse der Studie "Gesundheit in Deutschland aktuell 2009". Beiträge zur Gesundheitsberichterstattung des Bundes. Robert-Koch-Institut, Berlin 2011, 168.

[16] Kesmodel U, Wisborg K, Olsen SF, Henriksen TB, Secher NJ. Moderate alcohol intake in pregnancy and the risk of spontaneous abortion. Alcohol Alcohol 2002, 37(1), 87–92.

[17] Rasch V. Cigarette, alcohol, and caffeine consumption: risk factors for spontaneous abortion. Acta Obstet Gynaecol Scand 2003, 82(2), 182–188.

[18] Lum KJ, Sundaram R, Buck Louis GM. Women's lifestyle behaviors while trying to become pregnant: evidence supporting preconception guidance. Am J Obstet Gynecol. 2011, 205(3), 203.e1–7. doi: 10.1016/j.ajog.2011.04.030.

[19] Drogenbeauftragte der Bundesregierung. Förderschwerpunkt "Neue Präventionsansätze zur Vermeidung von Suchtmittelkonsum in Schwangerschaft und Stillzeit". 2015, available online at: http://www.drogenbeauftragte.de/drogen-und-sucht/alkohol/ alkoholund-schwangerschaft/kurz-und-abschlussberichte-der-zweiten-foerderphase-und-derevaluation-des-foerderschwerpunkts-neue-praeventionsansaetze-zur-vermeidung-vonsuchtmittelkonsum-in-schwangerschaft-und-stillzeit.html.

[20] Clarren S, Salmon A, Jonsson E. Prevention of Fetal Alcohol Spectrum Disorder FASD. Who is Responsible? In: Jonsson E (ed). Health Care and Disease Management, 1st edn. Wiley-Blackwell, Weinheim 2011, 369.

[21] Bundesausschuss der Ärzte und Krankenkassen, Richtlinien des Bundesausschusses der Ärzte und Krankenkassen über die ärztliche Betreuung während der Schwangerschaft und nach der Entbindung ("Mutterschafts-Richtlinien"). Bundesanzeiger AT 04.05.2015 B3, 2015.

[22] Siedentopf JP, Nagel M, Büscher U, Dudenhausen JW. Alkohol konsumierende Schwangere in der Schwangerenberatung. Prospektive, anonymisierte Reihenuntersuchung zur Abschätzung der Prävalenz. Deutsches Ärzteblatt 2004, 101(39), A2623–A2626.

[23] Burns E, Gray R, Smith LA. Brief screening questionnaires to identify problem drinking during pregnancy: a systematic review. Addiction 2010, 105, 601–614.

[24] Neumann T, Bergmann RL, Spies CD, Dudenhausen JW. Fragebögen zur Identifikation eines riskanten Alkoholkonsums in der Schwangerschaft und kurze Anleitung zur Entwöhnung. In: Bergmann RL, Spohr HL, Dudenhausen JW (eds). Alkohol in der Schwangerschaft. Häufigkeit und Folgen. Urban & Vogel, München 2006, 121–126.

[25] Nagel M, Hüseman D, Siedentopf JP. Berliner EvAS – Evaluation von Alkoholkonsum in der Schwangerschaft. Suchttherapie 2011, 12(4), 186–191.

[26] Landgraf M, Heinen F. S3-Leitlinie; Diagnostik des Fetalen Alkoholsyndroms. AWMF-Registernr: 022-025, 2012.

[27] Mullay A, Cleary BJ, Barry J, Fahey TP, Deirdre JM. Prevalence, predictors and perinatal outcomes of peri-conceptional alcohol exposure retrospective cohort study in an urban obstetric population in Ireland. BMC Pregnancy Childbirth 2011, 11, 27. doi: 10.1186/1471-2393-11-27.

[28] Cannon MJ, Dominique Y, O'Leary LA, Sniezek JE, Floyd RL. Characteristics and behaviours of mothers who have a child with fetal alcohol syndrome. Neurotoxicology and Teratology 2012, 34, 90–95.

[29] Garbutt JC, Kranzler HR, O'Malley SS, Gastfriend DR, Pettinati HM, Silverman BL et al. Efficacy and Tolerbility of Lng-Acting Injectable Naltrexone for Alcohol Dependence. JAMA 2005, 293(13), 1617–1625.

[30] Jones HE, Chisolm CM, Jansson LM, TerplanM. Naltrexone in the treatment of opioiddependent pregnant women: the case for a considered and measured approach to research. Addiction 2013, 108(2), 233–247.
[31] Ballard MS, Sun M, Ko J. Vitamin A, folate, and choline as a possibe preventive intervention to fetal alcohol syndrome. Medical Hypothesis 2012, 78, 489–493.

17 Awareness and support of persons with FAS in other European countries: governmental policy and social law

This chapter describes the current situation of patients suffering from FASD and their legal, social, economic and medical problems and conflicts exemplarily in three different countries: The Netherlands, the United Kingdom and Germany.

17.1 Fetal alcohol syndrome in the Netherlands

Martha Krijgsheld

17.1.1 Current status – December 2016

In The Netherlands, research on prevalence, prevention methods, and help for people with FASD is only just beginning. Thus, to date, most information and support has been provided by parent-run groups, the first and largest of which is the FAS Foundation of the Netherlands. This organisation was founded in 2002 by an adoptive mother and a foster mother, both raising children affected by FASD. According to the statutes, the aims of the foundation are as follows:
1. to provide information about FAS to the broad public;
2. to provide information about FAS and give support to families and carers;
3. to represent the interests of the FAS foundation in government institutions and industry;
4. to promote scientific research.

To reach these goals, the foundation
1. gives training sessions;
2. shares information in the broadest sense of the term;
3. offers the possibility for contact with other persons affected by FAS and for their families.

In 2005, the Health Council of the Netherlands advised the government that no amount of alcohol can be considered safe during pregnancy. According to the Health Council, there is only one safe advice: neither the man nor the woman should drink during the conception period, and the woman should not drink during pregnancy or breastfeeding [1]. This advice was repeated in another official report on pre-conception counselling [2]. Shortly after the appearance of the first report, a short awareness

https://doi.org/10.1515/9783110436563-017

campaign was carried out by the National Institute for the Promotion of Health and Prevention of Disease, but this was not continued. Neither was any research instigated into prevention, prevalence, or care of affected persons. Recent research suggests that drinking during pregnancy has declined in the past few years. A study by the TNO showed that while 17% of pregnant women reported drinking in 2007, that figure had declined to 7% in 2015. Women with a higher education report drinking more often than women with a low level of education [3].

On another positive note, the Netherlands boasts three specialised FAS diagnostic clinics (Gelre ziekenhuizen in Zutphen, Lentis in Winschoten en Groningen and Inter-Psy in Groningen). These clinics provide diagnostic services, initially just for children, now for adults as well. Furthermore, they increasingly offer some support and care. Diagnosis in these clinics is according to the 4-Digit Code method of Susan Astley.

As of the end of 2016, the picture looks more positive: The Secretary of State for the Health Ministry has commissioned a report on the status of FAS in the Netherlands and has called for more research.

17.1.2 Support and care for persons with FASD

There is no specific support or care for persons with FAS or FASD in the Netherlands. Doctors, psychologists, and education specialists receive no information on FASD during their training. There exist no protocols for diagnosis, education or support. However, in 2017 the first accredited training session for pediatricians, psychologists, and educational psychologists is to be held. This course is being organised by the FAS Foundation of the Netherlands in collaboration with the University of Utrecht, the Gelre Hospitals and the educational psychology group Zo-zorgoplossingen.

17.1.3 Care of children with a disorder or handicap

In 2015, child and youth social services was completely re-organised, with all care being transferred from central administration to the local communities. The communities also manage the budget for care out of the mental health services (GGZ). Thus, persons in need must ask for care at the local community administration rather than requesting care via the health care system. Each year, the client must present a new request for care to the community administration. The community then decides how much care can be offered. Persons with FASD and a very low IQ may receive a subsidy from the Long-term Care Law (Wet langdurig zorg, WLZ). This law regulates heavy and intensive care, which may be required lifelong. Adults with FASD can also ask for a subsidy from the Social Support Law (Wet maatschappelijke ondersteuning) so that they can buy care from their own chosen care providers.

There are several disadvantages to this system. Firstly, the care provided varies widely among communities. Secondly, since FASD is little understood, the need for care can be underestimated by inexperienced decision-makers. Finally, the need for care is often based on IQ, so that persons with FASD and a normal IQ may be denied the support they need.

17.1.4 Education

In 2014, a law was passed with the goal to guarantee educationadapted to the needs of each child (Wet op passend onderwijs). Under this law, each school is responsible for guaranteeing that each child finds a proper place in the educational system. This law means that as many children as possible should be placed in the normal school system rather than in special education. Thus, this law may lead to difficulties for children with FASD, who often need specialised attention in school.

17.1.5 The Law on Participation

The Law on Participation, that is, participation in work, was passed with the goal to encourage unemployed and handicapped persons to engage in paid work to the maximal level of which they are capable. Application of this law also falls under the responsibility of the local community administrations. The goal of this law is to encourage communities to evaluate the possibilities of each person and thus to give tailored advice. For example, youth with FASD with only a grade school diploma can be coached into a regular, paid job, as much as possible in a normal company.

One effect of this law has been the reduction of government support to organisations that traditionally provided a sheltered working environment. Here also, the availability of help is often based only on IQ, rather than on the secondary problems in areas of planning or social skills. Thus, youth and young adults with an IQ in the near-normal or normal range often cannot receive help in finding and keeping a job.

17.1.6 Conclusion

Awareness of FASD and support of persons with FASD has a long way to go in the Netherlands. The Netherlands is fortunate to have three excellent diagnostic clinics, so it is no longer difficult to obtain a good diagnostic work-up. However, nothing is known about the prevalence of FASD, and the government has not invested in either research or support. Up to now, the primary sources of information and support for families living with FASD are the FAS Foundation and several other smaller parent-run groups. The recent re-organisations of the social services and work laws have not led to better support for persons living with FASD and their families.

Bibliography

[1] Gezondheidsraad. Risico's van alcoholgebruik bij conceptie, zwangerschap en borstvoeding. Den Haag: Gezondheidsraad, 2005; publicatie nr 2004/22. ISBN 90-5549-000-8. https://www.gezondheidsraad.nl/nl/taak-werkwijze/werkterrein/gezonde-voeding/risicos-van-alcoholgebruik-bij-conceptie-zwangerschap-en.
[2] Gezondheidsraad. Preconceptiezorg: voor een goed begin. Den Haag: Gezondheidsraad, 2007; publicatienr. 2007/19. ISBN 978-90-5549-657-0. https://www.gezondheidsraad.nl/nl/taak-werkwijze/werkterrein/preventie/preconceptiezorg-voor-een-goed-begin.
[3] Alcoholgebruik tijdens zwangerschap en borstvoeding, TNO, January2016. https://www.trimbos.nl/actueel/nieuws/bericht/?bericht=1830.

17.2 Fetal alcohol spectrum disorders in the United Kingdom

Susan Fleisher and Sandra Butcher

17.2.1 Statistics

The Lancet Global Health places the UK among the top five countries in the world for the highest alcohol use during pregnancy [1] in a new study by the Canadian Centre for Addiction and Mental Health (CAMH) published in 2017 – Their estimates show that more than 40% of pregnant women in the UK drink alcohol while pregnant. Earlier studies indicated that drinking during the first trimester in the UK may be as high as 69–79% [2]. The data is inconsistent, but alarming. The study also indicates that the UK has one of the highest rates of fetal alcohol syndromein the world, with an estimated 61.3 cases per 10000 births [3] – significantly higher that the global average of 15 out of 10000. This is, however, only a rough estimate, albeit predicted using advanced statistical analysis. It is important to keep in mind that these figures are, according to the study, only "the tip of the iceberg" since they deal only with fetal alcohol syndrome and not the full range of fetal alcohol spectrum disorders.According to experts, the rate of FASD may be as much as 9 or 10 times higher.

There is an urgent need for UK-based methodologically sound studies on prevalence and more comprehensive data collection. The 2016 British Medical Association report noted, "There is currently no reliable evidence on the incidence of FASD in the UK…" [4] "More research is required to better understand the prevalence of FASD in the UK, which should include meta-analysis of existing data as well as population specific prevalence studies. A key complication in determining the incidence of FASD is the absence of robust and routine data collection.... . The lack of accepted diagnostic criteria may explain why data on FASD are not routinely collected in the UK, and, where data are collected, are restricted to FAS."

17.2.2 Official guidance

In 2016, the Chief Medical Officers from across the UK issued new guidance [5] after a public consultation. The latest advice from the UK's chief medical officers is clear, but it has not yet filtered through to all levels of UK society:
–   "If you are pregnant or think you could become pregnant, the safest approach is not to drink alcohol at all, to keep risks to your baby to a minimum.
–   "Drinking in pregnancy can lead to long-term harm to the baby, with the more you drink the greater the risk.
–   "The risk of harm to the baby is likely to be low if you have drunk only small amounts of alcohol before you knew you were pregnant or during pregnancy.
–   "If you find out you are pregnant after you have drunk alcohol during early pregnancy, you should avoid further drinking. You should be aware that it is unlikely in most cases that your baby has been affected. If you are worried about alcohol use during pregnancy do talk to your doctor or midwife."

Prior to this announcement, England and Wales lagged behind Scotland in terms of providing clear recommendations. "The new guidelines bring the rest of the UK in line with Scotland on advice for pregnant women. Previously, Scotland was the only country in the UK to advise women that there is no 'safe' amount of alcohol that can be drunk during pregnancy so the best approach is not to drink at all. That advice is now reflected UK-wide" [6].

Fetal alcohol syndrome is noted in the 2016 British Medical Association Report as "the leading known cause of non-genetic intellectual disability in the Western world." Fetal alcohol syndrome is one of a range of conditions caused by exposure to alcohol in utero that fall under the umbrella of fetal alcohol spectrum disorders (FASD), which some experts call a "hidden epidemic" [7] in the UK. The costs to society are high. "Based on data from the US, it is estimated that the annual cost of FASD in the UK is over £2 billion" [4].

17.2.3 Diagnosis and training

According to the 2016 BMA report, FASD are commonly under-diagnosed due to a number of reasons, including:
–   "the lack of a specific diagnostic test";

- "an under-reporting of maternal alcohol consumption, or lack of maternal alcohol history";
- "the difficulty in detecting the defining features associated with FASD in neonates";
- "confounding factors (eg poor nutritional maternal status or polydrug use) ";
- "differing and poorly defined diagnostic criteria for FASD";
- "the lack of multidisciplinary neurodevelopmental teams to complete comprehensive assessments needed to evaluate the full range of FASD";
- "A lack of knowledge and understanding of FASD among healthcare professionals also means they often may not feel competent to make a diagnosis" [4].
- "There is no clear pathway in the UK for the referral of individuals with suspected FASD to specialist services, to allow a complete diagnostic evaluation. Nor are there adequate specialist services to support these referrals. There is inconsistency in where individuals are referred; and the services to which they are referred may not necessarily have the skills required to diagnose and manage FASD effectively."

Efforts have been underway for decades to change this. The National Organisation for Foetal Alcohol Syndrome-UK (NOFAS-UK) established the first FASD Medical Advisory Panel at the Royal Society of Medicine in November 2004. World experts on FASD were brought together with British doctors to set the FASD agenda in Britain.

For example, "The BMA 2015 Annual Representatives Meeting unanimously passed a resolution calling for improved services and referral pathways for the diagnosis, management and support of individuals and families affected by PAE." And the 2016 BMA report stated, "Guidance on the diagnosis of the full range of foetal alcohol spectrum disorders should be developed and made available to all healthcare professionals throughout the UK." "Diagnostic and referral services for FASD should be commissioned and adequately resourced throughout the UK. There should be sufficient funding for the development, training and maintenance of multidisciplinary diagnostic teams and clear pathways established for the referral of FASD across the UK" [4].

17.2.4 Policy debates

The first record of discussion of fetal alcohol syndrome in Parliament is a 23 January 1979 written response from the Minister of State (Department of Health and Social Security) Mr. Moyle to Mr. Lewis Carter-Jones: "My Department's consultant adviser on alcoholism, Professor Kessel…concluded that in this country FAS was unlikely to be a great problem numerically; that it should neither be ignored nor seen out of perspective; and that regular excessive drinking should be discouraged in everyone." [8]

Thankfully, things have moved forward since then, though policy still lags behind science in this field. Over the past few decades efforts have progressed to address FASD in policy circles.

Working with NOFAS-UK, Lord Mitchell in the House of Lords raised the issue in Parliament on May 2004. In September 2004, Ross Cranston, MP sponsored a NOFAS-UK Press Conference in the House of Commons and put FAS on the governmenta-genda. Over the years, Parliament has debated issues such as warning labels (including a special effort on this led by Lord Mitchell in 2008), the lack of adequate statistics, and other related issues. On 14 October 2014, a pivotal Westminster Hall debate [9] on fetal alcohol syndrome was sponsored by Bill Esterson, MP.

Information provided by NOFAS-UK was extensively quoted during this debate. In September 2015, Bill Esterson, MP established an All-Party Parliamentary Group for Fetal Alcohol Spectrum Disorder [sic] [10] with 13 members (as of February 2017) and with secretarial support provided by the FASD Trust. The APPG's initial report in December 2015 laid out a series of recommendations for further progress [11].

17.2.5 "A scandalous lack of support"

In the forward to the 2016 British Medical Association report, Professor Sheila the Baroness Hollins highlighted "a scandalous lack of support for these children, who live and grow up with the impact of their impairments without the educational, emotional and social support they require to fulfil their potential. Too often they go without a diagnosis, or are misdiagnosed. They are also frequently affected by a range of secondary comorbidities, including social and mental health problems such as substance abuse or sexual inappropriateness, educational difficulties, or crime and consequent incarceration."

"There are no frameworks for [FASD] clinical management in the UK." The BMA recommends, "A framework for the clinical management of individuals affected by the range of fetal alcohol spectrum disorders, as well as their birth mothers, should be developed and adequately resourced."

This is further complicated by the fact that "[i]t is thought that up to 80% of children affected by FASD are with foster or adoptive families." [12] There is a debate as to whether or not these families and carers are adequately informed of the risks and implications of possible prenatal exposure to alcohol and whether or not they are properly supported.

The UK rolled out nationally a new Adoption Support Fund in May 2015 (the ASF had been piloted prior to that in selected areas). Controversially, because the demand was "unprecedented" the ASF has been capped with a "fair access limit" at £5,000 per year (in exceptional cases this can be higher) at least until March 2017. While the data is not FASD-specific, "The kind of support most frequently provided are therapeutic parenting (27%), specialist assessments of need (21%), psychotherapy (20%) and creative therapies (15%)" [13]. Not surprisingly, "multidisciplinary packages of support are the most expensive and often cover a range of therapeutic needs in families including giving parents the skills they need to parent their children therapeutically, regular child and family therapy sessions, therapeutic life story work and work with schools and others working with the child and family to ensure a joined up approach." In other words, the most expensive kinds of support are those that could be very helpful for those with FASD.

There are a range of programs designed in theory to support people with disabilities. The challenge is that due to the above-mentioned problems in diagnosis and support accessing related financial support and services is often difficult and confusing. Quite often the requests are turned down because FASD is not adequately understood. For example, an adult with FASD known by one of the authors was recently turned down because he presented well in an interview and his verbal skills masked deeper executive functioning challenges. He must now appeal. The process is intimidating and unfriendly to those with the added challenges of living with FASD.

Families are in theory entitled to support via the Disability Living Allowance program "for children may help with the extra costs of looking after a child who is under 16 and has difficulties walking or needs more looking after than a child of the same age who doesn't have a disability." [14] Personal Independence Payments are available for adolescents and adults over 16–65. As of January 2017, weekly payments for both programs range from £21.80 to £139.75 per week. The Disability Living Allowance (DLA) is a tax-free benefit for disabled people who need help with mobility or care costs. For those over 65, an attendance allowance of £55.10 or £82.30 a week can help with personal care if someone is physically or mentally disabled.

17.2.6 Education

In educational settings, children with FASD are often misunderstood or left unsupported. This situation deepens as they age, and especially if they are undiagnosed they often find themselves excluded for behaviour and other secondary issues. "There is as yet no direct guidance from any government agency in the UK to teachers on how to educate students with FASD" [15]. The Training and Development Agency for Schools (TDA) supported the NOFAS-UK FAS-eD research project, which looked into effective teaching and learning approaches for children with FASD [16]. The 2010 Primary Framework: Teaching and Learning Strategies to Support Primary Aged Students with Fetal Alcohol Spectrum Disorders and the The Secondary Framework: Teaching and Learning Strategies to Support Primary Aged Students with Fetal Alcohol Spectrum Disorder prepared for NOFAS-UK's FAS-eD project by Project Researcher Dr. Carolyn Blackburn and Project Director Professor Barry Carpenter, OBE, remain among the most comprehensive teacher training and development documents available.

The main guidance for the education of children with FASD in England and Wales falls under the "Special educational needs and disability code of practice: 0 to 25 years" [17]. "This Code of Practice provides statutory guidance on duties, policies and procedures relating to Part 3 of the Children and Families Act 2014 and associated regulations and applies to England. It relates to children and young people with special educational needs (SEN) and disabled children and young people." This guidance clearly states:

"The Equality Act 2010 sets out the legal obligations that schools, early years providers, post-16 institutions, local authorities and others have towards disabled children and young people:
–   "They must not directly or indirectly discriminate against, harass or victimise disabled children and young people.
–   "They must not discriminate for a reason arising in consequence of a child or young person's disability.
–   "They must make reasonable adjustments, including the provision of auxiliary aids and services, to ensure that disabled children and young people are not at a substantial disadvantage compared with their peers. This duty is anticipatory – it requires thought to be given in advance to what disabled children and young people might require and what adjustments might need to be made to prevent that disadvantage".

The challenge is that too often children affected by FASD are undiagnosed, their learning disabilities are not clearly identified, and in the face of increasing budgetary pressures in UK school systems, parents have to fight hard to access even minimal services – even when a diagnosis has been made. The English government has changed educational policy to have an increased focus on standardised testing, which many believe will put children with FASD at a further disadvantage in mainstream educational settings.

All across England, Local Authorities list their "Local Offers". From September 2014, every Local Authority was "required to publish information about services they expect to be available in their area for children and young people from birth to 25 who have special educational needs and/or disabilities (SEND); and also services outside of the area which they expect children and young people from their area will use. This [is] known as the 'Local Offer'." The Local Offer includes education, health and care services, leisure activities and support groups [18]. The Local Offersare still unknown to many families with children with FASD, but provide a useful starting point for exploring services available generally to those with disabilities, since there are no specific FASD-focused services.

Education and Health Care (EHC) plans are a new system being rolled out in England and Wales "for children and young people aged up to 25 who need more support than is available through special educational needs support." These plans are supposed to help young people with disabilities access education through to the age of 25, and include a little-noticed provision for "supported internships," study programmes "specifically aimed at young people aged 16 to 24 who have a statement of special educational needs, a Learning Difficulty Assessment, or an EHC plan, who want to move into employment and need extra support to do so" [19]. Again, the process for securing an EHC plan is daunting and too often unsuccessful, even for those with an FASD diagnosis. There are Special Educational Needs and Disabilities Information Advice and Support Services (SENDIASS) across the country, who are there to help advise parents.

In Northern Ireland, the SEN Code of Practice is similar. The "main difference" in England is that "support is available for SEN from birth to 25 both in school, further education and in training" [20]. In Northern Ireland, pupils in school from 16–19 remain the responsibility of the Education and Library Boards. Those over 19 support receive support from a range of other Departments included the Department for Employment and Learning.

In Scotland, Additional Support Needs (ASN) are highlighted, rather than SEN. "ASN cover a broader spectrum than SEN and can include children and young people with behavioural and learning difficulties, those who have sensory impairments and those who are particularly gifted.

17.2.7 Justice system

One international estimate says that people with FASD are 19–40 times more likely to become involved in the criminal justice system [21]. It is reasonable, therefore, to assume that this is also a challenge in the UK, although research is needed in this area.

"Within correctional/confinement settings, screening in order to detect Foetal Alcohol Spectrum Disorders (FASD) or Alcohol-Related Neuro Developmental Disorder (ARND) is frequently lacking. The courts may not recognise FAS/ARND which leads to inappropriate sentences for this vulnerable group" [22]. There are examples from other countries that could serve as a starting point for the UK on this issue. For example, in Canada, the FASD Justice Committee has developed a comprehensive website [23] with funding from the Public Health Agency of Canada and the Department of Justice as a resource for justice system professionals. As a first step in the UK, an online course is available from the UK Learning College: FASD and the Criminal Justice System [24].

17.2.8 Pockets of excellence

The UK is home to some leading experts, who prove that there are ways to diagnose and support people with FASD – people like Dr. Raja Mukherjee at the National Clinic for Foetal Alcohol Spectrum Disorders, Professor Moira Plant, an expert on gender and alcohol at University of the West of England, Dr Maggie Watts, Director of Public

Health in the Western Isles who formerly served as Foetal Alcohol Spectrum Disorder Co-ordinator for Scotland, and Professor Barry Carpenter, OBE and Dr. Carolyn Blackburn who have done previously mentioned ground breaking work on education and FASD. These experts and many, many more, work in cooperation with families, birth parents, and those with FASD to help chart pathways to brighter futures.

The debate in Scotland about FASD has in many ways been more advanced than in England and Wales. For example, in 2013 the Foetal Alcohol Spectrum Disorder Awareness Toolkit was produced by the Scottish Government Child and Maternal Health Division [25]. NHS Scotland provides online educational materials about FASD for health professionals and students [26].

17.2.9 Third sector support

Founded in 2003 as a charity, the National Organisation for Foetal Alcohol Syndrome-UK (NOFAS-UK) developed programmes to support families and individuals affected by FASD. NOFAS-UK also provides information for health professionals, social services and government agencies. NOFAS-UK initiated debates in Parliament to clarify guidelines regarding the risks of alcohol use in pregnancy.

NOFAS-UK's has provided training and resources for over 15000 midwives across the UK while also raising the profile of FASD in the media and among relevant professions. NOFAS-UK is a member of the FASD UK Alliance (https://fasd-uk.net), a coalition of groups and individuals from across the UK and abroad who are united together for positive social change for those affected by Foetal Alcohol Spectrum Disorders (FASD). The FASD UK Alliance (https://fasd-uk.net) runs a vibrant online Facebook support group that engages more than 1100 affected individuals, parents, guardians and carers. They also sponsor a Facebook Support Group for FASD Professionals and the FASD UK Resources YouTube Channel collects some of the best videos available from many sources.

ELEN – UK & European Birth Mum Network offers support and offers peer mentoring to pregnant women and supports women and their children who may have FASD.

Other charities devoted to FASD work are the FASD Trust, the FASD Network UK in the North East, FASD Devon and Cornwall (FASDDAC).

These are just a few of the organisations and networks that are active. In the absence of a coherent national strategy, the wheels of change are being driven by those with FASD, their families, carers and committed professionals. Those who have been advocating over the decades for FASD prevention and awareness in the UK are encouraged by the many positive steps forward. Although there is still a long way to go, the world of FASD in the UK is changing and improving.

Bibliography

[1]   Popova S, Lange S, Probst C, Gmel G, Rehm J. Estimation of national, regional, and global pre-valence of alcohol use during pregnancy and fetal alcohol syndrome: a systematic review and meta-analysis. The Lancet Global health. 2017, 5(3), e290–e9.

[2]   British Medical Association. Report 2016, 11.

[3]   Supplement to: Popova S, Lange S, Probst C, Gmel G, Rehm J. Estimation of national, regional, and global prevalence of alcohol use during pregnancy and fetal alcohol syndrome: a system-atic review and meta-analysis. The Lancet Global health. 2017, 5(3), e290–e9, 33.

[4]   British Medical Association. Report 2016, 6.

[5]   UK Chief Medical Officers' Low Risk Drinking Guidelines, August 2016, available online at: https://www.gov.uk/government/uploads/system/uploads/attachment_data/file/545937/ UK_CMOs__report.pdf.

[6]   New alcohol guidelines, 8 January 2016, http://news.gov.scot/news/new-alcohol-guidelines.

[7]   Cook PA, Mukherjee R. "How foetal alcohol spectrum disorders could be a hidden epidemic., The Conversation, 13 January 2016.

[8]   HC Deb 23 January 1979 vol 961 cc106–7W, available online at: http://hansard. millbanksystems.com/written_answers/1979/jan/23/foetal-alcohol-syndrome#S5CV0961P0_ 19790123_CWA_228.

[9]   https://hansard.parliament.uk/Commons/2014-10-14/debates/14101476000001/ FoetalAlcoholSyndrome?highlight=foetal#contribution-14101476000022.

[10] http://www.appg-fasd.org.uk/home/4589489440.

[11] http://www.appgfasd.org.uk/reports/4589489444.

[12] Complex Learning Difficulties and Disabilities Research Project. Specialist Schools and Academies Trust, Briefing Sheet, available online at: http://complexld.ssatrust.org.uk/ uploads/1b%20fasd-briefing.pdf.

[13] Adoption Support Fund. Frequently Asked Questions, available online at: http://www. adoptionsupportfund.co.uk/FAQs.

[14] https://www.gov.uk/disability-living-allowance-children/overview.

[15] Complex Learning Difficulties and Disabilities Research Project. Specialist Schools and Academies Trust, FASD Information Sheet, p. 6. Available online at http://complexld.ssatrust. org.uk/uploads/1c%20fasd-info.pdf.

[16] See for example, the NOFAS-UK Teacher Toolkit, available online at http://www.nofas-uk.org/ ?cat=27.

[17] Department of Health. Special educational needs and disability code of practice: 0 to 25 years: Statutory guidance for organisations which work with and support children and young people who have special educational needs or disabilities, January 2015, available online at https: //www.gov.uk/government/uploads/system/uploads/attachment_data/file/398815/SEND_ Code_of_Practice_January_2015.pdf.

[18] http://www3.hants.gov.uk/parents-sen/send-localoffer.htm.

[19] Department for Education. "Supported Internships", p. 6, available online at: https://www. gov.uk/government/uploads/system/uploads/attachment_data/file/389411/Supported_ Internship_Guidance_Dec_14.pdf.

[20] Murphy E. Paper on a Possible Amendment to the Special Education Needs and Disability Bill, Northern Ireland Assembly, Research and Information Service Briefing Paper, Paper 52/15 15 April 2015 NIAR 68-2015, available online at: http://www.niassembly.gov.uk/globalassets/ documents/raise/publications/2015/del/5215.pdf.

[21] Popova S, Lange S, Burd L, Rehm J. Cost attributable to Fetal Alcohol Spectrum Disorder in the Canadian correctional system. International journal of law and psychiatry 2015, 41, 76–81,

quoted in Allely CS, Gebbia P Studies Investigating Fetal Alcohol Spectrum Disorders in the Criminal Justice System: A Systematic PRISMA Review. SOJ Psychol 2016, 2(1), 9 of 11, available online at: http://usir.salford.ac.uk/38695/1/Allely%20and%20Gebbia%20(2016).pdf.

[22] Allely CS, Gebbia P. Studies Investigating Fetal Alcohol Spectrum Disorders in the Criminal Justice System: A Systematic PRISMA Review. SOJ Psychol 2016, 2(1), 1–11, available online at: http://usir.salford.ac.uk/38695/1/Allely%20and%20Gebbia%20(2016).pdf.

[23] http://fasdjustice.ca.

[24] http://www.uklearningcollege.co.uk/foetal-alcohol-spectrum-disorders-and-criminal-justice-System-p-477.html.

[25] Fetal Alcohol Spectrum Disorder Awareness Toolkit, Scottish Government Child and Maternal Health Division, September 2013, available online at (an update is planned for 2017): http://www.gov.scot/Resource/0043/00435992.pdf.

[26] Fetal Alcohol, educational resource for health professionals and students, available online at: http://www.nes.scot.nhs.uk/education-and-training/by-theme-initiative/maternity-care/about-us/current-projects/fetal-alcohol.aspx.

17.3 FASD in Germany

17.3.1 Introduction

In November 2011, the Drug Commissioner of the German Federal Government commissioned a report on the social consequences for patients with FASD [1]. (G. Schindler published responses to these specific problems in detail (www.drogenbeauftragte. de)). The Drug Commissioner was interested in, among other things, answers to the following issues:

1. Which measures are necessary to enable people suffering from FASD to participate successfully in community life?
2. Which social benefits are particularly involved in FASD diagnosis?

Receiving a FAS diagnosis is an important condition for the participation in community life for affected people. Unfortunately, this remains an unsolved problem because FASD is often not recognised and, therefore, not correctly diagnosed. In Germany, the diagnostic ICD-10 system (International Statistical Classification of Diseases and Related Health Problems) is used. Within this classification system, there is a disease category for congenital malformation syndromes due to known exogenous causes (Q86.0). This diagnostic code stands for the "full blown" fetal alcohol syndrome. As there is no separate diagnostic code for pFAS and ARND under the "umbrella" of FASD available in ICD-10, patients with FASD are also diagnosed with the code (Q86.0).

A positive development towards more diagnostic safety in FAS was the establishment of the German S3-guidelines, initiated by the Drug Commissioner of the German Federal Government. These guidelines focus only on the classical presentation of FAS.

However, only a minority of those affected by fetal alcohol exposure suffer from the classical symptoms of the syndrome. Between 70 and 80% of people affected show no recognisable dysmorphic facial features and remain largely undiagnosed.

Therefore, an additional separate diagnostic category in the ICD-10 for pFAS and ARND is urgently needed. This would lead to an increased awareness of FASD amongst clinicians, as well as emphasising the importance of a correct FASD diagnosis.

According to §119 SGB V (Social Security Code, Book V), centres for social pae-diatrics present a special institutional form of interdisciplinary outpatient treatment. Centres for social paediatrics are tasked with the examination and treatment of children and adolescents up to 18 years of age. They are responsible in the child's social environment and provide caregivers with advice and guidance. Therefore, centres for social paediatrics offer the best conditions for the diagnosis, treatment and care of this complex disorder in Germany.

17.3.2 FAS in adults

Diagnosing FAS in adults is an even greater challenge because until now, the con-tinuing difficulties in adults suffering from FAS have been almost unknown and unre-cognised by clinicians. This is due to the fact that FAS is not generally regarded as a long-lasting disease continuing into adulthood.

Implementation of nationwide centres with specialised physicians, preferably psychiatrists, are crucial for these patients. After receiving a diagnosis of FAS in these special centres, it is important that service providers acknowledge and accept this syndrome. Unfortunately, youth welfare services, schools, social services, employ-ment agencies, as well as physicians, still hesitate to acknowledge this persisting neuropsychiatric disorder.

Definition of "disability"

According to §2 Abs.1, SGB IX (Social Security Code, Book IX) individuals may be defined as disabled, when their physical health, mental capacity or mental health deviate presumably for more than 6 months from their age appropriate development, resulting in their restricted participation in society. These persons are assigned to §53 SGB XII (Social Security Code, Book XII) and are eligible for integration assistance provided by social welfare institutions.

Mental illness according to §35a SGB VIII (Social Security Code, Book VIII)

In Germany, children and adolescents are entitled to integration assistance from youth welfare services as a result of mental disability.

1. Children and adolescents are entitled to integration assistance benefits if their mental health deviates from age-appropriate development and results in restricted participation in society.
2. Following the German social law, youth welfare services clearly require an assignment from either:
   a) a child and adolescent psychiatrist
   b) or a child and adolescent psychotherapist
   c) or a paediatrician who has sufficient experience in the field of mental health issues in children and adolescents.

Assistance for young adults according to §41 SGB VIII (Social Security Code, Book VIII)

Patients with FASD are especially vulnerable during the transition from adolescence to adulthood. The necessary switch from support by youth welfare services to social services for adults often is a significant problem. Youth welfare services are generally responsible up to the age of 18 years (the maximum is the age of 27). At the age of 18, youth welfare services often wish to terminate support and do not wish to have further responsibility. One reason is that social benefits are not always granted due to lack of acceptance of the FASD diagnosis. Aid for young adults according to §41 SGB VIII (Social Security Code, Book VIII) provides assistance in the development of their individual personality and in achieving an independent life.

Because FASD is a lifelong impairment in mental and physical health, a seamless transition from youth welfare services to social services is crucial and there is no doubt that social services are obligated to provide integration assistance.

However, if young adults have not received a clear FASD diagnosis in childhood or adolescence, they are wrongly considered to be persons unmotivated and obstinate, and their disability to participate in society is assumed to be due to their own fault. Integration assistance according to §53 SGB XII (Social Security Code, Book XII) will, therefore, be refused as a consequence of this misjudgement. There is thus an urgent need to educate responsible authorities, institutions, services and the employment agencies about FASD in adulthood. Applicants with suspected signs of FASD must be referred to clinical specialists for examination.

17.3.3 Severe disability

Classified as being severely disabled are humans with a degree of disability ("Grad der Behinderung") of 50% or more. Consequently, people are entitled to financial compensation, employment benefits, tax allowances, early retirement, etc. These benefits should be available to most adults with FASD; however, they are often not granted due to the lack of a correct diagnosis. Of particular relevance to people suffering from

FASD, are "Merkzeichen" (marks), which can be given in addition to the degree of disability ("Grad der Behinderung") by the pension office.

"Merkzeichen B" indicates free public transportation, including for an accompanying person to compensate for the lack of orientation of the patient and to assist in stressful situations.

"Merkzeichen H" is granted for helplessness and indicates that the person needs considerable support in regular daily life activities.

Unfortunately, in German pension offices FAS is not part of the official list of diseases to date, and, therefore, the legal right for integration assistance for patients suffering from FAS is often refused.

Bibliography

[1] Schindler G, unter Mitarbeit von Hoff-Emden H. Gutachten: "Fetale Alkoholspektrum-Störungen (FASD) in der sozialrechtlichen Praxis", November 2011, available online at: http://drogenbeauftragte.de/fileadmin/dateien-dba/DrogenundSucht/Alkohol/Downloads/11-11-30_Rechtsgutachten_FASD.pdf.

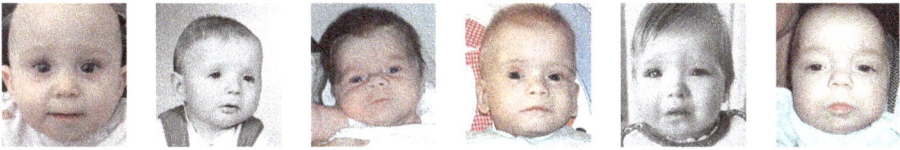

Part V: **Life stories**

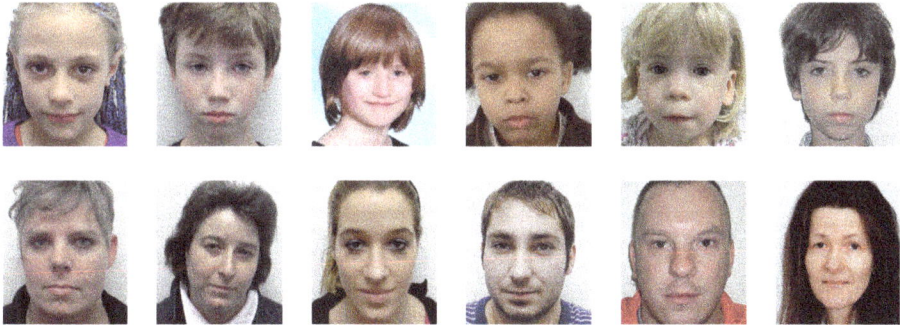

M.; born in 2009 (m); fetal alcohol syndrome (FAS); January 2013

Editor's note: This history of M's suffering by his foster mother is impressive, and it is remarkable how the entire foster family joins forces to provide a better life for M. He was medicated with melatonin and methylphenidate because of his severe sleeping disorder from a young age, and for his ADHD symptoms. The drug treatment was successful and provides an example that sometimes giving medication at an early age is indicated.

His foster mother reports:

"It all began nearly 3 years ago. M. was 2 years old. He moved from my mother after short-term foster care, and finally to me and my daughter. At that time, M. did not have any problems. For the first 6 months I stayed at home to make the transition easier. Then 2 years after he came into our family, M. was hospitalised with pneumonia.

M's problems began in the hospital, being away from his family and his familiar surroundings. Fortunately, he was back home after a few days. However, the first night he didn't sleep a wink and he cried inconsolably. I had to carry him in my arms throughout the night. The next morning he refused to eat, no matter what I offered him.

If I put him down he at once started to cry desperately. In the following weeks, this situation didn't improve. The continuous lack of sleep and his hunger caused an unstable mind, and his foster sister especially suffered from his aggressive behaviour. He bit and hit her and tore out chunks of her hair.

By this time, I couldn't live without M. anymore, but it became more and more exhausting for me. It was not possible to go to the bathroom without him or to sleep for more than one hour at night. Every evening it required up to 3 hours to comfort him before he was able to fall asleep, and then he didn't sleep for more than 30 minutes. Every attempt to burn off his energy failed and he was simply unable to sleep. I still hoped for a recovery.

M. had been in our family for 6 months when I had to return to work, hoping to regain some liberty. M. was supposed to go to kindergarten and I also expected some help in dealing with M.'s problems at home. But the period of adjustment turned out to be very difficult. M. was outgoing with everyone and didn't pay constant attention to me anymore, but if I only shifted on my chair, he freaked out, screamed and collapsed desperately. After about 6 weeks M. finally went to kindergarten and I returned to work.

However, the problems at home remained: the permanent lack of sleep and the daily struggle with M. strained my nerves. At the time, he maintained a low profile in kindergarten, but after only a couple of weeks M. started fighting tooth and nail against going to kindergarten as soon as getting out of bed. He went to kindergarten

https://doi.org/10.1515/9783110436563-018

kicking and screaming, but the nursery assured me that he always became quiet and happy again within 5 minutes after I left.

Unlike his peers, M. was not able to dress himself or participate in the activities at the kindergarten. When I picked him up in the afternoons, he was principally crying, sitting alone in a corner.

After M. was living with me for almost a year, he still did not sleep and was only eating under a lot of pressure. Due to the situation, my daughter was also suffering more and more. I couldn't take it anymore not knowing what to do next. Our paediatrician dismissed M.'s difficulties as being temporary and soon becoming better.

The doctors diagnosed regulatory disorder in infancy and ADHD and stated that M. was too young for any therapy. I was at a loss with this information, asking myself how to help and support him appropriately.

We did not receive any help from Child Services either; their statement that difficulties are common in foster children didn't get us anywhere.

I was very anxious about his first contact with his biological parents – what will happen, how will he react? Surprisingly, the visit passed well, but after leaving his parents he clung to me, scratching my arms. It took ages to put him into the car seat; he kept screaming and crying and kicking at the car window. At home he collapsed completely: whilst I was opening the door, M. started hitting his head repeatedly against the door. I tried to hold and to calm him, which did not work. He was bleeding and had many bruises on his forehead. He started to convulse and tremble. Once we were inside, he didn't calm down. My desperate call to Child Services fell on deaf ears. The uncertainty of knowing what was wrong with him was unbearable. Luckily, this was the only contact he ever had with his biological parents.

Afterwards M. was a different child: he didn't listen to me, crossed the street all of a sudden and no longer had any limits. As soon as I would leave a room, he screamed uncontrollably, following me no matter where I was going or what I was doing. During grocery shopping he would start to steal and throw things on the ground. Conversations were not possible anymore, because M. started screaming, harming himself or biting. At home he destroyed many things and smiled after he managed to break something. He threw glasses on the floor and ripped my mail into little pieces. Trying to burn off his energy was worthless because he climbed on everything and jumped down, often resulting in severe injuries.

Totally desperate, I went back to SPZ. They just told me to be consistent in my education. This time he received medication (melatonin) for his sleep disturbance. I could not imagine medication would help. But after coming home, I gave him the pill and just half an hour later, he lay down on the sofa and said: "Mommy, M. bed". His words affected me deeply, I was so relieved, I put him down in his bed and he immediately felt asleep and the next morning he was more relaxed than ever before.

This moment raised hope and also the strength to continue to fight for M. and my family. I wanted to find out what was wrong with him and to help him to become a happy and content child.

Many discussions with my family and also with other foster parents and several doctors raised the question of whether M. possibly was suffering from FASD. I knew that his biological mother drank during pregnancy, but I couldn't believe that that was his problem. Wasn't he, except for his frequent tantrums, a normal boy, a little bit lazy perhaps and with his own peculiarities? I had gathered online information about FASD, and quickly I had to conclude that the problems described were very similar to M's difficulties. This frightened me and for several weeks I did not know what to do, and the struggle with daily difficulties did not end.

After M. attempted to run away from the kindergarten ending up with a big gash necessitating hospital treatment, I realised there was an urgent need to know whether or not M. was suffering from FASD. I needed reassurance whether I was incorrect with my assessment or whether he was simply unable to learn and to understand. I scheduled an appointment with Prof. Spohr (FASD-Zentrum, Berlin). He diagnosed FAS. I couldn't believe it. I had been so strict with M. and sometimes maybe unfair, but he simply was unable to understand; he wasn't disobedient, he was ill. I was so angry and disappointed about all the people who had argued that M.'s behaviour and bad temper were my own fault without considering other causes.

There are still daily struggles with M., but knowing his diagnosis allows me to think and act in a different way, to understand what is wrong with him and subsequently to cater more to his needs. I am now able to avert his aggressive tantrums and rebuild confidence in his ability to manage certain things on his own. Of course, there are problems with medication, and every day with M. is an experience on its own, never knowing what will happen next or how he will react to new situations, but it is getting better day by day. Finally, we are a happy family."

A.; born in 2000 (m); partial fetal alcohol syndrome (pFAS); March 2011

Editor's note: A.'s mother, a chronic alcoholic had admitted to alcohol consumption during pregnancy. She has been alcohol dependent since the age of 14 years and multiple clinical withdrawal treatments failed subsequent to discontinuing rehabilitation.

The foster parents report:

"A. was born prematurely in the 30th week, weighing only 1360 g. His mother had been alcohol dependent since the age of 14; during the pregnancy she had consumed alcohol on a daily basis. After his mother was repetitively alcohol intoxicated and unable to take care of her infant, A. was taken in charge and primarily placed in a children's home in 2002. One year later A. came into our family.

At that time, he was still unsteady walking, was not able to speak a single word, had no sensation of pain, and when he was unwilling to do a task for which he was asked, he thrashed around. When he was sad, he hid himself under the table. On certain days, A. stereotypically opened and closed all doors of our house the entire day or he collected shoes of the whole family or cleaned the house with a cloth. Lying in bed, A. hit his head against the wall or the bars of his bed. At night he screamed continuously, sometimes for more than 2 hours. He suffered panic attacks at night, necessitating bringing him to the pediatric hospital on several occasions. A. received special needs assistance in the children's home and also later, when he lived in our family. During the day, he was almost untamable; he was able to play a little bit more calmly outside, but inside he was unable to concentrate on a single game. He didn't accept any "no", but rather started to scream or to destroy his bed.

May 2004 – A. now attended kindergarten in a special integration class. He didn't mind who accompanied him. He was still unable to speak and still wet himself. He went along with the nursery teacher without any problems; he didn't care whether it was his nursery teacher or a stranger. However, when the nursery teacher wanted to introduce some of the kindergarten rules to him, he hit her in the face, and she hit back.

At the age of 4.5, A. finally started to speak, and when he was 5 years old, it was possible for us to understand most of what he was saying. At that same age he had stopped wetting himself during the daytime, but nocturnal enuresis persisted until the age of 7. Up to the age of 6, A. had several accidents. He fell off his chair and broke his finger and he fell down the stairs because he still toddled. A. climbed out of the window onto the roof and at the age of 6 years he started to play with fire inside the house.

A. was enrolled in a regular school in 2007. He cried for a long, long time, because he didn't want to go to school. Later he was hardly manageable and difficult to control; he consistently disrupted the class, became aggressive and started to steal. He didn't reach the required standard of the first grade and due to a special educational assessment he was transferred to a special school.

He was unable to observe the rules and disrupted the class severely also at this school. A. started to smoke cigarettes in the schoolyard and began to steal both at home and at school. He gave the stolen money, his cell phone and his game boy as presents to his schoolmates. A. also collects many things like shampoo, bandages, cameras, cell phones, cleaning tablets, etc., and hoards them in his room or outside. A. acts innocently and considers every person to be trustworthy.

He hitchhikes to school, but it is impossible to allow him to play outside alone, because he will go everywhere without returning home. Disregarding our warnings and cautions, he constantly goes with strangers.

He is easily fooled into doing mischief; recently he attached extreme right-wing stickers to cars in order to please a group of right wing extremists.

Now, in the last grade of the special school, his maths, writing and drawing skills are still at primary school level, and he is more adequate reading. Consultations with his teachers are unhelpful because they are convinced that A. is just unwilling to learn and to abide by rules. Furthermore, they don't accept that A. is still unable to go to school independently by bus. Diagnoses given by physicians and psychologists have gone unrecognised.

To our experience, A. is a sweet boy who is unable to behave and act appropriately instead of being unwilling to meet the demands of every day life. Finally we presented A. to Dr. Spohr in Berlin, but even his diagnosis of FAS didn't effect a better understanding of his difficulties and bad behaviour with his teachers."

S.; born in 2004 (f); partial fetal alcohol syndrome (pFAS); April 2007, fetal alcohol syndrome (FAS); 2012

Editor's note: S. was introduced to me for the first time at the age of 2.5 and she was diagnosed as having a partial fetal alcohol syndrome because of the less pronounced facial features. At the age of 8 she came for consultation again and at that time the typical facial dysmorphia was clearly visible. She finally received the diagnosis of a full-blown fetal alcohol syndrome. Despite an early foster care at the age of 5 months, stable living conditions and an early diagnosis of FAS, together with intensive and competent support and an early treatment with methylphenidate, her deficits and problems increased with age according to greater demands in her daily routine.

The foster mother reports:

"The call from child and youth services came on a sunny morning before noon: a five-month-old infant needed to be taken into foster care. So we took our suitcase stored with sweets, coloring pens and further bits and bobs. In this particular case, we also took a bottle of milk, a rattle and a baby book along, thinking, hopefully, that it might be easier to make contact with the baby by feeding it with a bottle of milk.

When we saw her for the first time, we got scared: wide eyes and a blank look, thin little arms and legs, unnaturally fair skin – and she was dressed with clothes that were way too small.

When I put my arms around her, she became stark and stiff, and my words obviously failed to reach her. She did not make any eye contact and refused the milk bottle we offered her. At the age of 5 months she only weighed 4500 g.

From that day on, almost nothing was like it used to be in our family. She was reported to be a quite "normal" baby, but after 5 hours it was clear to us that nothing was "normal" at all. At this time we did not know anything about FAS and the resulting consequences. We were actually short-term foster parents and, therefore, it was planned that she would stay in our family only until a long-term foster family was found.

After the first 3 days, I slept on average 2 hours during the night because of my foster daughter's feeding problems. She was only able to drink 40–50 ml per meal. I started to feed her almost every hour because I was worried that otherwise she would starve. Each meal was like a battle, and out of 10 meals, 4 of them were lost because if I tried to give her 60 ml milk per meal instead of 50 ml she vomited the whole meal. Afterwards it took almost 20 minutes until she was able to take some food again and everything started all over again. If a healthy child of the same age needs about 1000 ml per day, this little child was surviving on only 500 ml. These feeding problems lasting through the night also caused permanent sleep deprivation. Therefore my husband and I took turns feeding her during the night so that one of us could sleep while the other tried to feed and calm down our frequently crying child.

During the first 3 months, S. did not make any contact and never smiled at us. Up to that time the child services still hadn't found a new foster family, and S. was supposed to stay with us for another 3 months. Meanwhile we received the information that her mother was a chronic alcoholic, but we still were unknowledgeable about possible consequences for the child. Feeding and sleep problems remained unsolved and torturous for both the child and for us.

One day S. suffered from an episode of acute vomiting and diarrhoea; within hours she was seriously ill and was admitted to the hospital. We informed the nursing staff about her eating behaviour and her sleep problems, as well as her continuous crying and restlessness if she experienced physical closeness. The nurses sneered at us, tried to comfort us and finally sent us back home. This was the first night we were able to sleep through the night in 4 months.

When we arrived at the hospital at 7 am the next morning, we were immediately informed about the turbulent night. Obviously, the nursing staff unsuccessfully had tried to comfort her, thus she had not slept that night.

When we came into her room, S. turned towards us. This was the first time that she consciously looked at us and smiled. From this day onward, one of us always stayed with her in the hospital. Now, S. cried only on rare occasions, and she put her thin little arms through the bars of her bed trying to touch us.

S. had finally "arrived" and we wanted her to stay with us. It was unbelievable what her smile had triggered; 2 months later she became our long-term foster daughter.

During this time period, a physician suggested the possibility of FAS for the first time. Some time later we went to see Dr. Spohr; from my point of view, he was the only one who was able to tell us about the consequences of living with a child suffering from FAS: no treatment will cure her, she will always need help and support, and we would often be stretched to our limits. But now it was our self-imposed task to raise her in order to help her to live.

After about 1 year we started with sensory integration therapy and we were lucky to find a therapist familiar with FAS. She instructed us about different proprioceptive techniques and the need of a consequently structured daily routine. At the same time we went to an outpatient clinic for eating disorders. S. still suffered from being underweight and growth deficiency. Afterwards we felt reassured because the doctor told us due to her low weight and small stature she was only able to eat small quantities of food at each meal. Now S. is 8 years old and she still eats like a bird.

Our large family, with many older foster siblings, helped her to have social contacts. Her speech abilities improved more than we had expected, but difficulties concerning her speech comprehension still remained. She was well coordinated and had a gift for sports, so we decided to find a gymnastics club for her. Unfortunately, nobody took sufficient time to work with her appropriately to her abilities. They seemed to be persuaded that she was too small, too thin and stupid, but fortunately we found a new club after some time and it provided the opportunity for exercise until adulthood. Athletics has now become an important and essential part of her life, and she has succeeded in a number of tournaments. We hope that gymnastics will support her further development, giving more self-confidence and stability.

As part of her FAS, she was diagnosed with ADHD. For various reasons, we initially had difficulty in accepting the recommendation for pharmaceutical treatment; we were increasingly surprised about the improvements caused by stimulant treatment with methylphenidate.

S. generally likes to go to school, but over the years her deficits became more evident in school achievement and in social relationships, and she sometimes is less motivated to go to school.

Obviously, she has her own and special attitude and norms!"

E.; born in 2001 (f); fetal alcohol syndrome (FAS); January 2006

Editor's note: E. is the fourth child of an alcohol-dependent woman, whose alcohol abuse was known already at the time of birth; her mother died from chronic alcohol abuse at the age of 34 in 2004. E. was a preterm hypotrophic newborn, suffered from a cleft palate and a congenital heart defect. Because the mother was unable to take care of her, E. was placed in her current foster family.

The foster parents report:

"E. was born in the 37th week of pregnancy and was small for dates with a weight of 1900 g, a height of 40 cm and a head circumference of 30 cm. After the infant's first physical examination, a median cleft palate was diagnosed. Additionally she suffered from a pulmonary stenosis, an artrial septal defect and also a suspected hearing impairment. Therefore, she was moved to an intensive care nursery. This was her fortune!

There she got professional care and treatment instead of living in the birth family under difficult and neglectful circumstances. Child services knew about the severe alcohol dependency and homelessness of the birth mother and, therefore, E. was placed immediately under guardianship, and an appropriate foster family was looked for.

E. came into our family at the age of 4 weeks. We had been previously informed about her physical conditions and the severity of her health impairment.

At that time, we were a family living with four children; the youngest child was 15 months old. Although handling a baby was still fresh in our mind, this time everything was completely different.

E. was just as small as a baby doll, her crying was scarcely audible, she was constantly shivering from cold and was always hungry. Because E. was so small and weak she was only able to drink 50 g per meal, which meant that for the first 4 months, we had to feed her 12 times during the day, and each meal took about 30 minutes.

At the age of 5 months her hearing impairment caused by middle ear fluid was ascertained, and finally surgical treatment was necessary. Despite ear tube insertion, her hearing impairment only improved slightly, and finally a sensioneural hearing loss was suspected. Furthermore, it became clearly recognisable that E. had limited awareness of her surroundings and social interaction, which is the reason why she received support in the form of early intervention.

Thanks to constant physiotherapy, her gross motor development improved and was almost age appropriate. E. was able to sit alone at the age of 7 months, to stand alone and crawl at 10 months and to walk alone at 18 months. In spite of all her limitations, her further development was positive, and she was a very small but agile little girl.

In November 2002, her cleft palate was surgically closed. She overcame all these troubles without any lamentation or complaints – as always. She was a fragile little person with so much strength and perseverance!

At the age of 2, E. attended nursery school. She was still unable to speak at that time, and although it was a nursery school for disabled children, there was no special group for children suffering from hearing impairment. Thus, at the age of 3 she was transferred to a support centre, specialised for children with speech and hearing impairments. With the help of occupational therapy as well as hearing and speech therapy, she progressed steadily.

After an extensive search, we finally found a specialised physician for children with FAS in 2004. I will never forget our first conversation with Prof. Spohr. Unambiguously he told us that our foster daughter would need our parental care, our help and further professional support for the rest of her life. At the age of 5, E. was diagnosed with severe FAS.

Her continuing developmental delay raised the question of what might be the best time for school enrolment.

A neuropsychological test was conducted to determine her current performance abilities, taking into account her hearing and speech disorder, and revealed an IQ of 74. She clearly had learning disabilities and she started school at a special needs school at the age of 7.

To her, going to school was an arduous path, and mathematics was a major difficulty; on the other hand, she was good in reading and copying. However, because she attended school, she reached her physical limits more often.

Her everyday life activities were only manageable with family support 24 hours a day. She was unable to grasp the sense of time, date, and the four seasons, and she was unable to remember them.

She is easily fooled into doing anything stupid without being able to realise dangers or consequences of her irresponsible behaviour. She is now in the fifth grade of a school for children with special needs. She is able to read and copy but without understanding the sense of it. She is only able to calculate numbers up to 10 by using her fingers and she is only able to solve all other tasks with difficulty and with a lot of support. We decided to transfer her to a school for children with mental disability. At this school she feels accepted and learns, according to her abilities, everyday practical skills. She will never receive a high school diploma, but that is not so important for us.

Currently, E. is 11 years old, but she looks and behaves like a 6-year-old. Her various difficulties are a continuing part of our daily life, and we are hardly able to handle the resulting problems. Because of her mental disability she often misses the point, and in these situations, she reacts by using profanity for verbal assaults and slanders, or she suddenly becomes stark and stiff. In these situations, it is impossible for us to communicate with her, and there is nothing helpful to change the situation but only to leave her alone; after a while her problems are gone.

It is important for us that she lives a happy life, with people loving and protecting her. She is such a sweet, affectionate girl with so much strength and perseverance, which demands great respect from us. She fell on hard times and, therefore, deserves to live happily. We do the best to make sure that our 'little angel' will be well protected, even if we once are unable to take care of her.

In fact, it can be said that living with a FAS child is completely different. Children with FAS need specialised care, professional support and medical treatment, if indicated.

All of what Prof. Spohr told us 10 years ago became true. His words always stick in our mind: 'you can only try to limit the damage. The most important aim for the future of your child is to be content and to be happy'."

N.; born in 2008 (f); partial fetal alcohol syndrome (pFAS); May 2012

Editor's note: N. is a 4-year-old girl adopted from Russia in December 2011. She had lived in a children's home after she was removed from her birth parents due to severe neglect by her alcoholic mother.

The adoptive mother reports:

"Imagine a toy duck which you can't switch off, which moves across the carpet without braking. Imagine that this duck squeaks incessantly, talks way too loudly or shrieks with a shrill voice. Imagine that this duck constantly asks questions, but is not really interested in the answers. Just imagine a very loud, hyperactive, four-and-a-half year-old girl who comes across as a 2-year-old and moves across the room with crooked movements, speaks incessantly and doesn't have the slightest idea of distance and proximity. When you imagine all that, you have an idea of what my daughter N. is like.

Prior to her adoption, I was evaluated by the adoption agency. A psychiatric expert closely examined my motives and abilities to raise a child; salary and tax certificates were screened in order to prove my financial eligibility. Then it finally happened: after paying an administrative fee of 10000 Euro, the Russian government permitted my entry into the country. I had already received a proposal for the adoption and a photo showing a small, pale girl.

The first time we saw her, N. was way too thin and small for her age. She looked like a little doll with her burgundy velvet dress and white lace collar. Dark blonde, wanton curls and wide, brown eyes – the dearest little girl! When we asked the paediatrician of the children's home why N. was way too small for her age, she referred to the probably small size of her birth parents. When I asked inquisitively if her mother possibly had been an alcoholic, the paediatrician responded: 'No, otherwise she would have been registered; she neglected her child, and N. got only one bottle of milk per day.'

I was informed that N.'s father was in jail for murder, and that legal guardianship was removed from the mother due to her severe alcoholism, but not until the adoption was complete and N. already lived with us.

N. needed attention every single second: when I went to the bathroom, she stood in front of the door, cried excessively, drumming with her fists on the door or kicked it with her feet until I came out. Watching a kid's movie with her meant that she cheerfully bounced and chattered without interruption, that she poked at my eyes and kicked at my partner's stomach, until we stopped the movie and we again paid full attention to her. When we tried to set limits, she always became aggressive.

In the nursery school, her behaviour was similar. She clung to the nursery teachers and regarded most of the other children as her competitors. If she liked a child, she was wild with excitement, screaming and firmly flinging her arms around his or her neck. Finally, no child wanted to do anything with N. anymore. On the one hand, she solicited our permanent attention, and, on the other hand, she seemed to be autistic and lacking any empathy.

She was unable to make friends and had difficulties interpreting emotions from other's faces. Her paintings were only a scribbling, and she was hopeless at handicraft work. At first we thought that was due to a lack of guidance in the children's home, but it didn't explain why she destroyed paintings of other children when the nursery teachers focused their attention on others.

Later on, we learned that her eye–hand-coordination impairment caused by prenatal alcohol exposure was the reason for her disability in painting and in performing handicraft work. She had a very low frustration tolerance, immediately starting to cry or go on a rampage if something didn't work out successfully or if she didn't like to do what was expected of her.

She played very simple games. Most of the time, N. put her dolls to bed. But when N. was annoyed with herself or with us, she was unable to engage in fantasy. For example, after she accidentally locked herself into a bathroom in a holiday apartment and needed to be freed by a handyman, she claimed that I had locked her up. She cut her bangs completely crooked with a pair of children's scissors and then told the babysitter that I had cut her hair as punishment. Once, youth services were even involved, since N. said that I had hit her.

On the other hand, N.'s speech ability was impressive. She was able to learn German within 4 months and had an above average result in a test comparing her to children who were born and raised in Germany. Since N. spoke German so fluently, no one could understand my suspicion that she might suffer from fetal alcohol syndrome.

Finally, we visited Prof. Spohr, at Charité Berlin, who diagnosed partial FAS, and this diagnosis lead to clarification. "Partial" only because the typical facial features were not as pronounced. Her main symptoms were growth retardation and microcephaly without mental retardation. Alcohol consumption in pregnancy was confirmed, so she received a 4-Digit Diagnostic score of 4/3/4/4 – all the criteria for a partial fetal alcohol syndrome!

The diagnosis 'partial' FAS however, did not make things any easier for us. On the contrary! Because you wouldn't notice anything unusual about N. on first glance and since most people – even many paediatricians – have absolutely no clue about the consequences of fetal alcohol exposure, everyone was appalled that N. could suddenly be seen as disabled. Many said: 'She will grow out of it!' Her kindergarten, which used to be very supportive, was now of the opinion that I was to blame for the problems: my attitude and wrong methods of upbringing were making N. ill. They became even more convinced of that after I informed them that N. received Ritalin from the Charité.

Currently, N. is attending an integrative kindergarten where her problems with other children have improved a little. Furthermore, the daily dose of 12.5 mg methylphenidate makes the situation a little easier for all of us. However, even with medication, N. remains constantly hyperactive. N. is unable to think logically or to adjust behaviourally to a changing environment if necessary. Everything must always happen in exactly the same way; otherwise she gets really confused and upset.

She always forgets procedures such as coming home, taking off her shoes, putting her coat down, and washing her hands. Due to her poor concentration she is unable to accomplish these routines appropriately. On the way from the door to the bathroom, N. may forget that she wanted to wash her hands. Instead, she might unroll metres of toilet paper, strangle the dog and chatter continuously. Only things of personal interest are remembered by a photographic memory. The rest she will forget immediately.

We don't know how things will continue. That's for sure that there is a system behind adoptions from Russia! The Russian government utilises the ambition of individuals to adopt a child due to childlessness. They pass the costs for treatment and upbringing of the multitude of prenatally alcohol exposed children on to trustful and well-off foreigners and the medical and social institutions. Now, the German youth services have to pay € 2550 per month only for N.'s placement in the specialised kindergarten!

Adoption applicants are checked comprehensively for their eligibility in quite a degrading manner, and they can't imagine that someone will deceive them but rather believe in a legal certainty. It would be more equitable to inform future adoptive parents that the child they are willing to adopt is severely disabled. However, the Russian government doesn't have to comply with obligatory standards or quality control in the adoption process.

I was informed by the child service that about every fourth child adopted from Russia or Kazakhstan suffers from FAS, and I am sure that the estimated number of cases is considerably higher.

However, all persons concerned remain silent for shame of fraud, fear of the child services or because they want to protect their disabled and innocent children. Because nobody dares to oppose this, the German government implicitly accepts these adoption procedures of the Russian government. When I asked the head of youth services in southern Germany, why our government accepts the Russian adoption policy, he was stuck for an answer. He assured me that he had stated this question repeatedly to several governmental committees and the answer was always the same: 'in order not to jeopardise economic cooperation between Russia and Germany'!"

F.; born in 1996 (f); fetal alcohol syndrome (FAS); August 2012

Editor's note: In August 2012, F. came for diagnostic investigation with her foster mother to our clinic. Due to confirmed prenatal alcohol exposure and characteristic symptoms, FAS was diagnosed (4-Digit Diagnostic Code: 4/4/4/4). Her biological mother had been severely alcohol-dependent for years and, therefore, her four older siblings had already been taken into care and were growing up in a children's home. F. and her younger sister remained in the family despite of her mother's persisting alcohol abuse. After a fire at home they finally were placed into foster care in 2006.

Her foster mother reports:

"F. came into our family at the age of 9 years. She was very small and thin. First I supported her in daily routines: I had to shower her, help her to tidy her room, and we did homework together, memorising poems and songs and teaching her the multiplication tables and much else. Her teachers made sure that she knew what homework was to be done, and it was possible to keep school things and her sport clothing at school; this helped her not to always forget important things. With increasing age, the demands of daily life continued to rise, leading to more behavioural difficulties. Seemingly without any reason, she could become very aggressive. When we urged or criticised her, she would literally explode. Mostly she directed her aggression only towards me. At first, I was very strict, thinking I cannot accept her disrespectful behaviour, but this approach was without any success. Angry outbursts occurred at regular intervals, and she insulted me with words like: 'You can't tell me anything, you're not my mother' or 'that is my business, I will leave soon anyway'.

Once, she was in such a rage that she started to destroy her room behaving like a wild animal. She kicked me, tried to bite me, ripped my sweater, attempted to pinch and scratch me and was constantly screaming. I held her firmly and dropped her down. At that moment, I felt certain that I had to stay close to her. After what felt like an eternity, she suddenly collapsed; she wept and sobbed softly and I released my grip gently and caressed her. She snuggled up against me, lying on my lap for a while. Then I looked straight in her eyes and asked: 'Is everything okay again?' She nodded, and we got up. After that she never became physical again, and our relationship improved appreciably.

... Today, she is mostly good-tempered; from time to time she hurts others indiscriminately and then the next day everything is fine again. After 2 years of psychotherapy, she learned to talk about her problems and she became more open minded.

Now, at the age of 16, she has great memory problems, she easily becomes lost outside her home environment and cannot grasp the sense of time. She particularly forgets verbal agreements and contents of conversations easily. With the growing demands in her daily life, her fear of failure is increasing.

In order to structure her daily life, everything has to be in its proper place in her room. We labelled the drawers of her desk with corresponding school subjects and she has a large wall calendar where she checks off each previous day. She has spare outfits for physical education in case she loses one of them, and we put every important event or appointment into her diary lying on her desk. We clean her room and wash her clothes together on a fixed day. When we go out, we have to write down where we are, because she easily forgets everything.

Since three years of age our daughter uses an alarm clock that allows her to get up in the morning by herself, and she has a list with an exact time schedule to catch the school bus on time. One morning I got up and saw her sitting at the kitchen table. I asked why she wasn't eating breakfast. She answered that it wasn't 5.40 am yet. When she gets up earlier, the entire list needs to be adjusted ...."

"... At the age of 14 years F. ought to manage the route to her weekly psychotherapy session independently. Because we live in a small village, F. is used to taking public transportation to get to school, but for therapy sessions – located in another town– the way is different. Hence, she had to learn to connect different stages and, therefore, we made a second list. Initially, we taught her the first step, going from school into town by train. This presented a lot of difficulties; it was a Tuesday and her school bus left an hour later. Therefore, F. concluded that the train to therapy session would also be 1 hour later. After three weeks, she understood that she has to follow the exact dates on her list. So she had learned the first step.

Then she had to find the right tramline and take this line in the correct direction. It also took several weeks until she at least was able to do it correctly. Taken all together, our training continued from the end of August until December, when she finally was able to manage the entire route by herself without contacting us for any questions...

We finally learned that she was often furious and aggressive because she felt misunderstood. Since we changed our conservative view of education and learned to interpret her behaviour adequately to given situations and requirements, her aggressive behaviour lessened.

Our principal aim is to provide F. social security for her future life She will never be able to live an independent life without support, like other adolescents will do. We want to create the prerequisites for a dignified and happy life."

D.; born in 2007 (f); fetal alcohol syndrome (FAS); August 2008

Editor's note: According to the former partner of D.'s biological mother, she started drinking at the age of 14 years and soon became a chronic alcoholic. The older siblings were removed from the family care due to severe neglect. D. lived with his biological family for the first 3 months of life, largely under the father's care. Because the maternal and paternal grandparents also had problems with alcohol, living with them was not possible. Therefore, D. was placed into a foster family at the age of 3 months. She was diagnosed as having FAS at the age of 11 months.

Her foster mother reports:

"D. is currently 3 years old:

'What are you doing?' and 'what is that?' are the favourite sentences of our little D. at the moment. We all are extremely proud of these sentences.

Six months before we doubted whether D. would learn to speak at all, and any kind of effort we made seemed ineffectual. A class supporting parents with children suffering from severe speech and developmental delay was helpful, and we gained hope.

D. is a child severely impaired by prenatal alcohol exposure and she came into our family at the age of 3 months. Because D. came to us without an appropriate diagnosis, we worried a lot about her strange abnormalities. We made an appointment with Prof. Spohr (FASD-Zentrum, Berlin), who finally diagnosed FAS. The long-term prognosis seemed to be frightening, but our close relationship with this lovely little girl helped us to remain patient. We wanted to enjoy the beautiful moments and be happy about the progress she made and not focus on her difficulties. Because we are unable to cope with the task of her education by ourselves, we sought support and help. At the moment D. visits the kindergarten for only 3 hours a day, and sometimes it is a great challenge for her. Because our own children developed totally differently, we are often stretched to our own limits of knowing how best to educate her. In particular, her enormous hyperactivity requires a great deal of strength. Even complete strangers look favorably on our nice and open-minded child, who would obviously go along with anyone, even strangers. Her mood changes rapidly; peaceful game situations all of a sudden turn into uncontrollable aggressive tantrums. D. gets frustrated easily and she subsequently throws her toys or hits her head on the floor. With the help of a psychologist, we are more and more able to defuse these situations, by holding and comforting her, instead of scolding her for bad behaviour, which was our previous reaction. D. needs clearly structured routines, short and precise statements, lots and lots of outside activities and mainly one-on-one care for behaving more within normal limits. Despite these difficulties, living with her is a worthwhile effort because we have learned to appreciate life in a different way and set new priorities. We are still amazed and astonished about her development from a little baby to a young human."

C.; born in 1996 (m); fetal alcohol syndrome (FAS); August 1996

Editor's note: When his foster mother presented C. at our clinic for the first time, he was 8 months old. Based on confirmed alcohol exposure during pregnancy and characteristic symptoms, we diagnosed "full blown" fetal alcohol syndrome (4-Digit Diagnostic Code: 4/4/4/4).

In the following years, we saw him regularly in our clinic. Since 3 years he proudly participates in my lecture for first-year medical students at the university, answering questions about his life with FAS. He is still unable to grasp the sense of numbers and is unable to calculate but with his charming nature he is able to impress the students by the fact that he knows the metro lines of Berlin by heart. C. still suffers from a significant growth deficiency. At the age of 18, his weight and height was equivalent to those of an 11-year-old child.

His foster mother reports:

"C. was the 11th child of a 33-year old alcohol dependent woman. According to her own statement, she drank two bottles of hard liquor per day! His birth weight was 2740 g and his birth length was 46 cm.

C. was discharged from the hospital and lived with his biological mother for 4 weeks. But then he was given to a friend because his mother didn't want to take care of 'the little brat' anymore. He had to be admitted to the hospital and finally came into our family for long-term foster care. He was 5 months old; he weighed only 5600 g and was only 62 cm long.

C. was very restless at first, and feeding him was very difficult. Following a strict daily routine with little sensory input, C. became calmer. He started speaking surprisingly early. At the age of 12 months he was able to articulate properly. At 16 months he was able to walk alone.

In August 1998, at the age of two and a half, he was enrolled in a nursery school for remedial education. C. weighed 9.5 kg and was of 82 cm tall.

At preschool age, I had to keep a close watch on him. He was obtrusive and had no fear of strangers; he go along with anyone. Furthermore, he was still suffering from eating difficulties. He was sent to a special school for disabled children at the age of 7 years.

C. seems to be clever but he is unable to digest information and impressions properly. He suffers from bad dreams, is easily overtaxed and often imitates others without being able to sense the meaning of words or behaviour. C. is a very anxious child and is easily irritated by every new situation. He often covers up his anxieties verbally. For a long while, dental visits were impossible. He suffered from atopic eczema, which became worse at school age.

At school age, C. is still obtrusive, unstructured and breaks all appointment. He is unable to grasp the sense of time and needs fixed daily and weekly routines.

On the other hand, he is very gifted in music, sings very often, and at his own wish he started playing the trumpet in October 2004.

C. mostly plays outside, but we had to limit the radius of his freedom because he would disappear easily. Among his school mates he is by far the smallest, but on the other hand very dominant. Others barely get a chance to speak in his presence. His school class consists of nine children. The teacher who is a foster father himself, is able to handle him very well. During the third grade C.'s poor arithmetic became clearly evident.

At the age of 11 years, C. still had difficulties to concentrate and he behaves obtrusively. His problems getting along with peers increased and he was unable to coordinate his appointments. He often agreed to meet with several people at the same time and, finally, he often broke every appointment. It is necessary that he follows my simple and clear instructions promptly, otherwise I have to start from scratch.

At the age of 12, C. weighted 23.5 kg and was 125 cm tall. Fortunately, he now was considered to have a degree of disability of 70%.

We have to organise his leisure time because he has no idea for activities spontaneously. Instead of playing the trumpet, he now takes piano lessons. With the help of a prepaid cell phone he is able to move independently further from home, and his cell phone timer will remind him to get in touch with me or to return home on time. This normally works quite well.

He needs support with his daily hygiene; I have to stay right next to him while he is showering or brushing his teeth or otherwise nothing happens. His self-esteem is very limited, but he uses his good verbal abilities to cover it up.

At the age of 14, C. has a height of only 131 cm. He generally is oriented towards younger children and still playful. Because of his small stature, nobody will notice that he is much older than his friends.

Now, at the age of 16, C. is still only 145 cm tall and needs a lot of support and help. He still imitates others and is unable to have an opinion. During conversations, he changes his mind according to the opinion of his partners' conversation and he often fabricates or exaggerates stories or happenings.

C. has not lost his peculiar charm over the years; he still is a very lovable person."

Report of family S. about their four adopted siblings with FAS

Editor's note: I met the family in Erfurt in 2012, when they participated in the annual German FASD conference. Their story is deeply moving.

"We are an exceptional family. Father and mother, married 25 years ago, living with 8 children aged between 19 and 24 – four biological and four adopted children. Four girls and four boys– all together in our large family since 1997 without having any knowledge about the disability of our adopted children until March 2012.

On reading a detailed article on FAS in a scientific journal I was immediately reminded of our adoptive children and our family's life. For me this finally explained for us the inappropriate and for us incomprehensible behaviour of our adoptive children, although all of our children were educated equally. What a relief!

When we adopted the four siblings from Brazil in 1997, they were already between 3 and 9 years of age and had a horrific life history of physical and sexual abuse and further traumatisation, which we didn't know at that time. We began integration of our four adopted children into our family with great commitment and without any fear or favour because we did receive reports and court records about our children's previous life in Brazil not until later years. At the time of adoption we were quite experienced in raising children, because our four children were already 4 to 8 years old. Furthermore, we had been successful in integrating three foster children into our family, who finally went back to their biological families a couple of years ago.

Our 'new children' were unable to speak even Portuguese when arriving in our family; they had experienced a miserable existence in a forested area under neglectful and deplorable conditions. Only the oldest child, aged 10, was able to put two or three words together but did not know any colours, numbers or letters.

We faced this enormous challenge with patience and inventiveness. Our attempts to provide structure and to support the children and to create a sense of togetherness resulted in an active everyday family life. In addition to studying language, our adoptive children had to learn arduously most of the requirements of daily life, which are quite natural for children raised under normal conditions. With the help of our biological children, they learned to use a bathroom, complying with table manners and conforming to rules in kindergarten or at school. Thinking retrospectively, our biological children were the best peer group for the adopted siblings; they are of same ages and were willing to play and live together with them.

Despite our pedagogical experience, we were unable to handle the constantly recurring difficult behaviour of our adopted children. I guess there is no gene for stealing and lying! All of our children were raised according to the same principles, but our Brazilian children did not learn from the resulting consequences of their behaviour. They repeatedly lied, stole and defrauded us. They had no idea of emotions and personal needs of others, and already familiar structures and routines of daily life had to be repeated and trained again and again.

Many dangerous and forbidden things happened in secret, unknown to our own biological children, who were unfamiliar behaviouring of a nature like this. Over time, our adopted children repeatedly committed different offences (theft, damage to property, etc.) but negative consequences and even sentences from a court of law did not have any effect on them.

During the last 16 years we implemented various therapies, consulted different child and adolescent psychiatrists, medical specialists and psychological experts. The children were diagnosed with auditory perception disorder, ADHD, ADS, borderline

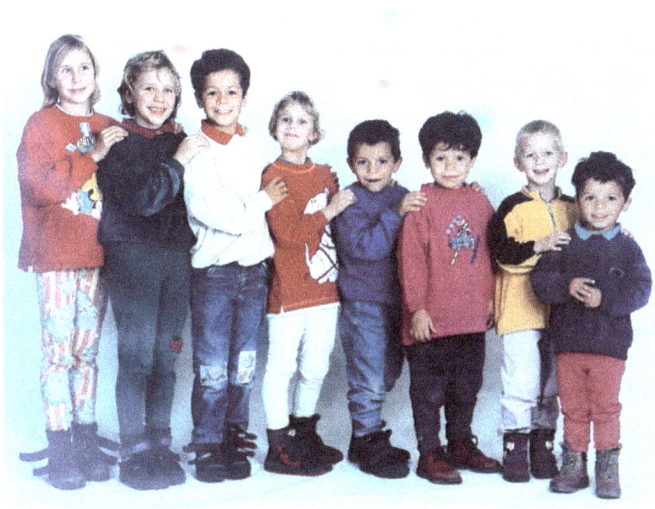

Fig. 17.1: The children of family F. at the time of the adoption of their four Brazilian siblings.

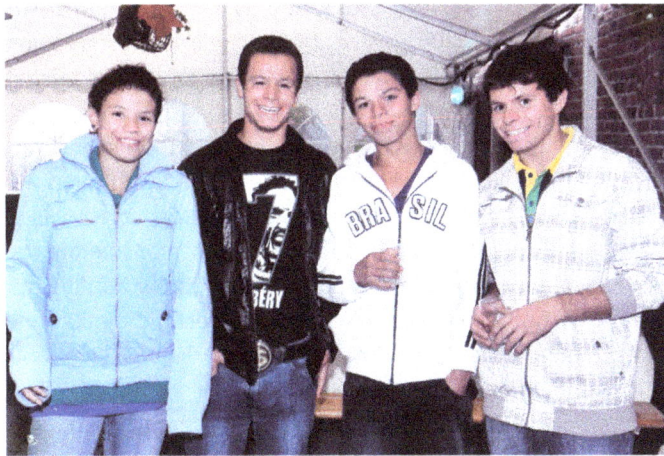

Fig. 17.2: Photo of the adopted children in adulthood.

personality disorder, dissociative personality disorder; the list got longer and longer, but no one diagnosed FAS or even thought about it.

Today, all four of our adopted children have received a confirmed diagnosis of FAS with a disability certificate of 70% and qualifiers G, B and H, acknowledging their highly limited competence in everyday life.

Our family suffered from the consequences of the unidentified FAS disability. Former friends, acquaintances and family members distanced themselves, condemning our educational methods and procedures. Although these people didn't know anything about the actual problems in our daily family life, we felt compelled to constantly justify ourselves.

We are convinced that every one of our eight children should have the same rights and duties, but this concept didn't work at all. Our adopted children demanded freedom but were then unable to deal with it. Despite our intensive support and help, they didn't succeed in graduating from school and or with vocational training. They still ran away from home, committed criminal offences and finally went to the bad side of life. Due to his criminal offences, the oldest adopted son was imprisoned for 2 years and later became homeless. The ones still living at home, had to be supervised constantly – going out with friends, spontaneous visiting of friends or just going out for diner, had to be well planned and would not have been possible without the help of our biological children, who were now studying in different cities and countries.

Only the confirmed diagnosis of FAS in March 2012, followed by socio-legal support finally changed our situation for the better. Our young adults returned home because institutional placement failed due to their delinquent behaviour. Inbetween this time, all of them received a full disability pension and finally took up employment in sheltered workshops. The oldest one is living in a closely supervised residential home, since living more independently was not possible; this was the only option to get him out of his homelessness, which had already lasted for 7 months. For more than a year we now have been looking for supervised living places for the three younger adopted siblings, but it always fails due to a lack of knowledge of FAS and the lack of related concepts to supervise our children adequately.

They are constantly faced with exaggerated expectations from their social surroundings due to their seemingly good abilities. They are well educated and mostly behave courteously and politely, they are gifted in language and well mannered. Based on their IQ-scores they are classified as being mentally disabled persons before the law. But a legal claim cannot create a proper living place for our young adults, and thus, we still have to take responsibility for them. This is a very demanding task; we can't fulfil all the needs of our adopted children. They require an adequate social environment for their future lives in order to leave home as soon as possible.

Due to his inability to comply with agreements our youngest adoptive son often ends up in real despair. He cannot understand why it is so difficult for him to behave adequately with respect to the requirements and circumstances in daily life. He is trapped in his disability.

It is sure we facilitated surrvival of our adopted children, but our dream to enable them to live an independent life with a driver's licence and children of their own was drowned by alcohol; it is a bitter fate.

My son asked me: 'So, if this woman hadn't drunk alcohol during pregnancy, I wouldn't be like this?' I answered: 'Yes, that's how it is'.

Despite their antisocial attitude and their inability to notice our suffering caused by their destructive behaviour, we managed to become a successful family. We live with our children and providing a secure home for them. Our children are charming and endearing as well, and we learned to protect ourselves from great disappointments and sorrow in the case that they cannot accept our love.

We always accepted and loved them like they are, never minding that they are now diagnosed with FAS; they are still the same children.

I hope with all my heart that we will find a place for them to live a comfortable and content life."

A family report

Editor's note: The contribution of this family is impressive. On the one hand, they took on three "healthy" children into foster care and had to struggle for a correct diagnosis of their children for a long time. On the other hand, I was touched by their courage in dealing with this unexpected challenge with such joy and humour.

The foster parents report:

"In April 2014, we went to the FASD clinic of Prof. Spohr with our then 2.5-year-old foster daughter. She suffered from developmental delay, and we supposed similarities to children with FAS. At the time, however, we didn't have any information on maternal alcohol consumption during pregnancy.

We were staggered by the clarity of the diagnosis of FAS and the statement of Prof. Spohr, who told us that there is nothing worse for intrauterine development than alcohol. We were not prepared for this unexpected diagnosis despite the fact that we both have pedagogical professions. FASD was, however, only discussed very briefly during our course of studies; especially the whole variety and peculiarity of this 'invisible' disorder remained unmentioned. We had had the impression that alcohol consumption during pregnancy is only a problem for a few chronically alcohol-dependent women.

The more we learned about FAS, the more we became aware of the 'brutality' of this diagnosis. We were also confronted with stigmatisation and the fact that the consequences of alcohol consumption during pregnancy are still trivialised or largely tabooed. It took up to half a year before our application for early intervention training was granted. The wide dimension of difficulties and impairments is just not recognised, and the difficulties and the impairments of our foster daughter were belittled by nursery teachers and our social surroundings.

Living with a child with FAS means struggling with difficulties every day, and in addition we had to do lobby work for affected children and their families and to cope with the youth welfare office because they didn't want to give us information about any alcohol consumption in the pregnancy of the biological mother of our foster daughter due to her personal rights. However, after we exerted pressure on them, the files were reviewed and, indeed, a reference to alcohol consumption during pregnancy was found.

Within a year, three of our five foster children received a FASD diagnosis! Again and again, we had to justify ourselves because we initiated the diagnostic procedure. We were accused of stigmatising our children, but I think we have had no other choice because without a confirmed diagnosis we would not be eligible for any special help or support. Further, even with a FAS diagnosis, you have to fight for everything.

Our daily routine must be structured and organised uniformly; even at the weekend, activities such as getting up in the morning, playing, being outside or partaking of meals proceeded unchanged in order to avoid complete chaos.

Despite our attempts to always structure daily routine to avoid children's tantrums, compulsiveness and anxieties are unavoidable. On the one hand, because we are sometimes exhausted and thus a little inattentive, and, on the other hand, because we wanted to keep up some flexibility in our daily routine. But changes in daily routine need to be arranged carefully and calculated; without prior notice, our children are unable to cope with new situations.

Nonetheless, we will go ahead happy and joyfully with our children, only pre-staging where we will end up one day."

M.; born in 1995 (m); fetal alcohol syndrome in adulthood (FAS adult); February 2013

Editor's note: According to his foster mother, M.'s biological mother suffered from a borderline personality disorder and consumed alcohol extensively throughout her pregnancy. At that time, his current foster mother took care of him during the day as a childminder. Due to his birthmothers' continuing and severe psychiatric symptoms, he moved into the family of his former childminder at the age of 5 years.

From the very beginning, M. suffered from sleep disturbances. As an infant he was very restless and his behaviour was sometimes quite risky. Psychotherapy in childhood improved his behaviour but his extreme chronic fatigue remained. Until today, M. has difficulty getting out of bed in the morning and is continuously tired during the day. An extensive examination in a sleep clinic did not reveal a diagnosis for his hypersomnia, and to date an effective treatment was not identified.

We always have to pull him out of bed in the morning; otherwise he would continue to sleep. Currently, he additionally suffers from a light depressive episode with anhedonia, loss of interest, sadness and a feeling of emptiness. Medical treatment with Escitalopram 20 mg did not improve his symptoms. An attention deficit syndrome was diagnosed in childhood, but an indicated medical treatment was not sustainable due to intolerable side effects.

His foster mother reports:

"…After 16 hours of sleep he was as tired as after 6 hours. We left him in bed for 4 days. He did not get up by himself. He urinated into plastic bottles and hid his food. He did not take his medication. He forgot to clean himself, and he was unable to get out of bed by himself to go to work, although he likes his job. Without our help he will never reach his goal. We have to check and control every little detail…"

Conclusion: This report illustrates the problem of sleep disturbances, often seen in patients with FAS. Apart from severe difficulties falling or staying asleep, the rarely seen hypersomnia in patients with FAS also results in difficulties to meet the demands of a daily routine.

A.; born in 1973 (f); fetal alcohol syndrome in adulthood (FAS adult); January 2013

Editor's note: We have reproduced the original letter and report after asking the patient for her permission not to expose her, but to show that despite her eloquence, like many other people with FASD, she still experiences a significant language deficit and apparent concentration difficulties while writing.

Letter from A.

"Dear Dr. Spohr,

… The trip went well and everything went according to plan. Was very exhausted and happy to be back home. So you may call me a fine friend…

Now I try next to describe my feelings from childhood and adolescence, which are not easy to describe.

Fears in different forms: So as you know, numbers are without meaning, why the numbers are x+ or x- etc. Small rooms and elevators; the elevator may crash or get stuck; I will be forgotten and will die. Large crowds, they are so inconsiderate and only think about themselves, parties with loud music, noisy noises, then everything contracts within me. To go straight up to people and to make contact frightens me.

I watch civilians very closely and simply say I am sceptical towards people. May sound melodramatic, but it is like that. Making a lot of contact, no thanks.

But also not being understood by civilians.

Sincerely,

A."

A. reports:

"I was born as a premature baby in 1973. Shortly after birth, I underwent gastric surgery. While I lived in an orphanage I met the family that adopted me. There I lived in a friendly and warm home. In first grade it became obvious that a large school class was an excessive challenge for me. Therefore the 'Michaelshof' (institute for handicapped children) was the next place to live and I went to school until the ninth grade. After leaving school, I did a traineeship in an old people's home for 1 year. There I learned housekeeping, for example, ironing and cleaning. Then I trained as a lumberman, while in the same time I finished my school qualification. I only managed it with great difficulty and private coaching.

After many years of unemployment and temporary traineeship, I got two labor contracts. After a short while I was discharged; I was too unstable. Inbetween I had to suffer as a martyr with doctors and a failed trial, which was actually supposed to help me to get employment in a sheltered workshop. Now the job centre is putting inhumane pressure on me."

Letter of a 21-year-old FAS-patient from England

Editor's note: Susan F., a politically active foster mother in the United Kingdom who initiated the support group 'NOFAS-UK' sent me this impressing letter and a photo of her 21-year-old foster daughter.

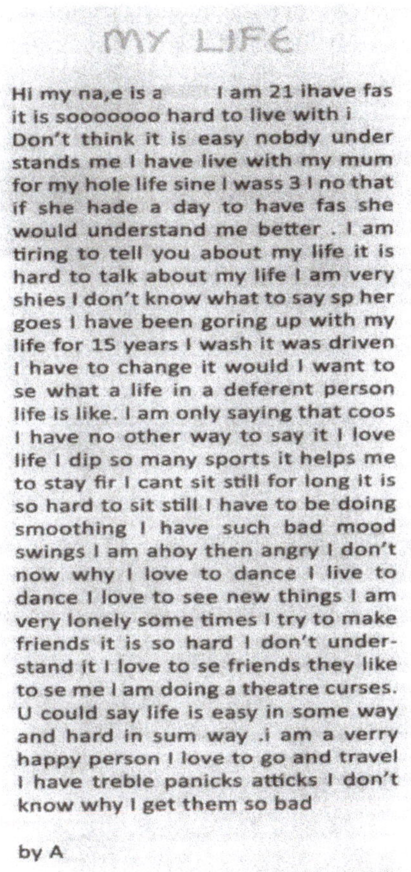

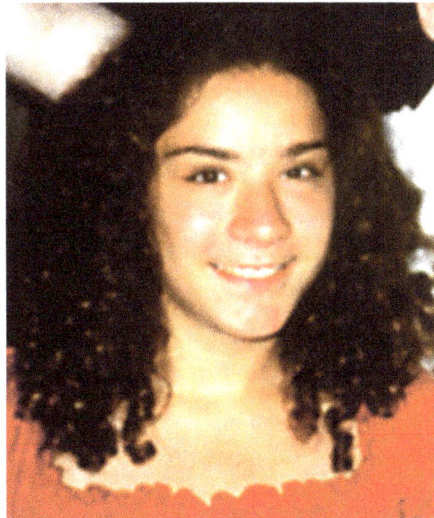

MY LIFE

Hi my na,e is a   I am 21 ihave fas
it is sooooooo hard to live with i
Don't think it is easy nobdy under
stands me I have live with my mum
for my hole life sine I wass 3 I no that
if she hade a day to have fas she
would understand me better . I am
tiring to tell you about my life it is
hard to talk about my life I am very
shies I don't know what to say sp her
goes I have been goring up with my
life for 15 years I wash it was driven
I have to change it would I want to
se what a life in a deferent person
life is like. I am only saying that coos
I have no other way to say it I love
life I dip so many sports it helps me
to stay fir I cant sit still for long it is
so hard to sit still I have to be doing
smoothing I have such bad mood
swings I am ahoy then angry I don't
now why I love to dance I live to
dance I love to see new things I am
very lonely some times I try to make
friends it is so hard I don't understand it I love to se friends they like
to se me I am doing a theatre curses.
U could say life is easy in some way
and hard in sum way .i am a verry
happy person I love to go and travel
I have treble panicks atticks I don't
know why I get them so bad

by A

Fig. 17.3: A.'s letter.

Fig. 17.4: A., 21-years-old FAS patient.

G.W.; born 1973 (f); fetal alcohol syndrome in adulthood (FAS adult); November 2011

Editor's note: Ms. W. came to Berlin for a diagnostic assessment for FAS in November 2011. She grew up with foster parents due to severe neglect and the chronic alcohol dependency of her biological parents. Her development was not age appropriate; she suffered from dystrophy, was ill often and has a congenital heart defect. At the time of her visit in Berlin, she actually lived in a supervised home. She wrote a book about her experiences with FAS and sent the following letter to the editor.

"Dear Professor Spohr,

Today I would like to tell you how I am doing. I have been suffering from FASD since birth and, therefore, I struggle daily with my disability. In my nice apartment I am very active, often cooking and baking. At home I feel entirely secure and content. My foster parents and I still have a good relationship.

Until December I was under the care of a social welfare organisation, but I cancelled their support because I was totally dissatisfied with them. Since January 2013, I receive support from a social worker for 1 hour a week, which is helpful for me because I can talk to her and she comforts me.

I'm often emotionally and mentally unstable and in November 2012 I was admitted to a psychiatric unit for 1 week followed by outpatient treatment for 4 weeks. I was very content with the clinical treatment and I was discharged from the clinic in better condition. Now I am continuing with the outpatient treatment.

In the hospital the physicians and nurses mentioned my book and asked me, if I would report about my problems and experiences with FAS next autumn. I gladly agreed because I want to assist in preventing alcohol consumption during pregnancy.

I have read a lot about FASD. Many symptoms apply to me.

Dear Professor Spohr, I want to thank you.

Your G."

Excerpt from G.W.'s life story

My problems and weaknesses:
1. Anxiety and panic disorder – usually manifest by sudden swelling of the larynx and a contraction of the chest.
2. I am mentally unstable; I quickly lose courage or patience. Related to this, I have stomach problems and my whole body trembles. These symptoms are triggered if somebody laughs or sneers at me.

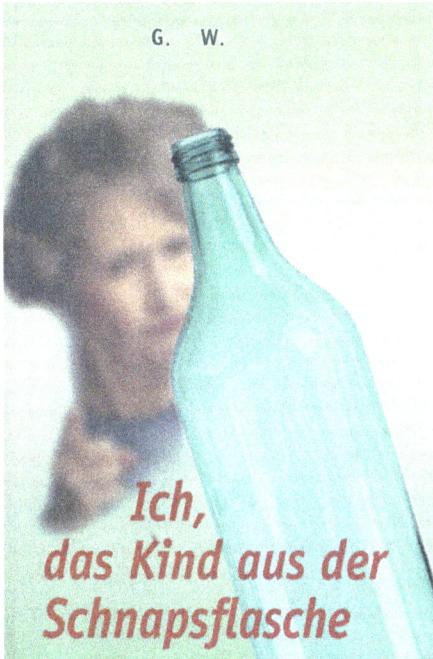

Ich, das Kind aus der Schnapsflasche

Fig. 17.5: Biography of G.W. 2012 ("Me, the child born out of the bottle").

3. I need a lot of time to complete things. Procedures in my daily routine should always be the same. I need to finish something, before I start anything new. My fine motor skills need to be trained constantly. It is important that I follow a daily schedule.
4. I am hardly able to stay on top of things if I have to organise or structure household tasks. However, if I get support and help, I'm able to be successful.
5. In an unfamiliar surrounding I always need help. Reading different train or tram schedules is difficult. Visual–spatial orientation is a problem for me as I often mix up the directions left and right.
6. I need to check the time constantly because I lack any sense of time.
7. My mood changes very rapidly: up in one minute and down the next.
8. I often try to avoid any issues – "I'd rather bury my head in the sand".
9. I have difficulties in concentrating on doing something for a long period of time; and soon I find myself getting quite nervous.
10. I think my sense of justice is highly developed. I always wish for things to take a turn for the better and, therefore, I speak up for myself, which is not always well received; I'm often misunderstood, ignored or people laugh at me.

L. born 1989 (w); fetal alcohol syndrome in adulthood; 2007

Editor's note: The adoptive mother's report about her adult daughter is quite exceptional; not only is it very detailed but also expansive beyond the given scope. The report is particularly impressive in describing very well problems adoptive parents face with their adoptee in both childhood and adulthood.

The adoptive mother reports:

Adoption: difficulties and problems
"About 13 months after the placement of our first adopted child, L (now age 23 years) was introduced to us. At that time she was 8 weeks old.

When the social worker in charge of this adoption, Mrs. A, first presented L. to us, she informed us that her mother was a smoker. She also indicated her suspicion that the birth mother might possibly have an alcohol problem, followed by the general remark that mothers normally are not willing to give detailed information about their history of alcohol use. However, we didn't pay any closer attention to this indication as the baby had been presented to us as a healthy child. The copy of the medical bulletin we received during the process of adoption also described L. as a well developing infant without deficits or signs of developmental retardation. Meanwhile, the former pediatrician who did this examination assured us in writing that he would not have given such an assessment without reservations, if he were to have had knowledge about the alcohol abuse of the mother. Even at that time the evaluating pediatrician was fully aware of the consequences of drinking alcohol during pregnancy.

Our original concern that this child might have a higher risk of developing an addiction to alcohol was deemed irrelevant after we considered that there are alcoholics in many families. Little did we, the hopeful adoptive parents, know about brain damage caused by consumption of alcohol during pregnancy. Our lack of concern was especially because the pediatrician confirmed in writing that L. developed normally.

Before the placement was initiated Mrs.A. had written a memorandum about a conversation with the birth mother, in which the latter had quite frankly spoken about her excessive drinking during her pregnancy. This important information was withheld from both of us and the attending physicians. It appears that Mrs. A in collaboration with her new colleague Mr. B., intentionally deceived all people involved.

The youth welfare department had not informed us about the mother's alcohol abuse during her pregnancy nor had they told us about the expected consequential damages of FAS even to this day.

Our own personal investigations when our daughter was almost 18 years old led us to the next higher communal youth welfare department to whom the file had meanwhile been assigned, and whom we requested to make all medical records about the mother and child available to us, including her alcohol abuse during pregnancy as well as her stay in psychiatry while being pregnant.

Had we had access to all of this information that Mrs. A. already had before placement even started, we would have been alarmed. We would never have considered proceeding with this child's placement, nor have been introduced to her, and most likely would not have decided to adopt L. as a part of our family.

The diagnosis and what follows?
A friend of us introduced us to FAS, when L. was almost 18 years old.

Immediately we contacted Prof. Spohr in Berlin for an examination and diagnosis. He asked us to check with the youth welfare department if there was any recorded information of alcohol abuse during the birth mother's pregnancy.

We were shocked to learn the results. The communal youth welfare department to which the file had been assigned gave us the protocol of the conversation between Mrs. A and the birth mother. It contained the information given by the mother that she had been drunk every day of her pregnancy and consequently had been hospitalised. All through the years we were denied this significant information although the youth welfare department was updated regularly on L.'s major problems and developmental retardation. So our right, not only to obtain a diagnosis of FAS but also to learn of specific treatment, was denied us for years. As a result of this modus operandi, not only L. but the whole family suffered from serious psychological and physical damage, as well as financial loss.

When she was 18 years of age, L. was diagnosed with FAS in Berlin. Thereafter she received her ID Card for the severely disabled (degree of disability 70%), which officially confirmed that she did not suffer from psychological disorders because of a hearing impairment, as we had always assumed, but even worse, suffered from FAS. Her associated lack in everyday competence paired with innocence and being easily influenced, plus her permanent urge to be entertained, had led to a continuous 24/7 supervision and guarding.

Over 5 years have passed since we took the pension office to court to fight for the missing recognition of L.'s disability at birth. We need an acknowledgement of her disability in order to deduct our personal expenses in our tax and pension declaration.

Partnership and relationship
L. easily makes friends but has difficulties in retaining friendships. She has had sex with frequently changing partners.

On her 18th birthday she went on a 'blind date' with someone she met online. They were supposed to meet in vacant barracks outside the city. None of my arguments could stop her from meeting a stranger at 7 pm on a November night. Only when I told her that the police would await her in front of the barracks and bring her to a home for the disabled did she refrain from going.

Another time we received an invoice from a doctor in a neighboring city. As we questioned L. about it, she frankly and without any signs of guilt told us that she met a man (where?) … who picked her up at the railway station. At the end of the meeting he drove her to this doctor in order for her to receive a prescription for the morning-after pill.

Sex education is a real problem. We had L. take several pregnancy tests as well as HIV tests. Finally we decided in favor of the contraceptive coil, which was quite an undertaking as it required the assistance of a caring gynecologist as well a trusting head physician in the hospital. The decisive factor in achieving this means of contraception was her sister's support, as she managed to convince L. of the necessity, as well as the advantage of the coil.

In the meantime, L. is dating her third steady boyfriend. Her first long-term relationship started after several largely sexual motivated affairs at the age of 19.

The young man X. shared the same history of an alcoholic birth mother and dedicated adoptive parents. Like L., the same aged X. suffered from uncontrolled outbursts. He barely managed to complete junior high and finish a 5-year internship under the guidance of a relative. Meanwhile, he is unemployed. Misunderstandings between L. and X. frequently led to losses of impulse control of both parties, sometimes even resulting in violent fights. X. also wasn't able to keep his needs appropriately under control and couldn't recognise L.'s limits. L., of course, suffered from the same deficiencies but in the nature of things with a smaller impact on her partner. She rather scratches, bites and kicks in self-defense. We were continuously concerned about how to explain such injuries, in the event of needing to consult the emergency unit.

After 18 months L. left X. for another man

The new man, Y., was trained pedagogically. He presumed failure of parental education in her upbringing and chose a new approach. L. should immediately move to an apartment of her own ('your parents have to pay for that'), take driver's lessons and request the guardian's court to end legal supervision. In this context the court asked Prof. Spohr questions about her special problem and finally confirmed in full our honorary guardianship. After half a year we felt impelled to inform Y. about L.'s problems as he was continuously plotting against us parents in the background. Y. ended the relationship immediately thereafter.

L. took the separation easily and quickly found comfort in other young men. Those phases of wandering around searching for distraction and new friends are the worst for us, and would aptly be described as hell on earth!

Currently L. is dating a friend of her ex X. They are planning to get married and have children. At this point our question arises, what will happen to those children? Will they be healthy or eventually also suffer from FAS, like L. and her younger brother? He is seriously affected and lives in an institute for disabled children. He has a baby with a 14 year-old severely disabled girl. As things stand, it is to be feared that his adoptive parents have to pay alimony for the mother and child. At this point we learned that our responsibility is not only limited to our tremendous efforts for our daughter, but as a result of the intergenerational contract, we are also committed to support and care for our grandchildren.

Profession
After obtaining her intermediate high-school certificate at a school for children with special needs, L. started a program for professional integration of problematic adolescents as recommended by the federal labor agency. She started to steal, was encouraged to be disobedient, threatened and had to be withdrawn from the class. Several short-term internships were arranged, but from the very start all were without prospect of an apprenticeship afterwards. After that, she started an apprenticeship as a cook, which was supported by the integrational service. The training chef aborted this after only 3 months. We had to sue the federal labor agency before the social welfare court to pay for the costs of the assisted courses at the vocational college.

Finally, this vocational college offered L. a tailor's apprenticeship. This training, which was cut to 2 years, was especially for students without graduation who could learn this in addition to the professional training.

In our desperate efforts to give L. the opportunity of a successful apprenticeship, we set up a secondary residence on the site where we lived with her during the week. It was not possible for her to stay in a boarding school as their care didn't meet her special needs. In addition, there is a railway station next to the school, representing permanent temptation for L.'s search for distraction.

While working L. needs to be supervised, reminded and instructed continuously. She once puzzled friends with the statement that one metre equals 30 cm. As she has not developed any sense of time, we weren't surprised when she announced at Easter that the next school holiday would then be Christmas. When solving an arithmetic problem she defined a week as 4 days. These deficits in coping with everyday living prevent her from working independently.

L. successfully completed this intensively accompanied apprenticeship in a class with six students. Nevertheless, she is unable to shorten a pair of trousers on her own. It is very likely that at the end one leg is shortened by 3 cm, whereas the other is 5 cm shorter, or one leg hasn't been worked on at all.

After the apprenticeship L. started a 'voluntary year of ecological service' ('Freiwilliges Ökologisches Jahr'). This government-supported program is supposed to give disabled people a chance of occupational orientation. She was dismissed from the first assignment location, as she wasn't able to meet the demands. A second short-term assignment location was immediately limited to 2 months. So, we finally asked the department head of the state youth welfare department for his support to find a third one. The 'voluntary year of ecological service' was then changed to a 'voluntary year of social service' and extended by 6 months.

In the afternoons L. helped take care of children with limited or low vision in a boarding school for the blind. She assisted the chlidrens while they were playing and eating or accompanied them from point A to point B. The teachers were pleased with her work. They had been informed about L.'s problems and had prepared themselves accordingly. The head of the school managed to find her an internship in an integrative kindergarten with the goal that this could be developed into an integrative full-time job. A sheltered workshop, which is an official institution for work for disabled people, is supporting this process, considering it as an 'external' workplace. The costs are so far being borne by the jobcenter.

Official local administrative bodies feel overburdened in handling this creative and pragmatic approach to create a job for L., particularly as such special arrangements are not provided for by German law. Therefore, regional offices need to be included in order to get L. integrated into the labor market.

Following the standardisd procedure, the socio-medical service examined L. and concluded that she is not suited for the regular German labour market. The German pension insurance deemed her to be fully incapacitated; therefore, she can only be considered for a job in a sheltered workshop for the disabled or in a guarded job with merely auxiliary functions.

Meanwhile, we drive L. to work every day, like we did during her period of voluntary ecological and social work, in order to make sure that she arrives at the kindergarten. Further, we pick her up afterwards to ensure that she doesn't wander around the city or the railway station in her search for distraction.

Last summer, L. completed an internship in the sewing room of an "anthroposophical" sheltered workshop, only to thereafter express the clear message that she would never be willing to work in such an organisation."

A.; born in 1985 (f); fetal alcohol syndrome in adulthood (FAS adult); April 2012

Editor's note: The biological mother of A. was according to her own admission, a chronic alcohol drinker. Later, she told her daughter that she was never actually drunk during the pregnancy, but that she did drink beer and liquor on a daily basis. In addition, she had smoked intensively. A. was born as a premature, malnourished baby weighing 2100 g in the 37th week of pregnancy and after discharge she was admitted to a children's home.

The adoptive parents report:

"At 2½ years of age, A. came to our family after being put up for adoption by child services with the description of a 'healthy child'. Since she grew up in a children's home, we assumed that the hyperactivity, eat, sleep and concentration problems had developed there. Full of joy due to having a child in our family, we started full of love and patience but at the same time with clear rules and constant assistance with her upbringing.

It was difficult for A. to clean up on her own and to remember daily routines. From the beginning, her personal hygiene and compliance with ground rules were problematic, so that daily check-ups and even the usage of post-its were necessary.

Everything that we undertook together, she enjoyed and was not difficult for her. We always had to praise her a lot and provide incentives to trigger her motivation, concentration and patience. Each small success gave us hope and every setback resignation. A. needed clear boundaries, fixed routines and permanent control from the beginning.

Living with a child affected by FAS is very stressful, requires a lot of strength, patience and a steady optimism. Only with help of our 'extended family' were we able to survive the hard times and constant antics of our daughter. When we were at our wits end and did not have any strength left, we could always count on the support of our siblings and parents. Sometimes we had to take a small 'break' in order not to jeopardise our marriage and health. We have the feeling that we have fulfilled a big task in our lives by raising and supporting this child.

Now our daughter is 27 years old and still requires constant support and control, particularly regarding her personal hygiene, with keeping her home orderly and clean, with money management and her ever changing group of friends.

A. was in regular primary school until 6th grade, after which she changed to a special needs school until the end of 9th grade. Hence, she can read, write and count – though not without problems or easily. She has a friendly and open-minded manner, is honest, open and always willing to help, and we are proud that she is now able to live on her own in a rented apartment!"

S.; born in 1979 (f); fetal alcohol syndrome in adulthood (FAS adult); February 2012

Editor's note: S. was examined in the FASD centre in Berlin in February 2012 and was diagnosed with a fetal alcohol syndrome in adulthood (4-Digit Diagnostic Code: 4/4/4/4). The sister and sister-in-law of her mother both confirmed severe alcoholism of the mother even during the pregnancy. The mother of S. died due to her severe alcohol problems.

S. reports:

"My name is S. I am now 32 years old. I suffer from FASD because my mother drank during pregnancy.

At birth I was obviously too small even for a premature birth in the 8th month of pregnancy (length: 28 cm and weight: 1200 g).

I did not learn about FASD until 2011, and after more information about this syndrome, it became clear to me that many of my difficulties were associated with FASD.

My short stature was a constant problem and still is to this day. In many situations of my life I need facilities such as ladders to reach certain heights. I must buy clothes in the children's department and trousers usually have to be altered. During my first years at school I received a chair and table from the kindergarten, because normal seats were too large.

During my school years I displayed behavioural problems. I disrupted the class, was unable to keep still and was always fighting with others. Therefore, I was perceived as an outsider and mostly ignored.

Until I was confronted with the consequences of FASD, I thought my learning difficulties were due to my lack of concentration. However, both are symptoms of FASD! It is, for example, extremely difficult for me to pay attention to two tasks at the same time. Working appropriately is only possible under special conditions and for employment this may be quite problematic. Many people do not tolerate the fact that nowadays I don't understand things easily, and, therefore, I am regarded as being stupid or unwilling to learn.

My aggressive behaviour – I cannot deny it – is another personal character trait. All of a sudden I can get incredibly angry for no apparent reason. Even little things can get me into a rage. To my environment, this behaviour seems childish and immature.

If I'm criticised, I tend to start crying like a little girl instead of getting aggressive. People react with incomprehension because I take criticism so personally."

C.; born in 2005 (f); partial fetal alcohol syndrome (pFAS); November 2011

Editor's note: The biological mother of C. was chronically alcohol dependent and was living in a home for women suffering from an addiction. She is, similarly to her own mother and biological brother, mentally disabled. The biological father of C. met her mother when they both were homeless. He suffered from severe alcohol and illegal substance dependency and died about 2 years ago in his mid-thirties.

The adoptive mother reports:

"First year of life: C. came into our family for foster care at the age of 9 days. We were surprised at how tiny she was. I followed the advice of the children's hospital to feed her with high-quality milk only. Feeding her was very difficult, because she vomited after the meal, and I had to start feeding her again. This procedure quickly turned out to be an arduous task and, therefore, we decided to feed only a small quantity of milk per meal in short intervals. At the age of 11 months, C. was able to walk alone and even able to run.

Second year of life: A social worker of the child and youth welfare office informed us about the possibility of an adoption of C. even without the explicit consent of both of her biological parents. Her father, who was in prison at that time, finally signed the adoption papers; her mother could not be found. We expected that with the support and love of our family, C.'s development and behaviour would become almost normal. So finally we were very happy about a successful adoption in the Autumn of 2006. C. learned to speak, although her pronunciation was a bit unclear. Her extremely uncontrolled movements and her hyperactivity were very striking.

Third year of life: We noticed that she was squinting and went to an optician and got glasses to correct her hyperopia. Her food mainly consisted of baby milk because she spat out almost all solid food; obviously she was unable to swallow it. She was constantly very hyperactive, often throwing filled plates and glasses onto the ground; she was extremely fast in doing so, and we had no chance to prevent damage. Therefore, we often put her in her baby buggy just in order to get a little rest, and she accepted it without protesting.

At our mother–child-gymnastics classes she often pushed other children, so we had to change to a special gymnastic class supposedly tailored to children with special needs. But after a short time she was dismissed for unacceptable behaviour. Her gymnastics teacher could not handle her anymore, because C. always did dangerous and forbidden gymnastic exercises even beneath the roof of the gymnastic hall.

Fourth year of life: The paediatrician asked if we were contented developmentally, and we affirmed because we still believed that she would catch up in her development. Due to her extreme hyperactivity, it was impossible to potty-train her. Most of the time, she rather liked to pee directly on the floor, so we decided better to wait a bit with toilet training.

She started pulling down curtains and destroying everything. We had to cut short our holiday because she climbed on balconies, damaged furniture, and her screaming and inappropriate behaviour attracted negative attention. We lost any interest in going on holiday with her anymore.

Her main food was still milk from the bottle and porridge. She continued to spit out solid food right away.

Fifth year of life: The paediatrician diagnosed a severe form of ADHD and prescribed amphetamine juice. After the first dose of amphetamine juice she suddenly thought her plush toys were real animals and she immediately screamed extremely because she saw one of them was about to fly away. She screamed and screamed, and it was impossible to comfort her, until she suddenly collapsed and started sleeping. We never wanted to give her this juice again, but the paediatrician recommended us to increase the dose. We did as we were told. When I tried to do homework together with her she was astonishingly highly concentrated and was able to draw pictures much better than before. But all of a sudden she jumped up and started to destroy anything lying on the shelf. She rampaged so heavily that I never gave her amphetamine juice again. Another physician told us to change medications and prescribed Risperidone and, surprisingly, this was very successful. So, we finally experienced days that were more quiet and structured. For the first time in her life, she slept throughout the night.

Our attempt to register her for a regular kindergarten failed because right on the first day she wreaked havoc in the playroom.

Sixth year of life: There were always new attempts to get her dry but but it didn't work to date. Meanwhile, she ate normally – her favourite food remained porridge; probably due to the fact that she didn't have to chew it, something she still doesn't like to do. We always had to remind her to chew her food.

Regarding preschool: I tried to teach C. to read and write and I was surprised about the difficulties we experienced. I noticed severe learning difficulties in different domains; therefore, I undertook a special learning program in order to be able to help her adequately. Also I slowly realised that C. might be mentally disabled.

Seventh year of life: During an examination for school attendance she was totally beside herself. On the one hand, they noticed her excellent visual abilities but, on the other hand, they also recognised her inadequate behaviour. When she received a compliment on her nice pair of spectacles she pulled them off and destroyed them completely. After a short period of observation, the school director told me that C. was not yet ready to be enrolled in primary school. We suddenly realised that she would need to attend a school for children with special needs.

Personally, I liked our morning routines, just the two of us, and I felt good being with her. Problems started in the afternoon when the entire family was present. C. then is unable to behave appropriately anymore. As soon as she is unobserved, she destroys everything on which she can lay her hands. Only with constant one-on-one supervision is she able to notice what is right and what is wrong in daily routine.

The adoptive father reports:

Advantages: C. is able to cooperate and is obedient. Sometimes she is also social and fair. She is quick, agile and cute. She is keen on sports and very affectionate.

Disadvantages: She makes everything dirty. She is very impulsive and acts without thinking. When we go shopping she pretends to be an animal crawling on all fours and is hard to control. She teases her sister too much. She is only able to behave well in a one-on- one relationship.

The adoptive mother reports:

Advantage: She is often very cuddly and clingy. She looks so sweet and cute. Being with her in the morning is always a lot of fun. We do a lot of activities, painting and dealing with preschool homework. When we go shopping, she always reminds me to bring something along for her sister. She likes to help me with cooking, although I can't leave her alone for one second, otherwise something catastrophic might happen.

Disadvantages: She constantly steals at home and in shops and starts screaming excessively when we force her to give back the stolen goods. She starts biting without a clear reason – out of the blue, really. Sometimes she gets enraged, and it is difficult to comfort her – e.g. whilst getting dressed or undressed. That is why we, at night, put her in her clean clothes for the next 24 hours, so we need to dress her only once a day!

Although we have a close relationship, she will not listen to me at all if someone else is present. It often happens in combination with obtrusive behaviour towards others, which is often very unpleasant for me, and I am very angry with her at such moments.

J.; born in 2000 (f); fetal alcohol syndrome (FAS); August 2011

Editor's note: J. and her two younger siblings were removed from their family due to severe neglect. J. was placed first in a children's home and she has now been living with her current foster family since the age of 3. When she came to our FASD-centre in August 2011, she showed symptoms of 'classic FAS' and at the time of the second visit in 2013 she already had severe difficulties in executive function.

The foster parents report:

"Our foster daughter J. has been living in our family for 13 years. We were not able to anticipate the severe and persisting difficulties we would encounter before she came to live with us. It started with the fact that Child Services did not give detailed information about her medical problems. After consulting her former SPZ, we got the devastating information that she suffered from FAS.

At the age of two-and-a-half, her development was at the level of a 1-year-old child; she was hardly able to walk and to speak.

After a weekend full of tears, realising that we have to live with a child suffering from FAS, we asked ourselves if we would have enough strength and patience to educate such a child. But at least we consciously decided to live with her without ever having seen her before.

At our first meeting we were introduced to a little girl looking very distraught and small for her age. Despite minor difficulties in communicating with her at the very beginning, we had a nice day all together and immediately became fond of her. After some meetings we were allowed to take her home. Despite many problems with Child Services and struggles with public authorities, our foster daughter learned to deal with her problems.

It is simply incomprehensible why foster or adoptive parents don't receive information about the alcohol exposure of these foster children. That's why it is a jump into the deep end for many of these parents. It was a nightmare for all of us, because due to the lack of information we were unable to understand why our child is so 'different'. Furthermore, these children don't receive the intensive care and support they urgently need. Mostly I was accused of being a crazy foster mother who cannot accept in the end that her child is disabled.

Now our foster daughter attends a special school for the physically disabled and she will manage to graduate from high school. To break down barriers and overcome all obstacles you need patience, a fighting spirit and above all never-ending love.

Many are not aware that children with FAS are entitled to benefits associated with a severe disability. I lost my job due to our foster child and as such did not pay into my pension fund for many years. Thanks to the great help and support of Prof. Spohr, our foster daughter received support (care level II, and a disabled person's pass). Fortunately, I am now insured under a pension scheme again. All of these problems would be avoidable if Child Services were to act in a more supportive and helpful way."

A.; born in 1997 (f); fetal alcohol syndrome in adulthood (FAS adult); March 2017

Editor's note: This is an excerpt of a long report written from the perspective of a foster mother and edited by her foster daughter, A. Many difficulties occurring during childhood and school age are described from the time when she came into her foster family at the age of 5 months. An unusually memorable period of her life is described below.

The foster mother reports:

"A. changed from a regular school to our country school as a child with special needs in the 4th grade. We lived on the outskirts, and this school was well managed, but A. was not accepted by her schoolmates, and one day they started to bully her. The boys were clearly aggressive towards her and the girls irritated her in more subtle and nasty ways. Because of her gullible nature A. was unable to interpret the behaviour of the girls and thus she often walked right into a trap. Her social interaction was often inadequate and not age appropriate and she reacted very emotionally.

As a teenager, she started to dance ballet, which was relatively late for her age, but she really liked it and for the first time she made friends. The clearly structured lessons had been very helpful to her. She was hardworking and achieved good results but she was never really relaxed. Ballet was a sort of therapy for her in the following years and sometimes she exercised 5 days per week. I always had to take her to the ballet lessons because she was unable to get there by herself. She proudly even danced in large performances. I was always at the back of the stage, inconspicuously paying attention and making sure that she was drinking and eating enough and wouldn't forget her medication. I also had to pack her ballet clothes because she was unable to do it herself even with a reminder. But when she was about 16 years old, she didn't want me to help her at all and, therefore, I decided to pack another set of clothes in my own bag because I knew that sooner or later she would need my help. She was dancing in the "Jungle Book", "Sleeping Beauty", "The Little Witch" and in "Snow Queen". There she was a completely normal part of the group despite her difficulties because her coach, who knew about her disability, was able to handle her well. Her coach was also able to improve her self-esteem because she trusted her to be part of the group without diminishing the quality of performance. I was deeply touched, seeing her so proudly performing on the stage. Surely this is one of her most important childhood memories! Evening after evening she didn't think about her lifelong problems, being an ever present part of her life; she was just dancing.

In the 8th grade, we visited Prof. Spohr once again and he told us that A. will never be able to live independently or to work in a normal course of employment situation.

To be honest, I couldn't believe this assessment, thinking it's not that bad. In my opinion, there are good reasons to believe that our foster daughter would be an exception. I thought, I just have to trust in her abilities and never give up hope; but in reality it is only difficult to accept the truth.

At that time her biological parents both died. My foster daughter met her mother shortly before she died at a family visit initiated by the youth welfare services. At that time her mother didn't drink alcohol anymore and she expressed deep regret for what she had done to her daughter. She was very proud of her daughter because she is such a handsome girl, which is true indeed. But A. is unable to forgive her mother till this day. We went to the funeral of her mother for a final farewell.

She now attended a public secondary school and had to repeat the 8th grade. She performed well at school but her social environment was difficult. I noticed that A. was incapable of generalising details and had difficulties in thinking logically and, therefore, I simplified her subjectmatters. However, her language abilities were very good. In English she received an A for both exams and, contrary to every expectation, at the final secondary school qualification she was top of the class. She was very proud. And so were we.

She was still socially immature and infantile compared to her ballet companions and she feared to be shunned by the group, therefore she finished dancing ballet. A. still lives in a very childlike world, believing, for instance, that her guinea pigs have "the magic touch".

If I only had known that she would, indeed, be unable to live on her own independently one day, I would have preferred to teach her everyday practical activities instead of demanding knowledge acquired at school. Maybe she would have felt better emotionally then. She still seems to be a very competent and eloquent person, and nobody would think she is severely disabled.

I'm very annoyed, that there are very few living groups for adults with FASD. A. would like to move out of our family in 1 or 2 years. Therefore, she is practicing everyday-life skills step by step, again and again. Maybe this will help her to live in her own apartment with external support. I hope with all my heart that she will find a place to live independently to a certain degree, and that she will be content and happy. No matter what happens, she will always be my child and I will protect her as best I can."

N.; geb. 1996 (m); fetal alcohol syndrome (FAS adult); June 2017

Author's note: A single mother describes her long and always difficult way through N.´s childhood and adolescence. The birthmother was alcohol and drug-dependent, a fact she always denied, but she died from chronic alcoholism when N. was 2.5 years old. His father did not show any interest in him, N. was taken into charge from the child protective services at 8 months and resided in several different places in the following years until he finally came to his current foster mother at the age of 5 years.

The foster mother reports:

"Despite of his gentle nature, his aggressive behaviour became apparent very early. He suffered from enuresis and encopresis, biting his nails, and nocturnal nightmares plagued him for many years.

Although his microcephaly was known since early childhood, despite several medical examinations a diagnosis of FAS never was confirmed. His psychotherapist who was treating him since summer of 2013 suggested quite the opposite: N. suffered from a severe crisis in adolescence due to traumatisation in early childhood.

N. changed school many times and always had problems with his teachers, who blamed him for his refusal to work and his lack of motivation and although he had severe difficulties with his classmates; they bullied him all the years because of his "being different" and his aggressive behaviour. Nevertheless, with intensive help and due to his persisting energy he finally achieved the secondary school leaving certificate.

In January 2017, in his third attempt to find a job on the employment market, he started as a bricklayer in a family operated construction company. Initially, his performance seemed to be satisfying in the construction area. After only 2 weeks he had problems with the vocational school because of not carrying out the teachers' instructions and refusing performance. He received a disciplinary warning and a written reprimand. With his increasing absenteeism and his lack of endurance, my son may lose his place of employment; my concern that he will slip into criminality is not without reason.

As he becomes older N. suffers from strong impulsivity ('explosive episodes'), low frustration tolerance, an exaggerated opinion of himself together with feelings of inferiority, and a total absence of a sense of guilt combined with an increasing tendency of lying and stealing making life with him sometimes almost unbearable.

Transition into adulthood seems to be connected with unexpected and great difficulties.

Already by 15 years of age, he was talking about his anxiety of becoming an adult. Obviously he felt unable to cope with the challenges of adulthood when comparing himself with other people. The discrepancy between the social expectations of what young adults commonly have to do to perform in daily life and his own limited capability seemed to increase with age.

So it is not surprising that his family doctor recently referred N. to a psychiatrist, with suspicion of a beginning depression.

N. needs much guidance and support in coping with everyday life. I still have to control N.'s sketchy hygiene and draw attention to rules, order and cleanliness.

Dealing independently with public authorities is impossible without support, and he still can't handle money.

Because of these persisting difficulties in his life, I finally realised that N. might not suffer from developmental delay alone. After intensive information about this topic, we both decided to reattempt the diagnosis of FAS.

In July 2017, at the age of 21 years, Prof. Spohr (Charité University Clinic, Berlin) made the definite diagnosis: FAS adult despite normal intelligence and absence of growth failure.

This diagnosis was a great relief to N. and offered an explanation for all the trouble and difficulties, which had run like a golden thread through his life, and which he was often unable to understand.

He finally conceives the congenital disease as a relief because now he is not alone in being responsible for all the problems and doesn't have to suffer from the idea of being an inferior human being.

The new situation raises hope that N.'s environment will accept his diagnosis and respond to him in a suitable way. I hope that his charm and wit, his creativity, helpfulness and his sensibility will give him a chance to reconcile with his fate to open his eyes for life and to discover new horizons."

Part VI: **Appendix**

A Residential communities and assisted individual housing for adults with fetal alcohol spectrum disorders (FASD) and behavioural disorders

Gela Becker

For 20 years, the children's home Sonnenhof in Berlin Spandau has taken care of children, youth and adults with FASD. With our efforts we strive towards the following goals:
- First: to include the pupils in our care in social life through fostering integrative work and caregiving.
- Second: to sensitise professional public, state institutions, charitable institutions and FASD-associations through public relations work and information.
- Third: to pass our experience on to service for youth care, integration support and disabled assistance through advanced training courses in questions about case management, support and FASD-specific interventions and to motivate other carriers to offer qualified FASD care as well.

In the advancement of our work as a carrier of stationary and outpatient support for education (in education-residential groups and communities, in assisted single living, through ambulatory support of young adults, through psychotherapy and family therapy) we have specialised – consultative accompaniment by Prof. Dr. Spohr – in mental disability and cerebro-organic impairments, which are directly associated with fetal exposure to alcohol. These impairments show the typical spectrum of behavioural disorders, cognitive and mental impairment and developmental disorder, which often makes a journey to an independent existence impossible.

Our experience shows that the majority of children and adolescents suffering from FASD are not in a position to live independently and responsibly as adults, as confirmed by the 2007 longitudinal study of Prof. Dr. Spohr. Results show that only 12% of young men and women with prenatal alcohol exposure find a job, earn a living and can live independently [1].

The long-term consequences are still not being taken seriously enough in Germany. With the support of the Diakonisches Werk and the Senate, the Sonnenhof e.V. responded to the statistically obvious need for care and support by establishing the nation's first specialised residential community in 2007.

We established assisted individual housing in 2009 as well as the opening our second in 2012) and our third (in 2015) FASD residential community. Thus, we strive to help children affected by FASD who have grown up in our foster care and whose accommodation in existing facilities is difficult due to their unique and special needs. We give them the assistance they still depend on as adults.

https://doi.org/10.1515/9783110436563-019

Furthermore, in cooperation with other organisations we strive towards differentiated forms of care in the inpatient area. We welcome the development of projects that emanate from a long-term perspective: to start support as early as possible, give assistance in close proximity to home and to establish and keep the more than often hard to build up social relations.

A.1 The FASD residential community

One of our shared apartments is housed in a detached home in Spandau. Our more intensive assisted living community is located on the second floor of a three-story building on the edge of a multi-story housing estate with good infrastructure. Due to the limited group capabilities of people with FASD, both shared apartments are set out to accommodate a maximum of four residents. Our residential communities provide outpatient care for young adult women and men with intellectual disabilities/organic brain impairments caused by fetal alcohol exposure and serious behavioural problems, who are eligible to means of integration assistance in accordance with § 53.1 SGB XII.

The main objectives are individual support on the way to a possible self-determined and independent life, preventing the worsening of impairments and lending support in dealing with the consequences of these impairments.

This includes assistance in dealing with the patients' own biographical development and in the development and implementation of prospects for future life planning.

Each resident has a private room that he/she can set up on his/her own terms with the help of the supervisor or relatives. Common areas are the common room, the kitchen and the sanitary facilities. The residents are supported in home economics duties as required.

Due to the peculiarities of the impairments in FASD, we also offer our outpatient care in the morning hours. Residents must be able to be without care at night and sometimes even a few hours during the day. We offer support in finding skills relevant to obtain employment and accompany, if necessary, the work while patiently motivating to again and again seek a new beginning.

A.2 Assisted individual housing – FASD

Assisted individual housing is usually for residents of our FASD-residential communities and for young adultswho we have already cared for in the youth services area, for whom the continuity of care on their path to self-sufficiency should be ensured by their reference supervisor. Due to the very limited group capacity of people with FASD, this kind of care is the only realistic option for many residents. This is a problem for all cases where the so far developed independence does not comply with the requirements. The assisted individual housing is intended for people with intellectual disabilities, who – apart from periods of crisis – do not require around-the-clock care, although there may be the need for intensive advancement/guidance in some areas and comprehensive assistance.

The location of the individual apartments is situated in the district of Spandau and in close proximity to our FASD-living communities, which are also used as a support base.

Our support services include:
1. individual support in learning practical life tasks
2. daily assistance with the structuring of the day
3. ehancement of social and conflict resolution skills
4. resource-oriented support of personal progress
5. aid in conflict and crisis situations
6. care and provision as required
7. collaboration with relatives.

The focus of our care is to enhance each individual resident. With the help of neuropsychological diagnostics, we strive to provide the daily-oriented special support for each adult with the development of compensatory aids to compensate the cerebo-organic dysfunctions.

Case-oriented, we offer executive function training sessions. Over the years we have tried a variety of professional trainings (e.g. planning and memory training), feel-good training by external therapists, etc., and have found that our residents – who are often over-treated – have an "allergic" response to professionals. We have found that the same training is also available in the context of several games and the combination of fun and training is much more efficient – therefore we play a lot. This includes computer games, which for some residents, are excellent for stress relief.

We are also prepared to compensate and counteract impairments in the areas of impulse control, drive, affect regulation, maturation, etc., as those are the most common comorbid symptoms (comorbid disorders: depression, anxiety disorders, attachment disorder, ADD, ADHD). The same applies to the secondary disorders in the area of the spectrum of behavioural disorders.

The risks of developing a substance addiction were the reason for us to develop and test new intervention strategies within a research project, which was supported by the Federal Ministry of Health. We prospectively provide these new intervention strategies for other institutions.

Even though the sample in our pilot testing was small ($n = 16$), it still shows tendencies in which individualised and demand-orientated intervention can be given. The need for assistance varies from the ability to accept help between 5 and 30 hours per week. When differentiating between the subtypes of the FASD, our sample only showed a slight increase of the help needed by people with FAS (see Fig. A.1).

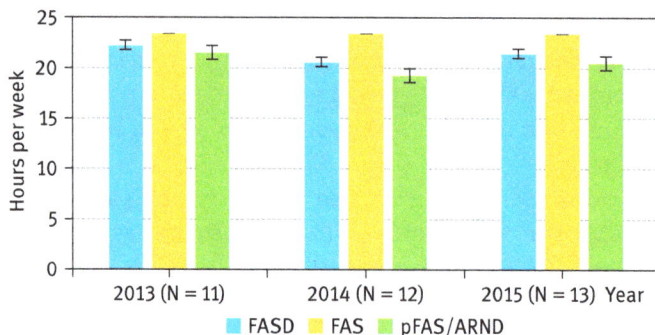

Fig. A.1: Average need of assistance of Sonnenhof residents with FASD in the years 2013, 2014 and 2015.

Research on the stress levels of those affected by FASD, rated with the SDQ (Strength and Difficulties Questionnaire, Goodman, 1997) by the caregivers, conducted by Frau Dr. Hoff-Emden indicates that the individual emotional distress is extremely high. The evaluation of our residents over a course of 3 years shows that secondary disabilities can be reduced (Figs. A.2, A.3).

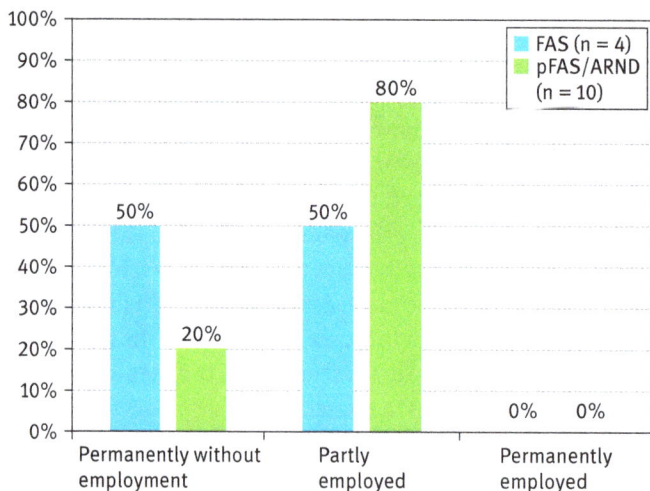

Fig. A.2: Problems with employment of Sonnenhof residents with FASD measured over the course of 3 years (2013–2015). A long-term concequence in adulthood for people with FASD (2015, $n = 14$).

Furthermore, our evaluation shows that the living situation of people with FASD can be significantly improved with demand-oriented individualised care and stability in caregivers. Especially concerning conflicts with the law such as sexual offences, crisis

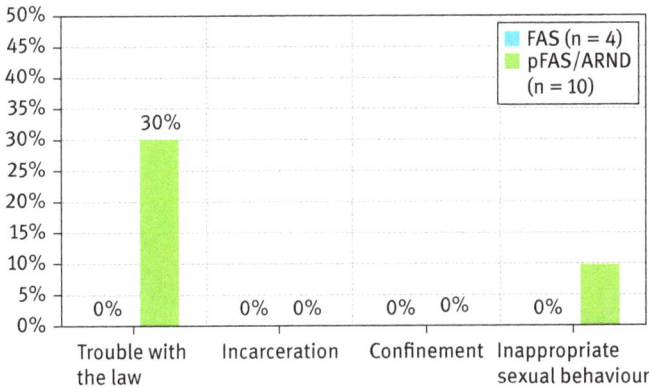

Fig. A.3: Secondary disabilities of Sonnenhof residents with FASD measured over the course of 3 years (2013–2015).

interventions and preventive detention can be reduced in comparison to American longitudinal studies with improved care.

Respecting self-determination rights, we often face a lack of compliance, partly due to the impairment itself, partly from the difficulty of dealing with this impairment, yet we set clear boundaries in the field of endangerment of self and others.

We do not move mountains; we smoothe the pathway, looking for creative solutions with the goal to further security and happiness for every individual as much as possible.

Bibliography

[1] Spohr HL, Willms J, Steinhausen HC. Fetal Alcohol Spectrum Disorders in Young Adulthood.
     J. Pediatr 2007, 150, 175–179.

Index

https://doi.org/10.1515/9783110436563-020

www.ingramcontent.com/pod-product-compliance
Lightning Source LLC
Chambersburg PA
CBHW081511190326
41458CB00015B/5339